Animal Health and Disease: The Role of Genetics

Animal Health and Disease: The Role of Genetics

Edited by Harrison Elliott

SYRAWOOD
PUBLISHING HOUSE
New York

Published by Syrawood Publishing House,
750 Third Avenue, 9th Floor,
New York, NY 10017, USA
www.syrawoodpublishinghouse.com

Animal Health and Disease: The Role of Genetics
Edited by Harrison Elliott

International Standard Book Number: 978-1-64740-374-4 (Hardback)

Cataloging-in-publication Data

Animal health and disease : the role of genetics / edited by Harrison Elliott.
p. cm.
Includes bibliographical references and index.
ISBN 978-1-64740-374-4
1. Animal health. 2. Animals--Diseases--Genetic aspects. 3. Animal genetics.
4. Veterinary genetics. I. Elliott, Harrison.
SF756.5 .A55 2023
636.082 1--dc23

TABLE OF CONTENTS

PREFACE

This book aims to highlight the current researches and provides a platform to further the scope of innovations in this area. This book is a product of the combined efforts of many researchers and scientists, after going through thorough studies and analysis from different parts of the world. The objective of this book is to provide the readers with the latest information of the field.

Certain animal populations are essential for humans as they provide a variety of products and services such as meat, milk, eggs, fiber and draught power. The genetic variation within animal populations is a major factor responsible for this diversity of function. Animal genetics plays a significant role in the development of animals in terms of animal health and disease. The traditional methods of animal selection and breeding were based on the phenotypic performance of animals. The application of omics technology can be potentially used to overcome the limitations of traditional breeding methods. There are several omics technologies such as genomics, metagenomics, metabolomics, proteomics, transcriptomics, epigenomics, and translatomics with a broad range of applications in animal health and disease. These omics tools allow rapid and effective detection of subtle phenotypic changes, dietary responses, and innate phenotypic propensities in animals. This book traces the significant advancements in the role of genetics in maintaining animal health and controlling diseases. It will prove to be immensely beneficial to students and researchers involved in this area of study.

I would like to express my sincere thanks to the authors for their dedicated efforts in the completion of this book. I acknowledge the efforts of the publisher for providing constant support. Lastly, I would like to thank my family for their support in all academic endeavors.

Editor

1

Selection for Favorable Health Traits: A Potential Approach to Cope with Diseases in Farm Animals

Guoyu Hu, Duy Ngoc Do, Janine Gray and Younes Miar *

Department of Animal Science and Aquaculture, Dalhousie University, Truro, NS B2N 5E3, Canada; gy494270@dal.ca (G.H.); duy.do@dal.ca (D.N.D.); Janine.gray@dal.ca (J.G.)

* Correspondence: miar@dal.ca

Simple Summary: The losses caused by the outbreak of diseases are disastrous for the animal farming industries. There is an urgent need for an efficient, economical, and permanent disease control method to cope with the adverse effects of diseases in farm animals. In this review, we have proposed that genetic/genomic selection for animals with favorable health traits provide potential methods to eliminate the adverse influences of diseases in farm animals. It is undeniable that the traditional methods for disease control (e.g., vaccination, treatment, and eradication strategy) and several other rising disease control and detection methods (e.g., genome editing, biosensor, and probiotics) are contributing to the prevention of diseases from farm animals, curing infected animals, and detecting sick individuals; however, the limitations and deficiencies of these methods cannot be ignored. Although genetic/genomic selection solutions are facing some challenges, the developments of selection-associated techniques (e.g., high throughput phenotyping and sequencing, and generation of big data) and the advantages of selection over the other disease control methods can provide animal farming industries the ability to cope with the issues caused by diseases through breeding for health traits.

Abstract: Disease is a global problem for animal farming industries causing tremendous economic losses (>USD 220 billion over the last decade) and serious animal welfare issues. The limitations and deficiencies of current non-selection disease control methods (e.g., vaccination, treatment, eradication strategy, genome editing, and probiotics) make it difficult to effectively, economically, and permanently eliminate the adverse influences of disease in the farm animals. These limitations and deficiencies drive animal breeders to be more concerned and committed to dealing with health problems in farm animals by selecting animals with favorable health traits. Both genetic selection and genomic selection contribute to improving the health of farm animals by selecting certain health traits (e.g., disease tolerance, disease resistance, and immune response), although both of them face some challenges. The objective of this review was to comprehensively review the potential of selecting health traits in coping with issues caused by diseases in farm animals. Within this review, we highlighted that selecting health traits can be applied as a method of disease control to help animal agriculture industries to cope with the adverse influences caused by diseases in farm animals. Certainly, the genetic/genomic selection solution cannot solve all the disease problems in farm animals. Therefore, management, vaccination, culling, medical treatment, and other measures must accompany selection solution to reduce the adverse impact of farm animal diseases on profitability and animal welfare.

Keywords: diseases; farm animals; genetic selection; health traits

1. Introduction

Disease control is a global challenge for livestock industries and farmers, as diseases bring tremendous economic losses to farm animal production systems. The animal farming systems in both developed and developing countries are suffering economically from different infectious diseases. Direct economic losses from the outbreaks of disease can account for up to 20% of the revenue in developed countries and up to 50% of the revenue within the livestock sector of the developing world [1]. Basically, all farm animal production systems are vulnerable to disease. Many diseases, such as bovine viral diarrhea (BVD), Johne's disease, and bovine respiratory disease complex (BRDC) in cattle farming; bluetongue and sheep pox in sheep farming; porcine reproductive and respiratory syndrome (PRRS), and African swine fever (ASF) in the swine industry; Newcastle disease and Marek's disease in the poultry industry; and Aleutian disease in the mink industry, contribute to economic losses and cause serious animal welfare issues via persistent infection, increased mortality, reduced productivity and reproduction performance, and decreased product quality. Therefore, finding the effective solutions to combat diseases has become a top priority for all livestock industries.

To control diseases, many methods have been used with some level of success. Vaccination, medical treatment, and eradication strategy are common methods to control health issues caused by diseases. These methods, however, are facing some bottlenecks, such as the side effects of vaccination [2,3], public concerns about residual drugs and drug resistance after employing medical treatment [4–9], and financial cost and high recurrence rate of using eradication strategies [10,11]. Several other methods including genome editing, biosensor, and probiotics provide animal farming industries more options to enhance animal health. Unfortunately, the lack of effective legal oversight (e.g., genome editing) and technological immaturity (e.g., genome editing, probiotics, and biosensor) make these technologies not widely available for controlling diseases of farm animals. This makes seeking alternative solutions one of the main concerns for animal producers.

Breeding for favorable health traits is one solution that is highly anticipated. Health traits mainly include health body traits, disease susceptibility traits, and immune system traits. Selecting favorable health traits, which are complex traits influenced by many genes and environmental factors is a powerful tool against disease [12]. Host genetics is significant in controlling the health status of each individual in the same environment. Compared with the other methods of disease control in farm animals, the selection of animals with favorable health traits such as disease resistance, disease tolerance [13], and immunity responses [14] has many advantages. Classical genetic selection and genomic selection are playing important roles in genetically improving health and controlling diseases. Although many challenges exist in both selection methods, the great potential to genetically eradicate diseases from farming systems is still attracting the attention of many animal farming industries.

Given the importance of disease in farm animals and the dramatic development of technologies for disease characterization, it is crucial to have a comprehensive and holistic view about challenges and solutions for combating disease in farm animals. Therefore, this review paper was written: (1) to present an overview of common diseases in farm animals and the methods used to control them; (2) to highlight the advantages of coping with diseases by selecting for health traits through genetic or genomic selection, as well as the current stages of selection on major diseases in livestock industries; and (3) to discuss the major challenges of employing health trait selection and the potential solutions that can help improve selection.

2. Farm Animal Diseases: Influence, Prevalence, and Controlling Issues

2.1. *The Influence, Prevalence, and Controlling Issues of Common Diseases in Farm Animals*

Disease in farm animals is a significant challenge to farm animal industries worldwide. Cattle, sheep, swine, poultry, and fur-bearing animals such as mink are the most important farm animals for human society and provide the main resource of milk, meat, egg, wool, and fur. Unfortunately, all these important farming systems are vulnerable to disease (Figure 1).

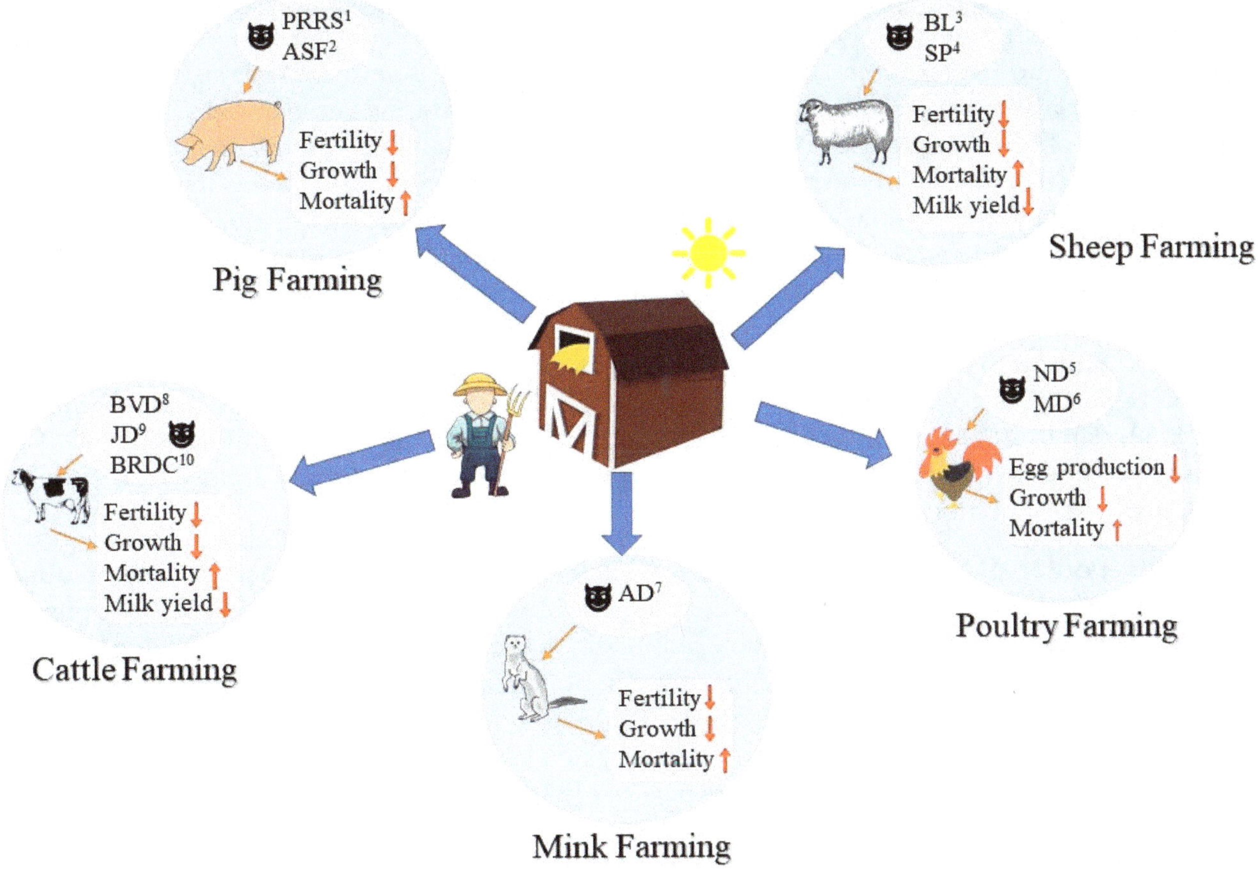

Figure 1. Economic consequences of common diseases in farm animals including pig, sheep, poultry, mink, and cattle. The upward-pointing arrows refer to increase, and the downward-pointing arrows refer to decrease (PRRS[1] = Porcine reproductive and respiratory syndrome; ASF[2] = African swine fever; BL[3] = Bluetongue; SP[4] = Sheep pox; ND[5] = Newcastle disease; MD[6] = Marek's disease; AD[7] = Aleutian disease; BVD[8] = Bovine viral diarrhea; JD[9] = Johne's disease; BRDC[10] = Bovine respiratory disease complex).

In cattle, BVD, Johne's Disease, and BRDC are the most costly and persistent diseases (Table 1). The BVD commonly causes respiratory and reproductive complications in the herd. The prevalence of BVD in Northern Ireland can reach as high as 98.5% in non-vaccinated dairy herds and 98.3% in beef herds [15]. The BVD causes the dairy industry to lose 40 to 100 thousand US dollars per herd in Canada and 10 to 40 million US dollars per million calvings in Europe [16,17]. Culling infected animals and vaccinations are employed as short-term strategies to control this disease; however, they do not effectively eradicate BVD from the dairy farms [18,19]. Johne's disease affects the small intestine of ruminant animals and results in weight loss, diarrhea, decreased fertility, and death. The current strategy of controlling Johne's disease is based on timely detection through *Mycobacterium avium* ssp. *Paratuberculosis* enzyme-linked immunosorbent assay testing and then culling infected animals as there is no effective vaccine or treatment. For this reason, Johne's disease is still rampant worldwide [10]. Approximately 68% of dairy operations in the USA were affected by this disease [20]. This disease causes economic losses of 15 million Canadian dollars per year to the dairy industries in Canada, and 200 to 250 million US dollars per year in the USA [21]. The BRDC, which is usually associated with infections of the lungs, causes pneumonia in calves and has been regarded as one of the primary causes of morbidity and mortality in beef farming [22,23]. In the USA, BRDC is the leading natural cause of death in beef cattle and causes financial losses of more than one billion US dollars annually [24]. The main method of controlling BRDC is using antibiotics; however, bacterial pathogen resistance to antibiotics for BRDC has caused the producers, practitioners, and the animal health industry to doubt the sustainability of using antibiotics to control BRDC [25].

In sheep, bluetongue and sheep pox are two common diseases in the sheep industry, causing significant economic losses (Table 1). Bluetongue causes huge economic losses to the sheep industry due to high mortality and morbidity, as well as the trading of animals associated with its outbreak. The prevalence of bluetongue was 19% in Italy [26], but in Sudan, the prevalence has been as high as 94% [27]. In 2007, the cost of the bluetongue disease for sheep breeding farms in the Netherlands was estimated at 12.6 million euros [28]. Vaccination has been regarded as the most viable method for the prevention and eradication of bluetongue disease; however, the expensive cost and potential side effects seriously influence the practicality and effectiveness of bluetongue disease vaccine [29]. Sheep pox is a serious, and often fatal infectious disease in sheep and causes a high mortality rate in sheep populations. Although live vaccines have been developed and are used worldwide, sheep pox still persists in regions where vaccination is routinely practiced, causing huge economic losses to the sheep industry [30]. Up to 22% [31] and 40% [32] of sheep in India and Ethiopia were infected by this disease, respectively. Annual economic losses from sheep pox disease in Maharashtra, India, were 2.4 million US dollars due to high mortality rates [33].

In swine, outbreaks of contagious diseases, such as PRRS and ASF, have not only resulted in significant economic losses for swine industries but have also caused animal welfare and environmental concerns (Table 1). The PRRS can cause anorexia, lethargy, hyperemia of the skin, dyspnea, hyperthermia, increased mortality rates, and reduction in average daily gain [34]. Up to 48% of swine farms in Ontario, Canada, were infected by PRRS from 2010 to 2013 [35]. In 2013, the total annual losses due to PRRS in the US were estimated at 664 million US dollars [36]. In Canada, the cost of PRRS was estimated at 130 million Canadian dollars per year [37]. Vaccination is considered the most feasible method for PRRS control; however, the high mutation rate and antigenic variability of the PRRS virus influences the effectiveness of controlling PRRS through vaccination. Meanwhile, the limited protection period of the vaccine against PRRS makes vaccination effective for only short time periods instead of eradicating the virus permanently [38,39]. The ASF is a viral disease that leads to high morbidity and mortality in swine and has drastic influences on global domestic swine production. The absence of an effective vaccine and available methods of disease control causes tremendous economic losses to the infected areas [40]. The ASF was reported in most provinces of China from August 2018 to July 2019 and resulted in an insufficient supply of pork products in China. The overall mean rate of incidence was 12.5%, and the highest incidence rate of 30% occurred in April–May 2019 [41]. In Russia, ASF has resulted in the loss of 800,000 pigs and 0.83–1.25 billion US dollars since its outbreak in 2007 [42].

In poultry, diseases such as Newcastle disease and Marek's disease have caused devastating economic losses worldwide (Table 1). Newcastle disease was regarded as one of the biggest threats to the poultry industry as this disease significantly affected poultry production throughout the world and has accounted for huge economic losses due to high mortality, high morbidity, and trade restrictions [43]. The average prevalence in adult birds was 85% in the breeding and wintering grounds of Michigan, Mississippi, and Wisconsin states of the US, and Ontario province of Canada from 2009 to 2011 [44]. The outbreak of Newcastle disease in California state of the US from 2002 to 2003, caused 3.3 million birds to be culled and cost 200 million US dollars to eradicate the virus [45]. With no effective treatment for Newcastle disease, vaccination is primarily used by the poultry industry to control the spread of disease. The multiple worldwide outbreaks of Newcastle disease in the past few years, however, have shown that the vaccination strategies are not fully effective in controlling this disease in different environmental conditions [46,47]. Marek is another disease that affects the poultry industry and is one of the most ubiquitous highly contagious viral avian infections affecting chicken flocks worldwide. Although the clinical Marek disease is not always apparent in infected flocks, the subclinical decrease in growth rate and egg production can significantly affect the economic benefits of chicken farms [48]. In Iraq, the overall prevalence of Marek disease was 49.5% with a range of 37% to 65% in different areas [49]. Even though mass vaccination is relatively efficient in controlling Marek's disease, the appearance of highly virulent strains that can decrease vaccine immunity results in Marek's disease virus continuing to cause a serious threat to the poultry industry [50,51]. The annual economic losses due to Marek's disease were estimated as high as 1–2 billion US dollars worldwide [52].

As the primary source of fur among all fur industries, mink farming also suffers from the serious economic losses caused by Aleutian disease (Table 1). Aleutian disease, a chronic and persistent viral infection can cause a decrease in litter size (2.5 kits per whelping), high adult and embryonic mortalities (30–100%), and poor fur quality [53–56]. From 1998 to 2005, 24% to 71% of farmed mink were infected in Nova Scotia province of Canada [57]. The test-and-remove strategy, which is the process used to remove mink tested positive for Aleutian Disease, is employed as the main method to control Aleutian disease because of the ineffective immunoprophylaxis and treatment [58]. The unsatisfactory outcome of the test-and-remove strategy, however, makes Aleutian disease still a major problem and results in tremendous economic losses for the mink industry in North America and Europe [57,59]. The annual economic losses to the mink industry were estimated at approximately ten million US dollars in Denmark during 1984 [60].

Table 1. Prevalence and economic losses of common diseases and their impacts on performance in farm animal species.

Species	Disease	Prevalence	Economic Losses	Milk Yield	Fertility/Egg Production	Growth Rate	Mortality	Vaccine Available?	Specific Treatment?
Cattle	Bovine Viral Diarrhea	Up to 98.5% and 98.3% in non-vaccinated dairy and beef herds, respectively [15]	40–100 thousand USD per herd in Canada [16] and 10–40 million USD per million calvings in Europe [17]	Reduced (~0.074 kg/day [61])	Reduced (21% abortion rate [62])	Reduced	High (~50% in calves [63])	Yes	No
	Johne's Disease	68.1% of US dairy operations were infected [20]	15 million CAD annually in Canada and 200–250 million USD in US [21]	Reduced (up to 25% [64])	Reduced (7% lower rate of conception [65])	Reduced	Culling infected individuals	Yes	No
	Bovine Respiratory Disease Complex	45.9% in UK dairy heifers	One billion USD annually in US [24]	N/A	N/A	Reduced	Moderate (~20% in calves [66])	Yes	No
Sheep	Bluetongue	19% in Italy [26] and up to 94.3% in Sudan [27]	In 2007, 12.6 million euros in the Netherlands [28]	Reduced (up to 42% [67])	Reduced (25% abortion rate and 50% decrease in fertility [68])	Reduced	High (up to 41.5% [69])	Yes	No
	Sheeppox	Up to 22% [31] in India and 40% in Ethiopia [32]	2.4 million USD annually in Maharashtra, India [33]	N/A	N/A	Reduced	High (up to 40% [70])	Yes	No
Swine	Porcine Reproductive and Respiratory Syndrome	Up to 48% of pig farms in Ontario, Canada [35]	664 million USD annually in US [36] and 130 million CAD annually in Canada [37]	N/A	Reduced (up to 40% abortion rate [71])	Reduced	High (up to 100% [72])	Yes	No
	African Swine Fever	12.5% in China from August 2018 to July 2019 [41]	1.25 billion USD from 2007 to 2017 in Russia [42]	N/A	Reduced (54% abortion rate [73])	N/A	High (30–70% [74])	No	No
Poultry	Newcastle Disease	85.2% in eastern North America between 2009 and 2011 [44]	200 million USD from 2002 to 2003 in California, US [45]	N/A	Reduced (55% of egg production [75])	Reduced	High (up to 100% [76])	Yes	No
	Marek's Disease	49.5% in Iraq [49]	1–2 billion USD annually worldwide [52]	N/A	Reduced (decrease 5% egg production [77])	Reduced	Moderate (10–30% [78])	Yes	No
Mink	Aleutian Disease	Up to 71% in Nova Scotia, Canada between 1998 and 2005 [57]	10 million USD in Denmark during 1984 [57]	N/A	Reduced fertility (~2.5 kits per whelping [56])	Reduced	High (30–100% [55])	No	No

2.2. *Current Methods to Control Diseases in Farm Animals*

Many disease-controlling methods are contributing to help farm animals cope with diseases. Vaccination, treatment, and test-based culling strategies are common approaches for the livestock industry to treat diseases and reduce the economic losses caused by subsequent health issues. Meanwhile, the development of genome editing, biosensor, and probiotics have provided more options for solving the economic and animal welfare issues caused by disease in animal farming systems. These methods have made great contributions to the control of diseases, but their deficiencies exposed in the application process cannot be ignored (Table 2).

Table 2. Strengths and weaknesses of common non-selection disease control methods in farm animals.

Controlling Method	Advantages	Disadvantages
Vaccination	▪ Prevent and mitigate various diseases in livestock ▪ Provide solutions to control diseases which have complex, limited or no treatment options available ▪ Decrease the antimicrobial resistance	▪ Only administered to healthy subjectsMay cause adverse reactionsBring expensive cost for large-scale use
Medical treatment	▪ Treat many common diseases in livestock species ▪ Increase in feed efficiency and performance	▪ Increase the occurrence of drug residues ▪ Increase the risk of drug resistance
Culling	▪ Main method used to control highly contagious and inextirpable diseases	▪ Fail in permanently eradicating some diseases from livestock farms ▪ High reinfection rate in some cases ▪ Very costly in large-scale farms
Genome editing	▪ Offer solutions to control untreatable diseases at affordable costs ▪ Has high efficiency and low cost in controlling diseases	▪ No legal regulations have been established to supervise genome editing animals ▪ Is not mature enough for large-scale use ▪ Public's concerns
Biosensor	▪ Effective in disease detection and isolation, and health monitoring	▪ Not effective in practical livestock health management ▪ Not widespread and promoted due to the lack of investment
Probiotics	▪ Have great potential to reduce the risk of intestinal diseases ▪ Have the potential to replace some antibiotics	▪ Lacking adequate related research ▪ Unable to apply in large-scale livestock farming

2.2.1. Vaccination

Vaccination has long been a key tool to reduce disease in livestock and maintain the health and welfare of livestock. Vaccines are contributing to preventing and mitigating many livestock diseases (e.g., Johne's Disease and BRDC in cattle, bluetongue and sheeppox in sheep, PRRS in swine, and Newcastle and Marek's diseases in poultry), which have complex, limited or no treatment options available, as well as reducing the use and misuse of antibiotics [79–82]. Vaccines play a significant role in preventing livestock diseases, but they also have some unsatisfactory side effects. First, vaccines are only administered to healthy subjects because they aim to prevent, not to treat. This means the vaccine can only protect the animal from disease, instead of eradication of disease [83]. Second, vaccination may cause adverse reactions in vaccinated animals. This means a vaccine may cause some adverse side effects (e.g., anaphylaxis, decrease in production traits) to a recipient [2,3]. Third, mass vaccination campaigns can be very expensive and may be unprofitable for some livestock farmers [84].

2.2.2. Medical Treatments

Medical treatment is one of the main typical treatments for coping with diseases in farm animals. Veterinary drugs not only play a crucial role in controlling the diseases-related risks but also make contributions to higher agricultural productivity and a steady livestock supply [85,86]. The overall economic benefit can be increased by using the medical treatments because their applications can increase feed efficiency and performance (growth rate, egg production) for 1% to 15% more than animals that do not receive antibiotics or medical treatments [87]. Although veterinary drugs have played an important role in the field of animal husbandry and agro-industry, the increasing occurrence of residues and resistance have become issues worldwide [4–9].

2.2.3. Culling

Culling infected animals and carrying strict hygiene practices are also commonly applied to control many highly contagious and inextirpable diseases in farm animals by reducing the transmission of disease. High culling rate and cost of culling make it expensive to control some diseases by culling strategy. The overall annual culling rate of 590 randomly selected dairy herds from New Zealand for BVD was 23.1% in 2002, and the cull cost for each cow was 324 US dollars [61]. About 200,000 pigs were culled from August to October of 2018 due to the outbreak of ASF in China. The direct damage from culling was estimated at about 37.8 million US dollars [88]. For controlling PRRS in Vietnam, the government needs to provide a subsidy to encourage pig farmers to voluntarily cull infected pigs [89]. This strategy, however, still cannot eradicate some of the viruses in some cases, such as Aleutian disease in mink and Johne's disease in dairy cattle [10,11,57]. Many potential reasons such as the variability of the virus genome, ineffectiveness of biosecurity failure, viral transmission from wild animals, and persistent virus on the farms lead to the failure of culling strategies [57,90,91].

2.2.4. Genome Editing

Genome editing is a powerful technology that can precisely modify the genome of an organism. The main genome editing tools are zinc-finger nucleases, transcription activator-like effector nucleases, and CRISPR/Cas9, which have been successfully employed to many farm animal species including swine, cattle, sheep, and poultry to cope with diseases at affordable costs by creating farm animals with disease-resistant genes [92–99]. There are clear opportunities especially in cases where conventional control options have shown limited success. For PRRS, the in vitro research has shown that the macrophage surface protein CD163 and specifically the scavenger receptor cysteine-rich domain 5 (SRCR5) of the CD163 protein mediate entry of PRRS virus into the host cell [100]. Based on this information, a genome-edited pig with increased resistance to PRRS virus infection could be generated with a disruption to the *CD163* gene. The genome-edited pigs created by completely knocking out the *CD163* gene [98,101] or by removing only the SRCR5-encoding genome section [102,103] showed resistance to PRRS virus infection. However, such studies did not deliver the complete resistance in the pigs in which the endogenous *CD163* gene was edited. The effectiveness of genome editing in disease control will be influenced by many factors, such as the proportion of gene-edited animals in the population and how these gene-edited animals are distributed within and across farms [96]. The disease-specific epidemiological models, however, are missing in helping with defining the exact proportion of gene-edited animals needed for each species/disease. Meanwhile, the limited shelf-life of genome editing needs to be considered. Genome editing shares the potential risk of vaccines, as the efficacy might be time-limited due to the emergence of escape mutants [96]. Especially for some RNA viruses with extremely high mutation rates, like the PRRS virus [104], this concern is justified. So far, no legal regulations have been established to supervise genome-editing animals, and all previous examples are at a preliminary stage. This means that applying this technology to farm animal production still needs a large amount of research and comprehensive monitoring systems to ensure biosafety [96]. On the other hand, public concerns about genome-edited farm animal products are also a factor that cannot be ignored, and directly determines whether genome-edited farm animal products have market value [95].

2.2.5. Biosensor

A biosensor is used to quantify physiological, immunological, and behavioral responses of farm animal species through detecting specific interaction results to a change in one or more physico-chemical properties (pH change, electron transfer, mass change, heat transfer, uptake or release of gases or specific ions) [105]. This technology is applied in disease detection and isolation, and health monitoring in cattle, swine, and poultry [106–112]. Although the biosensor can detect abundant precise data, the data is currently not being effectively transferred into practical information that could be used for the decision-making process in farm animal health management. At the same time, the lack of investment by individual farmers has also limited the widespread application and promotion of this technology [108].

2.2.6. Probiotics

The use of probiotics is also believed to have great potential to reduce the risk of the diseases of farm animals especially intestinal diseases and to replace the use of some antibiotics [113,114]. Creating a bacterial competition using probiotics, which are live microorganisms that provide a health benefit to the host when administered in adequate amounts, is a strategy to maintain health and prevent and treat infections in animals [114]. Many probiotic products are available for farm animals to improve their health and prevent them from disease [115–117]. Lack of statistical analysis, unclear experimental protocols, lack of precise identification of microorganisms, and missing data related to the viability of the organisms make it difficult to assess the studies associated with probiotics based on earlier research [118]. Meanwhile, the lack of an appropriate government regulatory framework and safety studies slow the industrial exploitation of novel probiotic genera and delay the large-scale application of this technology in animal farming [119].

3. Selection for Animals with Favorable Health Traits

3.1. Health Traits in Farm Animals: Definition, Classification, and Components

Historical emphasis on farm animal selective breeding programs were only focussed on profitability, and the most easily measured traits such as milk yield in dairy cows or bodyweight in swine. Recently, selection between and within breeds for health traits is attracting more attention from farm animal producers. The farmers realize that only by having a more comprehensive assessment of animal performance, the level of productivity can be maintained or improved [120].

Health traits could simply be the traits related to the health status of animals, and therefore, they could be disease traits or host immune status. According to the Animal Trait Ontology [121,122], health traits are a part of animal welfare traits. The traits could be further divided into three main groups including health body traits, disease susceptibility traits, and immune system traits. For each group, several subgroups are also included such as immune system traits which could include acquired immune system traits and innate immune systems traits. Health traits are defined by the interaction between host genetics and environment which includes the management factors as well as the pathogens. Host genetics play important roles in animals, which decide the health status of each individual in the same environment. Selection for host genetics often involves selection for disease resistance or tolerance as well as their immune systems. To maximize the host genetic potentials, it is important to study the gene by environment interaction. Genomic selection for gene by environment interaction might become more feasible using the big data [123].

Health traits could be reported at different levels as within (individual variations) or between populations. The heritabilities of health traits depend on many factors such as the nature of the traits or the method of records; however, they are known to be low-to-moderate. For instance, the estimated heritabilities for the susceptibility of cattle to Johne's disease infection were ranged from 0.06 to 0.18 [124–126]. Therefore, selection for health traits can be achieved but might require quite longer time compared to the other production traits with higher heritabilities.

3.2. The Benefits of Selecting Farm Animals with Favorable Health Traits

Genetic improvement of animal health brings many benefits to the farmers, such as increase in production, reduction in the cost of treatment, enhancement of product quality and fertility (Figure 2). Overall, it improves animal welfare as less animals suffer from disease, as well as improving environmental health and human health by reducing the potential disease transmission to humans. Breeding animals with health traits for controlling disease offers several advantages over the other methods of disease control. Selecting health traits, such as disease tolerance, disease resistance, and immune response, can be an inexpensive and relatively simple way to improve animal health, welfare, and productivity. Breeding for health traits appears more and more attractive as the infectious organisms evolve resistance to the drugs and vaccines used to control them, as the costs of treatment and veterinary care increases faster than the value of the animals, and as a result of the huge economic loss caused by the culling of animals with positive disease tests results.

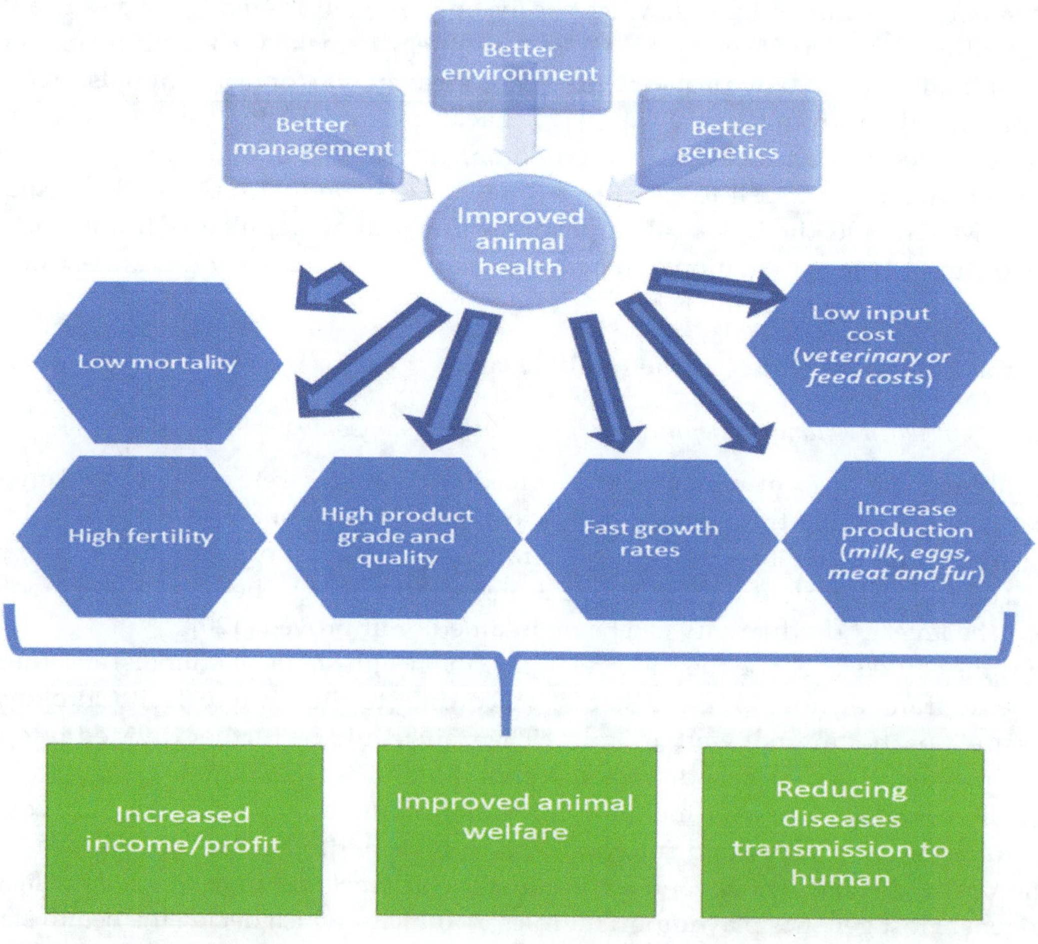

Figure 2. Overall benefits of selection for improved animal health.

Protecting farm animals by vaccination or drug treatment has been the major method used to protect at-risk farm animals; however, the public concern about vaccination or drug treatment is increasing due to the drug residues and the resistance of pathogens and parasites to drugs and vaccines [127]. The intense selection pressure, which evolved into the resistance of parasites to drugs, can be imposed on the parasite population by treating farm animals with drugs such as antibiotics or anthelmintics [128]. Genetic improvement of the health of farm animals through selecting disease resistance may reduce the need for treatment with antibiotics and reduce the risk of residues in farm animal products. The worldwide control strategies to cope with helminths are entirely based on the frequent use of dewormers, which are anthelmintic drugs [129]. These control strategies have been increasingly regarded as unsustainable given the emergence of multiple drug-resistant parasites [130]. Each time an anthelmintic is employed, the resistant parasites will be selected for and will pass their resistant genes onto the next generation of worms [129]. As a result, breeding for genetic resistance is a significant component in integrated parasite management programs [131]. The genome-wide selection strategies are playing an important role in selecting animals for nematodes resistance traits [129]. The most frequent reason for using antibiotics in lactating dairy cattle is mastitis [132]. In the earlier research of bovine mastitis in Finland, the proportion of coagulase-negative Staphylococci resistant to at least one antibiotic drug increased from 27% in 1988 to 50% in 1995 and from 37% to 64% for S. aureus strains [133]. Significant increases in the antibiotics resistance were also observed in France as tetracycline resistance in *Streptococcus uberis* isolates increased from 15.7% to 20.4% and third-generation cephalosporin resistance in *Escherichia coli* isolates increased from 0.4% to 2.4% in the period from 2006 to 2016 [134]. The issues of antibiotic resistance make a permanent improvement in mastitis resistance for cow through selected breeding [135]. Vaccination can be regarded as an alternative strategy for genetic improvement of mastitis; however, a single vaccination can only provide a short-term protection instead of a permanent protection from generation to generation. Although it may be more cost-effective in the short run by using effective low-cost vaccination, genetic improvement in disease resistance has more advantages in the long run [135].

Selection for health traits can reduce the production costs associated with disease control in farm animals [136]. Culling, or test-and-remove strategy, is one of the common approaches to control highly contagious diseases such as PRRS in swine and Aleutian disease in mink. It can cause huge economic loss to farmers due to the expensive cost in replacing a diseased animal and the loss of farmed animals. Bovine tuberculosis, caused by the bacterium *Mycobacterium bovis*, is an endemic disease with zoonotic potential in many parts of the world, notably in the UK and Ireland [1]. The primary method used to control this disease is compulsory testing of cattle followed by the slaughter of test-positive animals at a total cost exceeding GBP 227 million in the UK and Ireland in 2010–2011 [137]. Highly tolerant animals still have good performance in an environment with significant virus exposure, and thus genetic selection for disease tolerance has the potential to reduce the production costs associated with culling diseased animals and eliminating the disease virus. In some developing countries, the majority of poor farmers cannot afford or do not have access to therapeutic and vaccine control, and thus the selection for healthy animals is critical for effective disease control [136].

Selection for animals with health traits (e.g., disease tolerance and disease resistance) has the potentials to bring positive economic impacts to animal farming industries. The disease-resistant animal has the ability to prevent the entry of a pathogen or inhibit the replication of the pathogen [138]. Therefore, selecting the disease-resistant animal has the potential to save the cost of medicine treatment and eliminate the economic losses caused by disease (such as reduced production, high mortality, and low fertility). The disease-tolerant animal has the ability to limit the influence of infection on its health or production performance [138]. Hence, selecting the disease-tolerant animal has the potential to minimize the adverse influence caused by disease during the production period.

3.3. *Methods of Selection for Health Traits*

Artificial selection is the process used for determining the parents for the breeding program, the number of offspring the selected parents produce, and the duration that the selected parents remain in the breeding population [139]. Artificial selection is commonly used in farm animal selection to maximize the benefits by selecting favorable characteristics and excluding the features that are not sought after by the market. The principle of selection is choosing the individuals with the best sets of alleles as genetic parents to reproduce so that the next generation has more desirable alleles than the current generation. The consequence of successful selection is genetically improving future generations of a population by increasing the proportion of desirable genes in the population over time [139]. The progress of selection for farm animal species can be viewed according to the development of molecular techniques as traditional genetic selection, marker-assisted selection and genomic selection.

3.3.1. Traditional Genetic Selection

Improvement of farm animals has focused on the selective breeding of individuals with superior phenotypes. With the development of increasingly advanced statistical methods that maximize selection for genetic gain, this simple approach has been spectacularly successful in increasing the quantity of agricultural output. Selections for certain health traits have been done for a long time when the ancient people tried to select animals with better health or resistance to certain diseases during domestication [140]. These selections were purely based on their observation of performance characteristics without any information about molecular genetics. Existing selection techniques, however, still rely on laborious and time-consuming progeny-testing programs and often depend on subjective assessment of the phenotype. The traditional genetic selection breeding program evaluates the genetic potential of animals, which is based on breeding value, for some important traits using phenotype and pedigree information observed on the animal [141]. Genetic selection has significantly increased the production levels of farm animal species. The high accuracy of breeding value estimation, the moderate-to-high heritability of most production traits, and the use of large databases containing production records of many farm animal species and their genetic relationships have been found to boost breeding programs based on genetic selection and have become quite successful [142]. The application of genetic selection in commercial farm animals based on aspects of output such as higher growth rate in poultry, less fat percentage rate in swine, and greater milk yield in cows has had significant effects on outputs in the farm animal industries [143]. Genetic selection for health traits has been applied in countries with routine health data records collected for a long time. For instance, health traits have been included in breeding programs in Scandinavian countries since the mid-1970s [144]. Mastitis, ketosis and displaced abomasum diseases records were included in the breeding programs of dairy cattle in Canada [145,146]. The impacts of genetic selection for health traits depend on the nature of the traits (heritability), sample size, methods of recording, the priority of selection (e.g., economic weight in the selection index), environments and species; however, the progress for genetic selection for health traits is often lower than production traits.

3.3.2. Marker-Assisted Selection

The molecular techniques such as Polymerase Chain Reaction (PCR), Fluorescence In Situ Hybridization (FISH), and Sanger sequencing were developed in the 1980s [147]. These techniques performed the amplification and sequencing of DNA and identification of markers linked to genes for economically important traits such as disease resistance. When available, these markers will provide animal breeders with an objective test system to identify the animals carrying desirable alleles at birth or even earlier such as an embryo or sperm [148]. The method allows the identification of genes or DNA markers for genetically engineering disease resistance and selection of enhanced production traits [148]. Quantitative trait loci (QTL) mapping is the first step to detect chromosomal regions affecting complex traits, which will be used in the fine mapping for identification of DNA markers for traits of interest. The QTL detection experiments in farm animals started in the 1990s when Andersson et al. [149] detected a QTL for fatness on chromosome four in pigs. Many QTLs were detected initially using initial linkage maps in either crossbreds for highly divergent traits of interest, or commercial populations where half-sib families were available. In the early 1990s, QTL experiments were based on resource populations with a few hundred animals; over time resource population size has increased to thousands of animals coupled with an increasingly large number of markers. Consequently, the number of detected QTLs has also increased rapidly in different farm animal species (Table 3). While genetic markers that are linked to the QTL could be used to choose animals for selective breeding programs, the most effective markers are the functional mutations within the trait genes. For instance, the QTL identified for milk yields and components in chromosome 14 of Holstein dairy cattle is linked to the Acyl-CoA: Diacylglycerol Acyltransferase 1 (*DGAT1*) K232A Polymorphism in Sweden [150], Germany [151], Canada [152], and China [153]. Strategies to identify markers for traits and the application of these markers are described with reference to examples of loci that control a range of different traits [154]. Detection of QTLs, and genes involving the traits of interest helps to develop the marker-assisted selection programs [155]. For example, Ruane and Colleau [156] found that the application of marker-assisted selection could increase 6% to 15% of the selection response for milk production in cattle that used multiple ovulation and embryo transfer in the first six generations of selection. However, most of the detected genes and markers only explain a small proportion of phenotypic variances, and therefore, they are not effective for the selection of quantitative traits. For instance, all genetic markers of 42k genotyping panel could only explain about 11% of phenotypic variation in mortality due to Marek's disease virus infection in layers [157].

Table 3. The number of quantitative trait loci (QTLs) detected in animal species by 7 July 2020.

Species	Number of Publications	Number of Traits	Overall	Health	Disease Suppressibility	Immune Capacity	Pathogens and Parasites	Blood Parameters
Cattle	1001	646	142,261	6380	2771	232	124	355
Chicken	328	430	12,246	820	739	NA	NA	294
Horse	94	56	2446	1128	1026	19	NA	1
Swine	698	691	30,580	6598	586	3230	81	2747
Sheep	173	262	3305	619	135	39	335	37

3.3.3. Genomic Selection

High-throughput genomic technologies especially high-throughput single nucleotide polymorphism (SNP) genotyping, genotype-by-sequencing, as well as the whole genome sequencing methods, have been commercially available for more than ten years. Genomic prediction/selection was the biggest change in the artificial selection of livestock species by adapting high-throughput genotyping technologies in the farm animal sector [158]. Genomic selection refers to making breeding decisions based on genomic estimated breeding values (GEBVs) obtained from SNP effects using various prediction methods [158]. The main approach for genomic selection is to determine the SNP effects from a reference population consisting of a subset of animals with both SNP genotypes and phenotypes for traits of interest, then to use the SNP effects to compute the breeding values (genetic merit) for other genotyped animals that are not yet phenotyped. The basic statistical method used for genomic prediction is similar to the traditional best linear unbiased prediction (BLUP) method that has traditionally been used in animal breeding for a long time, except that the relationship matrix is computed based on SNP genotypes or genomic information. The major advantages of genomic selection are the higher prediction accuracy (compared to traditional EBVs obtained using pedigree information) and the shorter generation interval [159]. The accuracy of GEBVs depends on the size of the reference population used to derive prediction equations, the heritability of the trait, the extent of relationships between selection candidates and the reference population, the relationship between test and reference populations, number of SNPs, number of loci affecting the traits as well as how close assumptions in genomic prediction methods are to the truth [160,161]. Genomic selection has been successfully applied in the farm animal sections and has accelerated the genetic gain not only for the production traits but also for many health traits [162].

3.4. *Selection for Different Types of Health Traits*

3.4.1. Selection for Disease Response Traits (Resistance, Tolerance, and Resilience)

Disease tolerance and resistance are the most common targeted disease response traits in farm animal breeding programs, as they are natural and distinct mechanisms of a host's response to infectious pathogens and could be targeted for genetic improvement [13]. Resistance is the ability of a host to prevent the entry of a pathogen or inhibit the replication of the pathogen. Tolerance is an ability of a host to limit the influence of an infection on the host's health or production performance without interfering with the life cycle of the pathogen [138].

To date, most efforts to control infectious disease focus on selecting disease resistance farm animals to improve the ability of the host to fight disease. The heritable differences of disease resistance between animals lead to opportunities to breed animals for enhanced resistance to the disease [163]. In cattle, the major focus on health traits selection is for mastitis resistance. Many different approaches have been proposed in order to increase the possibility of selection for mastitis [164]. Up to date, 2382 QTLs have been identified for mastitis resistance in dairy cows (Animal QTL Database, https://www.animalgenome.org/cgi-bin/QTLdb/BT/nscape?isID=1439). Not only increasing the number of QTLs, the genetic and genomic selection for mastitis has also achieved a certain level of success (reviewed by Weigel and Shook, [165]) because of the increasing accuracy of prediction for mastitis or the inclusion of different new methods of identification of mastitis incidence in the selection index. For instance, the accuracy of genomic prediction could reach as high as 0.50 to 0.55 for mastitis infection depending on the models [166]. Unlike mastitis, less progress is reported for selection for Johne's disease and BRDC resistance, which might be due to the lack of accurate measurements and their less serious impact on production. The heritabilities for Johne's disease (range from 0.07 to 0.16) and BRDC (range from 0.07 to 0.19) resistance and differences among breeds have been documented in the previous studies [20,124,167,168]. These heritability estimates and significant estimates of additive genetic variances indicate that computing traditional phenotype-based genetic evaluations for resistance to Johne's disease and BRDC is feasible in cattle populations. In swine, 43 QTLs for PRRS resistance have been mapped to 12 chromosomes (Animal QTL Database, https://www.animalgenome.org/cgi-bin/QTLdb/SS/traitmap?trait_ID=779). The major QTL region was located on chromosome four (SSC4) that explained 16% of the genetic variance of PRRS virus load with a frequency for the favorable allele of 0.16 and a heritability of 0.30 [169]. In poultry, a number of QTLs associated with Marek's disease resistance have been reported in various lines and breeds of chicken using SNP or microsatellite markers since 1998 [170–174].

The research focus associated with selecting health traits has expanded to increase the host's tolerance to reduce the harmful effects of infection on health and performance [13,175]. Genetic selections of disease tolerance are rare, as the genetics of disease tolerance and its measurement are more difficult to elucidate than disease resistance in farm animals [1,176]. Growing evidence, however, indicates the potential for genomic selection of disease tolerance. Genomic studies have been able to map the QTL for tolerance traits as Zanella et al. [177] identified a number of QTLs for Johne's disease and Hanotte et al. [178] detected 16 QTLs for trypanosomosis, in the cross of N'Dama and Boran cattle. Meanwhile, the results of genomic prediction (accuracy of 0.38) for facial eczema suggested that genomic selection for the facial eczema disease tolerance has the potential to help the New Zealand sheep industry to cope with the issues caused by facial eczema [179].

Although both resistance and tolerance traits may be under genetic control and could thus be targeted for genetic improvement, selecting tolerance for disease may have some advantages over selecting disease resistance [176]. Firstly, the resistance ability of a host can limit the replication of a pathogen within the host, and therefore, selecting host resistance has a potential to increase the selection advantages on pathogen strains that can withstand host resistance mechanisms and eventually result in a loss of selection advantage of the host [180,181]. It is the potential pitfall for a long-term breeding strategy which focuses on disease resistance if the disease virus has a high mutation rate such as the PRRS virus in swine [182]. It has been theoretically proposed that selecting tolerance might not motivate such selection pressure on the pathogen [181]. Secondly, compared with the resistance mechanisms which directly influence the life-cycle of the pathogen, improving host tolerance has the potential to provide cross-protection against other strains of the virus, or other prevalent infectious agents due to the mechanisms of tolerance which primarily target host-intrinsic damage prevention or repair mechanisms [175,183,184].

Resilience is another health trait that is attracting the attention of animal breeders. Generally, resilience is an ability of an animal either to minimize the influences caused by disturbances or to return to the body condition prior to exposure of a disturbance [185]. The capability of taking care of a larger number of animals is one of the requirements for the intensification of farm animal production. Selecting resilient animals can improve this capability of the farm animal industries because resilient animals are healthy and easy-to-care-for animals that need less attention time [186]. On the other hand, compared to the direct selection based on disease tolerance and resistance, the selection based on resilience is a more pragmatic way of keeping healthy animals, because it does not need the records on pathogen burden, which is the amount of pathogen in the animal's body [187–189]. Resilience, however, is not yet included in breeding goals due to the difficulty of phenotyping [13]. Fortunately, the current developments on the big data collection and new disease resilience indicators defined based on these data provide great opportunities to breed for improved resilience in livestock [190].

3.4.2. Selections for Immune Response Traits

Immunity response traits are also important health traits for animal breeders to select for improving the farm animals' ability to withstand disease. The immune system is important to control infections and diseases. The immune response traits have been recommended to be selected for decreasing the incidence and impact of the disease in farm animals [14,191]. In Holstein cattle, the lower occurrence of mastitis improved response to the commercial vaccine, and increased milk and colostrum quality are all observed in cows with superior or high immunity response [118]. Consequently, improving the inherent ability to cope with the diseases in dairy cattle through genetic selection for superior or high immunity response is feasible [192]. In cattle, the High Immune Response (HIR™) and the Immunity+, which are used to identify and select animals with naturally optimized immune responses, have been applied in the genetic selection of cattle for improved immunity and health [14]. In swine, the total and differential numbers of leukocytes, expression levels of swine leukocyte antigens I and II, and serum concentrations of IgG and haptoglobin are immunity traits that have been demonstrated to have additive genetic variation. These immunity traits, therefore, have the potential to be used as criteria to improve the selection of pigs for coping with clinical and subclinical diseases [193]. In poultry, the presence of genetic variability in immune response traits and the discovery of SNPs associated with immune response traits indicate that genetically enhancing antibody response and resistance to parasitism is feasible through genomic selection [194].

3.5. Challenges in the Selection of Health Traits

Health traits, such as disease resistance, disease tolerance, and immunity response level are usually quantitative traits which are influenced by many genetic and environmental factors. Although genetic selection has significantly increased the production traits in farm animal species such as higher growth rate, less fatness, and greater milk yield [143], selection for health traits is much more complicated and faces some challenging obstacles. The potential problems in selection for health traits can be classified under desirability, feasibility and sustainability [195].

3.5.1. Desirability

The desirability describes the importance of the disease relative to the other diseases or production traits. The correlations between health traits and economic traits are often negative, which means the health traits are potentially genetically antagonistic to production traits [196,197]. Milk yield in dairy cattle has unfavorable correlations with many disease response traits [198,199]. The genetic correlations between mastitis and milk production or high somatic cell score and milk production are moderate and positive [200]. In poultry, genetic selection for greater body weight can lead to decreased immunity to fowl cholera and Newcastle disease [201]. The opposite results, however, also occur in some research. For example, van der Most et al. [202] stated that selection for growth in poultry can compromise the immune function, while the selection for immune function does not consistently affect growth. Therefore, identifying the genetic correlations between health traits and production traits in farm animals is an important aspect of health traits selection. Applying the economic selection index is one of the solutions to deal with the antagonistic genetic correlation between traits. In 1943, Hazel [203] first presented the aggregate genotype, which was also called net merit of animals as a linear combination of breeding values for each trait weighted by the economic value of the traits. After that, the economic selection index for multi-trait selection has been used in animal breeding research fields and employed in animal agriculture industries. The breeding objective can be defined as the aggregate breeding value expressed by profit or economic efficiency, and it is the overall goal of breeding programs to increase the profits or economic efficiency for breeders and/or producers. In this way, multi-trait selection with the economic selection index can minimize the adverse influences caused by the antagonistic genetic correlations between target traits to achieve the overall goal of breeding programs [204].

3.5.2. Feasibility

Feasibility accounts for the tools available with which to perform the selection. The success of selection for health traits is highly dependent on correctly identifying the phenotype for traits associated with the host's abilities to withstand infectious diseases. Accurately identifying the phenotypes for health traits is expensive and difficult. An extensive data recording is required to enable an accurate genetic evaluation. High labor costs are required for long-term recording of large amounts of phenotypic and progeny data [12]. In a combined population of infected and healthy individuals, it is not correct to consider an individual with good performance to have favorable health traits, nor the sick populations to be genetically susceptible [205]. Some susceptible animals still show good performance because they may not have been sufficiently exposed to the pathogens. An animal displaying a healthy performance without clinical symptoms may have sub-clinical infections and represents a pathogen carrier. The clinical expression of a disease can be confounded by infection with one or more similar diseases such as pneumonia which can be confused with pulmonary adenomatosis, bronchitis, and pleuritis. Meanwhile, diagnosing a disease accurately and specifically is costly and time-consuming [196].

3.5.3. Sustainability

Sustainability means the enhanced resistance to the infectious disease in the farms or flocks is stable for a long period especially when the pathogens often evolve faster than the hosts [195]. The long-term success of selection involves not only the choice of the best animals with disease resistance but also the management systems with the ability to cope with the constant changes in the farming environment. For instance, hot environment caused by global warming could impair production and reproductive performance, metabolic and health status, and immune response [206]. The climate changes also cause changes in the pathogens or create novel pathogens which require the producers to constantly adapt new methods and treatments for their animals. Genomic selection of robustness and fitness traits could be a solution for this challenge [190,207].

3.6. *Promise of Selection for Health Traits*

3.6.1. High-Throughput Phenotyping and Sequencing, and Generation of Big Data

Big data is a mix of different sources of data (structured and unstructured) that comprises a large volume of information [208]. The major characteristics of big data include volume, velocity, variety, variability, veracity, validity, and volatility [209]. Big data has been adapted to the farm animal sector such as precision farming [210], biosensors [211], electronic feeding stations, and automatic milking systems [123]. Big data is also important for infectious disease surveillance and modeling [190,212]. It is clear that big data generated from high-throughput phenotyping will give unprecedented opportunities for combating diseases and selecting healthy animals [213,214]. For example, the mastitis and claw health can be recorded via high-throughput phenotyping devices such as real-time biosensors [215,216]. The use of big data for animal health care, however, needs a careful handling of the data [217] and selection of appropriate statistical methods [218,219]. High-throughput sequencing data, such as genomics, transcriptomics, proteomics, and epigenomics etc., have been adapted to improve animal health [220,221] as they could help to understand the biology of disease, computing EBVs, and pinpointing the biomarkers.

3.6.2. Data Sharing and International Corporations

Data sharing and international corporations can play crucial roles in the selection of healthy traits even those selections that take place locally. The major reason for this is that many diseases in farm animals are transboundary diseases. The outbreaks of diseases could potentially affect other farms in different countries such as the outbreaks of Avian Influenzas Virus that cause significant loss in many nations worldwide. Information sharing plays a crucial role in controlling diseases for nations on the same continent especially for developing countries [222]. It is also important to have a standard protocol for recoding the incidences, progress of the disease and consequences of diseases for better use of data. In cattle, for instance, the International Committee for Animal Recording provides a recording guideline for 1000 diagnoses that can be used toward the genetic improvement of health traits (ICAR GUIDELINES, https://www.icar.org/index.php/icar-recording-guidelines/). International corporations could work together in a joint effort for phenotyping or genotyping animals/disease to enlarge the resources and enhance the human capacity to deal with disease. For example, the use of automatic milking systems from different nations could improve the modeling of mastitis infections [165] or the sharing of omics data could better develop the statistical methods and enhance understanding about the disease biology [223]. The current 1000 Bull Genomes Project is a successful story regarding the sharing of genomic data for improving the prediction accuracy of future genomic EBVs [224]. It is important to indicate that increasing the capacity of cloud storage and computing could also support the sharing of data and corporations.

4. Conclusions

Selecting favorable health traits to cope with diseases in farm animals has increasingly become an attractive focus of animal farming industries. Given some limitations and deficiencies of current non-selection disease control methods and the advantages of genetic selection over the other methods, breeding for health traits is a promising solution for the sustainable development of livestock farming. Although some remaining challenges regarding the accuracy of phenotyping and low heritability of disease traits hinder the progress of breeding for health traits, the advancement of sequencing techniques and affordable cost of genotyping make selective breeding more beneficial as a method for disease control but also require more storage and computing power. With the development of cloud computing, big data analyses increase the feasibility of selection for animal health traits. Increasing threats, such as climate change, have caused changes in the environments that require international collaborations to deal with the disease on a global scale. Eventually, smart farming with healthy animals and clean environments will be achieved with the sustainable selection methods of favorable health traits. The genetic and genomic selection solution, however, cannot address all the problems caused by disease farm animals. Therefore, it is necessary to accompany selection solution approaches with other disease control and monitor methods (e.g., vaccination, culling strategy, biosensor, and genome editing) to help animal agriculture industries to reduce the economic losses and animal welfare issues caused by farm animal diseases.

Author Contributions: Conceptualization, G.H., D.N.D. and Y.M.; writing—original draft preparation, G.H. and D.N.D.; writing—review and editing, G.H., D.N.D., J.G. and Y.M.; supervision, Y.M. All authors have read and agreed to the published version of the manuscript.

Acknowledgments: Authors are thankful to the anonymous reviewers whose critiques and comments greatly improved the manuscript.

References

1. Bishop, S.C.; Woolliams, J.A. Genomics and disease resistance studies in livestock. *Livest. Sci.* **2014**, *166*, 190–198. [CrossRef] [PubMed]
2. Rashid, A.; Rasheed, K.; Asim, M.; Hussain, A. Risks of vaccination: A review. *J. Venom. Anim. Toxins Incl. Trop. Dis.* **2009**, *15*. [CrossRef]
3. Yeruham, I.; Yadin, H.; Haymovich, M.; Perl, S. Adverse reactions to FMD vaccine. *Vet. Dermatol.* **2001**, *12*, 197–201. [CrossRef] [PubMed]
4. Beyene, T. Veterinary drug residues in food-animal products: Its risk factors and potential effects on public health. *J. Vet. Sci. Technol.* **2016**, *7*, 1–7. [CrossRef]
5. de Jong, A.; Thomas, V.; Simjee, S.; Moyaert, H.; El Garch, F.; Maher, K.; Morrissey, I.; Butty, P.; Klein, U.; Marion, H.; et al. Antimicrobial susceptibility monitoring of respiratory tract pathogens isolated from diseased cattle and pigs across Europe: The VetPath study. *Vet. Microbiol.* **2014**, *172*, 202–215. [CrossRef]
6. Ibrahim, A.; Junaidu, A.; Garba, M. Multiple antibiotic residues in meat from slaughtered cattle in Nigeria. *Internet J. Vet. Med.* **2010**, *8*, 1–7.
7. Kehinde, O.G.; Junaidu, K.; Mohammed, M.; AbdulRahman, A.M. Detection of antimicrobial drug residues in commercial eggs using Premi®Test. *Int. J. Poult. Sci.* **2012**, *11*, 50–54. [CrossRef]
8. Rokka, M.; Eerola, S.; Perttila, U.; Rossow, L.; Venalainen, E.; Valkonen, E.; Valaja, J.; Peltonen, K. The residue levels of narasin in eggs of laying hens fed with unmedicated and medicated feed. *Mol. Nutr. Food Res.* **2005**, *49*, 38–42. [CrossRef]
9. Wilson, M.E. The afterlife of antibiotics. *J. Travel Med.* **2020**, *27*. [CrossRef]
10. Pritchard, T.C.; Coffey, M.P.; Bond, K.S.; Hutchings, M.R.; Wall, E. Phenotypic effects of subclinical paratuberculosis (Johne's disease) in dairy cattle. *J. Dairy Sci.* **2017**, *100*, 679–690. [CrossRef]
11. Themudo, G.E.; Østergaard, J.; Ersbøll, A.K. Persistent spatial clusters of plasmacytosis among Danish mink farms. *Prev. Vet. Med.* **2011**, *102*, 75–82. [CrossRef] [PubMed]
12. Holmberg, M.; Andersson-Eklund, L. Quantitative trait loci affecting health traits in Swedish dairy cattle. *J. Dairy Sci.* **2004**, *87*, 2653–2659. [CrossRef]
13. Doeschl-Wilson, A.B.; Villanueva, B.; Kyriazakis, I. The first step toward genetic selection for host tolerance to infectious pathogens: Obtaining the tolerance phenotype through group estimates. *Front. Genet.* **2012**, *3*, 265. [CrossRef] [PubMed]
14. Mallard, B.A.; Emam, M.; Paibomesai, M.; Thompson-Crispi, K.; Wagter-Lesperance, L. Genetic selection of cattle for improved immunity and health. *Jpn. J. Vet. Res.* **2015**, *63*, 37–44. [CrossRef]
15. Cowley, D.B.; Graham, D.A.; Guelbenzu, M.; Doherty, M.L.; More, S.J. Aspects of bovine herpesvirus 1 and bovine viral diarrhoea virus herd-level seroprevalence and vaccination in dairy and beef herds in Northern Ireland. *Ir. Vet. J.* **2014**, *67*, 18. [CrossRef]
16. Carman, S.; van Dreumel, T.; Ridpath, J.; Hazlett, M.; Alves, D.; Dubovi, E.; Tremblay, R.; Bolin, S.; Godkin, A.; Anderson, N. Severe acute bovine viral diarrhea in Ontario, 1993-1995. *J. Vet. Diagn. Invest.* **1998**, *10*, 27–35. [CrossRef]
17. Houe, H. Economic impact of BVDV infection in dairies. *Biologicals* **2003**, *31*, 137–143. [CrossRef]
18. Brownlie, J. BVD—Why vaccination alone is not the complete answer to eradication. *Livestock* **2014**, *19*, 221–224. [CrossRef]

19. Pinior, B.; Firth, C.L.; Richter, V.; Lebl, K.; Trauffler, M.; Dzieciol, M.; Hutter, S.E.; Burgstaller, J.; Obritzhauser, W.; Winter, P.; et al. A systematic review of financial and economic assessments of bovine viral diarrhea virus (BVDV) prevention and mitigation activities worldwide. *Prev. Vet. Med.* **2017**, *137*, 77–92. [CrossRef]
20. Attalla, S.A.; Seykora, A.J.; Cole, J.B.; Heins, B.J. Genetic parameters of milk ELISA scores for Johne's disease. *J. Dairy Sci.* **2010**, *93*, 1729–1735. [CrossRef]
21. Cho, J.; Tauer, L.W.; Schukken, Y.H.; Smith, R.L.; Lu, Z.; Grohn, Y.T. Cost-Effective Control Strategies for Johne's Disease in Dairy Herds. *Can. J. Agric. Econ.* **2013**, *61*, 583–608. [CrossRef]
22. Gershwin, L.J.; Van Eenennaam, A.L.; Anderson, M.L.; McEligot, H.A.; Shao, M.X.; Toaff-Rosenstein, R.; Taylor, J.F.; Neibergs, H.L.; Womack, J.; Bovine Respiratory Disease Complex Coordinated Agricultural Project Research Team. Single Pathogen Challenge with Agents of the Bovine Respiratory Disease Complex. *PLoS ONE* **2015**, *10*, e0142479. [CrossRef] [PubMed]
23. Miles, D.G. Overview of the North American beef cattle industry and the incidence of bovine respiratory disease (BRD). *Anim. Health Res. Rev.* **2009**, *10*, 101–103. [CrossRef]
24. Neibergs, H.; Neibergs, J.; Wojtowicz, A.; Taylor, J.; Seabury, C.; Womack, J. Economic benefits of using genetic selection to reduce the prevalence of bovine respiratory disease complex in beef feedlot cattle. In Proceedings of the 2014 Beef Improvement Federation Annual Meeting and Convention, Lincoln, NE, USA, 18–21 June 2014; pp. 82–87.
25. DeDonder, K.D.; Apley, M.D. A literature review of antimicrobial resistance in Pathogens associated with bovine respiratory disease. *Anim. Health Res. Rev.* **2015**, *16*, 125–134. [CrossRef] [PubMed]
26. Carvelli, A.; Sala, M.; Autorino, G.L.; Scicluna, M.T.; Iacoponi, F.; Rombola, P.; Scaramozzino, P. A cross-sectional serosurvey in a sheep population in central Italy following a bluetongue epidemic. *PLoS ONE* **2019**, *14*, e0208074. [CrossRef] [PubMed]
27. Elhassan, A.M.; Fadol, M.A.; El Hussein, A.R.M. Seroprevalence of bluetongue virus in dairy herds with reproductive problems in Sudan. *Int. Schol. Res. Notices (ISRN) Vet. Sci.* **2014**, *2014*, 595724. [CrossRef]
28. Velthuis, A.G.; Saatkamp, H.W.; Mourits, M.C.; de Koeijer, A.A.; Elbers, A.R. Financial consequences of the Dutch bluetongue serotype 8 epidemics of 2006 and 2007. *Prev. Vet. Med.* **2010**, *93*, 294–304. [CrossRef]
29. Kyriakis, C.S.; Billinis, C.; Papadopoulos, E.; Vasileiou, N.G.; Athanasiou, L.V.; Fthenakis, G.C. Bluetongue in small ruminants: An opinionated review, with a brief appraisal of the 2014 outbreak of the disease in Greece and the south-east Europe. *Vet. Microbiol.* **2015**, *181*, 66–74. [CrossRef]
30. Boumart, Z.; Daouam, S.; Belkourati, I.; Rafi, L.; Tuppurainen, E.; Tadlaoui, K.O.; El Harrak, M. Comparative innocuity and efficacy of live and inactivated sheeppox vaccines. *BMC Vet. Res.* **2016**, *12*, 133. [CrossRef]
31. Hota, A.; Biswal, S.; Sahoo, N.; Venkatesan, G.; Arya, S.; Kumar, A.; Ramakrishnan, M.A.; Pandey, A.B.; Rout, M. Seroprevalence of Capripoxvirus infection in sheep and goats among different agro-climatic zones of Odisha, India. *Vet. World* **2018**, *11*, 66. [CrossRef]
32. Hurisa, T.; Jing, Z.; Jia, H.; Chen, G.; He, X. A Review on Sheeppox and Goatpox: Insight of Epidemiology, Diagnosis, Treatment and Control Measures in Ethiopia. *J. Infect. Dis. Epidemiol.* **2018**, *4*, 2474–3658. [CrossRef]
33. Garner, M.; Sawarkar, S.; Brett, E.; Edwards, J.; Kulkarni, V.; Boyle, D.; Singh, S. The extent and impact of sheep pox and goat pox in the state of Maharashtra, India. *Trop. Anim. Health Prod.* **2000**, *32*, 205–223. [CrossRef] [PubMed]
34. Lunney, J.K.; Fang, Y.; Ladinig, A.; Chen, N.; Li, Y.; Rowland, B.; Renukaradhya, G.J. Porcine reproductive and respiratory syndrome virus (PRRSV): Pathogenesis and interaction with the immune system. *Annu. Rev. Anim. Biosci.* **2016**, *4*, 129–154. [CrossRef] [PubMed]
35. Arruda, A.G.; Poljak, Z.; Friendship, R.; Carpenter, J.; Hand, K. Descriptive analysis and spatial epidemiology of porcine reproductive and respiratory syndrome (PRRS) for swine sites participating in area regional control and elimination programs from 3 regions of Ontario. *Can. J. Vet. Res.* **2015**, *79*, 268–278. [PubMed]
36. Holtkamp, D.J.; Kliebenstein, J.B.; Neumann, E.; Zimmerman, J.J.; Rotto, H.; Yoder, T.K.; Wang, C.; Yeske, P.; Mowrer, C.L.; Haley, C.A. Assessment of the economic impact of porcine reproductive and respiratory syndrome virus on United States pork producers. *J. Swine Health Prod.* **2013**, *21*, 72.

37. Mussell, A.; Oginskyy, A.; Grier, K.; Morin, M.; Lachance, M.; Whittington, L.; Friendship, R. *A Risk, Benefit, Strength, Weakness, Opportunity and Threat Analysis for the Control. and Possible Eradication of Porcine Reproductive and Respiratory Syndrome (PRRS) Virus Within the Canadian Swine Herd*; George Morris Centre: Guelph, ON, Canada, 2011.
38. Hess, A.S.; Islam, Z.; Hess, M.K.; Rowland, R.R.; Lunney, J.K.; Doeschl-Wilson, A.; Plastow, G.S.; Dekkers, J.C. Comparison of host genetic factors influencing pig response to infection with two North American isolates of porcine reproductive and respiratory syndrome virus. *Genet. Sel. Evol.* **2016**, *48*, 43. [CrossRef]
39. Sun, N.; Sun, P.; Lv, H.; Sun, Y.; Guo, J.; Wang, Z.; Luo, T.; Wang, S.; Li, H. Matrine displayed antiviral activity in porcine alveolar macrophages co-infected by porcine reproductive and respiratory syndrome virus and porcine circovirus type 2. *Sci. Rep.* **2016**, *6*, 1–13. [CrossRef]
40. Brown, V.R.; Bevins, S.N. A Review of African Swine Fever and the Potential for Introduction into the United States and the Possibility of Subsequent Establishment in Feral Swine and Native Ticks. *Front. Vet. Sci.* **2018**, *5*, 11. [CrossRef]
41. Liu, J.; Liu, B.; Shan, B.; Wei, S.; An, T.; Shen, G.; Chen, Z. Prevalence of African Swine Fever in China, 2018–2019. *J. Med. Virol.* **2019**, *92*, 1023–1034. [CrossRef]
42. USDA. *GAIN Report: Russia 2017 Livestock and Products Annual RS1757*; United States Department of Agriculture: Washington, DC, USA, 2017.
43. Bello, M.B.; Yusoff, K.; Ideris, A.; Hair-Bejo, M.; Peeters, B.P.H.; Omar, A.R. Diagnostic and Vaccination Approaches for Newcastle Disease Virus in Poultry: The Current and Emerging Perspectives. *Biomed. Res. Int.* **2018**, *2018*, 7278459. [CrossRef]
44. Cross, T.A.; Arsnoe, D.; Minnis, R.; King, D.; Swafford, S.; Pedersen, K.; Owen, J. Prevalence of avian paramyxovirus 1 and avian influenza virus in double-crested cormorants (Phalacrocorax auritus) in eastern North America. *J. Wildl. Dis.* **2013**, *49*, 965–977. [CrossRef] [PubMed]
45. Wise, M.G.; Suarez, D.L.; Seal, B.S.; Pedersen, J.C.; Senne, D.A.; King, D.J.; Kapczynski, D.R.; Spackman, E. Development of a real-time reverse-transcription PCR for detection of Newcastle disease virus RNA in clinical samples. *J. Clin. Microbiol.* **2004**, *42*, 329–338. [CrossRef] [PubMed]
46. Dimitrov, K.M.; Afonso, C.L.; Yu, Q.; Miller, P.J. Newcastle disease vaccines—A solved problem or a continuous challenge? *Vet. Microbiol.* **2017**, *206*, 126–136. [CrossRef] [PubMed]
47. Mayers, J.; Mansfield, K.L.; Brown, I.H. The role of vaccination in risk mitigation and control of Newcastle disease in poultry. *Vaccine* **2017**, *35*, 5974–5980. [CrossRef]
48. Morrow, C.; Fehler, F. Marek's disease: A worldwide problem. In *Marek's Disease*; Davison, F., Nair, V., Eds.; Elsevier Academic Press: London, UK, 2004; pp. 49–61.
49. Wajid, S.J.; Katz, M.E.; Renz, K.G.; Walkden-Brown, S.W. Prevalence of Marek's disease virus in different chicken populations in Iraq and indicative virulence based on sequence variation in the EcoRI-Q (meq) gene. *Avian Dis.* **2013**, *57*, 562–568. [CrossRef]
50. Boodhoo, N.; Gurung, A.; Sharif, S.; Behboudi, S. Marek's disease in chickens: A review with focus on immunology. *Vet. Res.* **2016**, *47*, 119. [CrossRef]
51. Reddy, S.M.; Izumiya, Y.; Lupiani, B. Marek's disease vaccines: Current status, and strategies for improvement and development of vector vaccines. *Vet. Microbiol.* **2017**, *206*, 113–120. [CrossRef]
52. Dunn, J.R.; Gimeno, I.M. Current status of Marek's disease in the United States and worldwide based on a questionnaire survey. *Avian Dis.* **2013**, *57*, 483–490. [CrossRef]
53. Farid, A.; Ferns, L. Aleutian mink disease virus infection may cause hair depigmentation. *Scientifur* **2011**, *35*, 55–59.
54. Hansen, M.; Lund, E. Pregnancy rate and foetal mortality in Aleutian disease virus infected mink. *Acta Vet. Scand.* **1988**, *29*, 271.
55. McDonald, R.A.; Lariviere, S. Diseases and pathogens of Mustela spp, with special reference to the biological control of introduced stoat Mustela erminea populations in New Zealand. *J. R. Soc. N. Z.* **2001**, *31*, 721–744. [CrossRef]
56. Reichert, M.; Kostro, K. Effect of persistent infection of mink with Aleutian mink disease virus on reproductive failure. *Bull. Vet. Inst. Pulawy* **2014**, *58*, 369–373. [CrossRef]
57. Farid, A.; Zillig, M.; Finley, G.; Smith, G. Prevalence of the Aleutian mink disease virus infection in Nova Scotia, Canada. *Prev. Vet. Med.* **2012** *106*, 332–338. [CrossRef] [PubMed]

58. Farid, A.; Daftarian, P.; Fatehi, J. Transmission Dynamics of Aleutian Mink Disease Virus on a Farm Under Test and Removal Scheme. *J. Vet. Sci. Med. Diagn.* **2018**, *7*, 2. [CrossRef]
59. Christensen, L.S.; Gram-Hansen, L.; Chriel, M.; Jensen, T.H. Diversity and stability of Aleutian mink disease virus during bottleneck transitions resulting from eradication in domestic mink in Denmark. *Vet. Microbiol.* **2011**, *149*, 64–71. [CrossRef]
60. Aasted, B.; Alexandersen, S.; Christensen, J. Vaccination with Aleutian mink disease parvovirus (AMDV) capsid proteins enhances disease, while vaccination with the major non-structural AMDV protein causes partial protection from disease. *Vaccine* **1998**, *16*, 1158–1165. [CrossRef]
61. Heuer, C.; Healy, A.; Zerbini, C. Economic Effects of Exposure to Bovine Viral Diarrhea Virus on Dairy Herds in New Zealand. *J. Dairy Sci.* **2007**, *90*, 5428–5438. [CrossRef]
62. Roeder, P.; Jeffrey, M.; Cranwell, M. Pestivirus fetopathogenicity in cattle: Changing sequelae with fetal maturation. *Vet. Rec.* **1986**, *118*, 44–48. [CrossRef]
63. Khodakaram-Tafti, A.; Farjanikish, G. Persistent bovine viral diarrhea virus (BVDV) infection in cattle herds. *Iran. J. Vet. Res.* **2017**, *18*, 154.
64. Losinger, W.C. Economic impact of reduced milk production associated with Johne's disease on dairy operations in the USA. *J. Dairy. Res.* **2005**, *72*, 425–432. [CrossRef]
65. VanLeeuwen, J.; Haddad, J.; Dohoo, I.; Keefe, G.; Tiwari, A.; Tremblay, R. Associations between reproductive performance and seropositivity for bovine leukemia virus, bovine viral-diarrhea virus, Mycobacterium avium subspecies paratuberculosis, and Neospora caninum in Canadian dairy cows. *Prev. Vet. Med.* **2010**, *94*, 54–64. [CrossRef] [PubMed]
66. Urban-Chmiel, R.; Wernicki, A.; Puchalski, A.; Dec, M.; Stęgierska, D.; Grooms, D.L.; Barbu, N.I. Detection of bovine respiratory syncytial virus infections in young dairy and beef cattle in Poland. *Vet. Quart.* **2015**, *35*, 33–36. [CrossRef] [PubMed]
67. Barnard, B.; Gerdes, G.H.; Meiswinkel, R. Some epidemiological and economic aspects of a bluetongue-like disease in cattle in South Africa-1995/96 and 1997. *Onderstepoort J. Vet. Res.* **1998**, *65*, 145–151. [PubMed]
68. Toussaint, J.-F.; Sailleau, C.; Mast, J.; Houdart, P.; Czaplicki, G.; Demeestere, L.; VandenBussche, F.; Van Dessel, W.; Goris, N.; Bréard, E. Bluetongue in Belgium, 2006. *Emerg. Infect. Dis.* **2007**, *13*, 614. [CrossRef]
69. Conraths, F.J.; Gethmann, J.M.; Staubach, C.; Mettenleiter, T.C.; Beer, M.; Hoffmann, B. Epidemiology of bluetongue virus serotype 8, Germany. *Emerg. Infect. Dis.* **2009**, *15*, 433. [CrossRef]
70. Limon, G.; Gamawa, A.A.; Ahmed, A.I.; Lyons, N.A.; Beard, P.M. Epidemiological Characteristics and Economic Impact of Lumpy Skin Disease, Sheeppox and Goatpox Among Subsistence Farmers in Northeast Nigeria. *Front. Vet. Sci.* **2020**, *7*, 8. [CrossRef]
71. Pena, R.N.; Fernández, C.; Blasco-Felip, M.; Fraile, L.J.; Estany, J. Genetic Markers Associated with Field PRRSV-Induced Abortion Rates. *Viruses* **2019**, *11*, 706. [CrossRef]
72. Pils, M.C.; Dreckmann, K.; Jansson, K.; Glage, S.; Held, N.; Sommer, W.; Länger, F.; Avsar, M.; Warnecke, G.; Bleich, A. Mortality Due to Porcine Reproductive and Respiratory Syndrome Virus in Immunocompromised Göttingen Minipigs (Sus scrofa domestica). *Comp. Med.* **2016**, *66*, 392–398.
73. Schlafer, D.; Mebus, C. Abortion in sows experimentally infected with African swine fever virus: Clinical features. *Am. J. Vet. Res.* **1984**, *45*, 1353–1360.
74. Sánchez-Cordón, P.; Montoya, M.; Reis, A.; Dixon, L. African swine fever: A re-emerging viral disease threatening the global pig industry. *Vet. J.* **2018**, *233*, 41–48. [CrossRef]
75. Van Eck, J.; Davelaar, F.; Van Den Heuvel-Plesman, T.A.; Van Kol, N.; Kouwenhoven, B.; Guldie, F. Dropped egg production, soft shelled and shell-less eggs associated with appearance of precipitins to adenovirus in flocks of laying fowls. *Avian Dis.* **1976**, *5*, 261–272. [CrossRef] [PubMed]
76. Sedeik, M.; Elbestawy, A.; El-Shall, N.; Abd El-Hack, M.; Saadeldin, I.; Swelum, A. Comparative efficacy of commercial inactivated Newcastle disease virus vaccines against Newcastle disease virus genotype VII in broiler chickens. *Poult. Sci.* **2019**, *98*, 2000–2007. [CrossRef] [PubMed]
77. Purchase, H. Clinical disease and its economic impact. In *Marek's Disease*; Springer: Berlin, Germany, 1985; pp. 17–42.
78. Biggs, P.M.; Nair, V. The long view: 40 years of Marek's disease research and Avian Pathology. *Avian. Pathol.* **2012**, *41*, 3–9. [CrossRef] [PubMed]

79. Bastida, F.; Juste, R.A. Paratuberculosis control: A review with a focus on vaccination. *J. Immune Based Ther. Vaccines* **2011**, *9*, 8. [CrossRef]
80. Buchy, P.; Ascioglu, S.; Buisson, Y.; Datta, S.; Nissen, M.; Tambyah, P.A.; Vong, S. Impact of vaccines on antimicrobial resistance. *Int. J. Infect. Dis.* **2020**, *90*, 188–196. [CrossRef]
81. Grubman, M.J.; Baxt, B. Foot-and-mouth disease. *Clin. Microbiol. Rev.* **2004**, *17*, 465–493. [CrossRef]
82. Zientara, S.; MacLachlan, N.J.; Calistri, P.; Sanchez-Vizcaino, J.M.; Savini, G. Bluetongue vaccination in Europe. *Expert Rev. Vaccines* **2010**, *9*, 989–991. [CrossRef]
83. Chen, R.T. Vaccine risks: Real, perceived and unknown. *Vaccine* **1999**, *17*, S41–S46. [CrossRef]
84. Tago, D.; Sall, B.; Lancelot, R.; Pradel, J. VacciCost—A tool to estimate the resource requirements for implementing livestock vaccination campaigns. Application to peste des petits ruminants (PPR) vaccination in Senegal. *Prev. Vet. Med.* **2017**, *144*, 13–19. [CrossRef]
85. Page, S.; Gautier, P. Use of antimicrobial agents in livestock. *Rev. Sci. Tech.* **2012**, *31*, 145–188. [CrossRef]
86. Wang, J.; Deng, Y.; Diao, H. Perceived Risk, Expected Benefits and Pig Farmers' Behaviors of Veterinary Drug Usage. *Int. J. Environ. Res. Public Health* **2018**, *15*, 1716. [CrossRef] [PubMed]
87. Council, N.R. *The Use of Drugs in Food Animals: Benefits and Risks*; National Academies Press: Washington, DC, USA, 1999.
88. Shao, Y.; Li, M.; Zhang, W.; Ji, Y.; Hayes, D.J. World's Largest Pork Producer in Crisis: China's African Swine Fever Outbreak. *Agric. Policy Rev.* **2018**, *2018*, 1.
89. Zhang, H.; Kono, H.; Kubota, S. An integrated epidemiological and economic analysis of vaccination against highly pathogenic porcine reproductive and respiratory syndrome (PRRS) in Thua Thien Hue Province, Vietnam. *Asian Austral. J. Amin.* **2014**, *27*, 1499. [CrossRef] [PubMed]
90. Canuti, M.; O'Leary, K.E.; Hunter, B.D.; Spearman, G.; Ojkic, D.; Whitney, H.G.; Lang, A.S. Driving forces behind the evolution of the Aleutian mink disease parvovirus in the context of intensive farming. *Virus Evol.* **2016**, *2*, vew004. [CrossRef]
91. Kashtanov, S.; Salnikova, L. Aleutian mink disease: Epidemiological and genetic aspects. *Biol. Bull. Rev.* **2018**, *8*, 104–113. [CrossRef]
92. Kalds, P.; Zhou, S.; Cai, B.; Liu, J.; Wang, Y.; Petersen, B.; Sonstegard, T.; Wang, X.; Chen, Y. Sheep and Goat Genome Engineering: From Random Transgenesis to the CRISPR Era. *Front. Genet.* **2019**, *10*. [CrossRef]
93. Lillico, S.G.; Proudfoot, C.; King, T.J.; Tan, W.; Zhang, L.; Mardjuki, R.; Paschon, D.E.; Rebar, E.J.; Urnov, F.D.; Mileham, A.J.; et al. Mammalian interspecies substitution of immune modulatory alleles by genome editing. *Sci. Rep.* **2016**, *6*, 21645. [CrossRef] [PubMed]
94. Proudfoot, C.; Lillico, S.; Tait-Burkard, C. Genome editing for disease resistance in pigs and chickens. *Anim. Front.* **2019**, *9*, 6–12. [CrossRef]
95. Ruan, J.; Xu, J.; Chen-Tsai, R.Y.; Li, K. Genome editing in livestock: Are we ready for a revolution in animal breeding industry? *Transgenic Res.* **2017**, *26*, 715–726. [CrossRef] [PubMed]
96. Tait-Burkard, C.; Doeschl-Wilson, A.; McGrew, M.J.; Archibald, A.L.; Sang, H.M.; Houston, R.D.; Whitelaw, C.B.; Watson, M. Livestock 2.0–genome editing for fitter, healthier, and more productive farmed animals. *Genome Biol.* **2018**, *19*, 204. [CrossRef]
97. Van Eenennaam, A.L. Application of genome editing in farm animals: Cattle. *Transgenic Res.* **2019**, *28*, 93–100. [CrossRef] [PubMed]
98. Whitworth, K.M.; Rowland, R.R.; Ewen, C.L.; Trible, B.R.; Kerrigan, M.A.; Cino-Ozuna, A.G.; Samuel, M.S.; Lightner, J.E.; McLaren, D.G.; Mileham, A.J.; et al. Gene-edited pigs are protected from porcine reproductive and respiratory syndrome virus. *Nat. Biotechnol.* **2016**, *34*, 20–22. [CrossRef] [PubMed]
99. Wu, H.; Wang, Y.; Zhang, Y.; Yang, M.; Lv, J.; Liu, J.; Zhang, Y. TALE nickase-mediated SP110 knockin endows cattle with increased resistance to tuberculosis. *Proc. Natl. Acad. Sci. USA* **2015**, *112*, E1530–E1539. [CrossRef]
100. Van Gorp, H.; Van Breedam, W.; Van Doorsselaere, J.; Delputte, P.L.; Nauwynck, H.J. Identification of the CD163 protein domains involved in infection of the porcine reproductive and respiratory syndrome virus. *J. Virol.* **2010**, *84*, 3101–3105. [CrossRef] [PubMed]
101. Yang, H.; Zhang, J.; Zhang, X.; Shi, J.; Pan, Y.; Zhou, R.; Li, G.; Li, Z.; Cai, G.; Wu, Z. CD163 knockout pigs are fully resistant to highly pathogenic porcine reproductive and respiratory syndrome virus. *Antivir. Res.* **2018**, *151*, 63–70. [CrossRef]

102. Burkard, C.; Lillico, S.G.; Reid, E.; Jackson, B.; Mileham, A.J.; Ait-Ali, T.; Whitelaw, C.B.A.; Archibald, A.L. Precision engineering for PRRSV resistance in pigs: Macrophages from genome edited pigs lacking CD163 SRCR5 domain are fully resistant to both PRRSV genotypes while maintaining biological function. *PLoS Pathog.* **2017**, *13*, e1006206. [CrossRef] [PubMed]
103. Burkard, C.; Opriessnig, T.; Mileham, A.J.; Stadejek, T.; Ait-Ali, T.; Lillico, S.G.; Whitelaw, C.B.A.; Archibald, A.L. Pigs lacking the scavenger receptor cysteine-rich domain 5 of CD163 are resistant to porcine reproductive and respiratory syndrome virus 1 infection. *J. Virol.* **2018**, *92*. [CrossRef]
104. Murtaugh, M.P.; Stadejek, T.; Abrahante, J.E.; Lam, T.T.; Leung, F.C.-C. The ever-expanding diversity of porcine reproductive and respiratory syndrome virus. *Virus Res.* **2010**, *154*, 18–30. [CrossRef]
105. Velasco-Garcia, M.N.; Mottram, T. Biosensor technology addressing agricultural problems. *Biosyst. Eng.* **2003**, *84*, 1–12. [CrossRef]
106. Luo, Y.; Nartker, S.; Miller, H.; Hochhalter, D.; Wiederoder, M.; Wiederoder, S.; Setterington, E.; Drzal, L.T.; Alocilja, E.C. Surface functionalization of electrospun nanofibers for detecting E. coli O157:H7 and BVDV cells in a direct-charge transfer biosensor. *Biosens. Bioelectron.* **2010**, *26*, 1612–1617. [CrossRef]
107. Montrose, A.; Creedon, N.; Sayers, R.; Barry, S.; O'riordan, A. Novel single gold nanowire-based electrochemical immunosensor for rapid detection of bovine viral diarrhoea antibodies in serum. *J. Biosens. Bioelectron.* **2015**, *6*, 1–7. [CrossRef]
108. Neethirajan, S.; Tuteja, S.K.; Huang, S.T.; Kelton, D. Recent advancement in biosensors technology for animal and livestock health management. *Biosens. Bioelectron.* **2017**, *98*, 398–407. [CrossRef]
109. Neitzel, A.C.; Stamer, E.; Junge, W.; Thaller, G. Calibration of an automated California mastitis test with focus on the device-dependent variation. *Springerplus* **2014**, *3*, 760. [CrossRef] [PubMed]
110. Schaefer, A.L.; Cook, N.J.; Bench, C.; Chabot, J.B.; Colyn, J.; Liu, T.; Okine, E.K.; Stewart, M.; Webster, J.R. The non-invasive and automated detection of bovine respiratory disease onset in receiver calves using infrared thermography. *Res. Vet. Sci.* **2012**, *93*, 928–935. [CrossRef] [PubMed]
111. Tarasov, A.; Gray, D.W.; Tsai, M.Y.; Shields, N.; Montrose, A.; Creedon, N.; Lovera, P.; O'Riordan, A.; Mooney, M.H.; Vogel, E.M. A potentiometric biosensor for rapid on-site disease diagnostics. *Biosens. Bioelectron.* **2016**, *79*, 669–678. [CrossRef]
112. Ye, W.W.; Tsang, M.K.; Liu, X.; Yang, M.; Hao, J. Upconversion luminescence resonance energy transfer (LRET)-based biosensor for rapid and ultrasensitive detection of avian influenza virus H7 subtype. *Small* **2014**, *10*, 2390–2397. [CrossRef]
113. Galyean, M.L.; Eng, K.S. Application of research findings and summary of research needs: Bud Britton Memorial Symposium on Metabolic Disorders of Feedlot Cattle. *J. Anim. Sci.* **1998**, *76*, 323–327. [CrossRef]
114. Reid, G.; Friendship, R. Alternatives to antibiotic use: Probiotics for the gut. *Anim. Biotechnol.* **2002**, *13*, 97–112. [CrossRef]
115. Corcionivoschi, N.; Drinceanu, D.; Pop, I.M.; Stack, D.; Ştef, L.; Julean, C.; Bourke, B. The effect of probiotics on animal health. *Anim. Sci. Biotechnol.* **2010**, *43*, 35–41.
116. Markowiak, P.; Śliżewska, K. The role of probiotics, prebiotics and synbiotics in animal nutrition. *Gut Pathog.* **2018**, *10*, 21. [CrossRef]
117. Roy, A.; Panja, A.S.; Maitra, M.; Bandopyadhyay, B. Isolation and Characterizations of Probiotics from Bovine (Cow) Milk. *Res. Rev. Biotechnol. Biosci.* **2019**, *6*, 24–32. [CrossRef]
118. Rautray, A.K.; Patra, R.; Sardar, K.; Sahoo, G. Potential of probiotics in livestock production. *Explor. Anim. Medical Res.* **2011**, *1*, 20–28.
119. Sanchez, B.; Delgado, S.; Blanco-Miguez, A.; Lourenco, A.; Gueimonde, M.; Margolles, A. Probiotics, gut microbiota, and their influence on host health and disease. *Mol. Nutr. Food Res.* **2017**, *61*. [CrossRef] [PubMed]
120. Haskell, M.J.; Simm, G.; Turner, S.P. Genetic selection for temperament traits in dairy and beef cattle. *Front. Genet.* **2014**, *5*, 368. [CrossRef]
121. Golik, W.; Dameron, O.; Bugeon, J.; Fatet, A.; Hue, I.; Hurtaud, C.; Reichstadt, M.; Salaün, M.-C.; Vernet, J.; Joret, L. ATOL: The multi-species livestock trait ontology. In Proceedings of the 6th Metadata and Semantics Research Conference (MTSR 2012), Cádiz, Spain, 28–30 November 2012; pp. 289–300.
122. Hughes, L.M.; Bao, J.; Hu, Z.-L.; Honavar, V.; Reecy, J.M. Animal trait ontology: The importance and usefulness of a unified trait vocabulary for animal species. *J. Anim. Sci.* **2008**, *86*, 1485–1491. [CrossRef]

123. Mulder, H. Is GxE a burden or a blessing? Opportunities for genomic selection and big data. *J. Anim. Breed. Genet.* **2017**, *134*, 435–436. [CrossRef]
124. Gonda, M.; Chang, Y.; Shook, G.; Collins, M.; Kirkpatrick, B. Genetic variation of Mycobacterium avium ssp. paratuberculosis infection in US Holsteins. *J. Dairy Sci.* **2006**, *89*, 1804–1812. [CrossRef]
125. Koets, A.; Adugna, G.; Janss, L.; Van Weering, H.; Kalis, C.; Wentink, G.; Rutten, V.; Schukken, Y. Genetic variation of susceptibility to Mycobacterium avium subsp. paratuberculosis infection in dairy cattle. *J. Dairy Sci.* **2000**, *83*, 2702–2708. [CrossRef]
126. Mortensen, H.; Nielsen, S.S.; Berg, P. Genetic variation and heritability of the antibody response to Mycobacterium avium subspecies paratuberculosis in Danish Holstein cows. *J. Dairy Sci.* **2004**, *87*, 2108–2113. [CrossRef]
127. Morris, C.A. A review of genetic resistance to disease in Bos taurus cattle. *Vet. J.* **2007**, *174*, 481–491. [CrossRef]
128. Nicholas, F.W. *Veterinary Genetics*, 1st ed.; Oxford Science Publications: New York City, NY, USA; Clarendon Press: Oxford, UK, 1987.
129. McManus, C.; do Prado Paim, T.; de Melo, C.B.; Brasil, B.S.; Paiva, S.R. Selection methods for resistance to and tolerance of helminths in livestock. *Parasite* **2014**, *21*, 56. [CrossRef] [PubMed]
130. Kaplan, R.M. Drug resistance in nematodes of veterinary importance: A status report. *Trends Parasitol.* **2004**, *20*, 477–481. [CrossRef] [PubMed]
131. Sayers, G.; Sweeney, T. Gastrointestinal nematode infection in sheep—A review of the alternatives to anthelmintics in parasite control. *Anim. Health Res. Rev.* **2005**, *6*, 159–171. [CrossRef] [PubMed]
132. Guterbock, W.M.; Van Eenennaam, A.L.; Anderson, R.J.; Gardner, I.A.; Cullor, J.S.; Holmberg, C.A. Efficacy of intramammary antibiotic therapy for treatment of clinical mastitis caused by environmental pathogens. *J. Dairy Sci.* **1993**, *76*, 3437–3444. [CrossRef]
133. Myllys, V.; Asplund, K.; Brofeldt, E.; Hirvelä-Koski, V.; Honkanen-Buzalski, T.; Junttila, J.; Kulkas, L.; Myllykangas, O.; Niskanen, M.; Saloniemi, H. Bovine mastitis in Finland in 1988 and 1995—Changes in prevalence and antimicrobial resistance. *Acta Vet. Scand.* **1998**, *39*, 119–126. [PubMed]
134. Boireau, C.; Cazeau, G.; Jarrige, N.; Calavas, D.; Madec, J.-Y.; Leblond, A.; Haenni, M.; Gay, É. Antimicrobial resistance in bacteria isolated from mastitis in dairy cattle in France, 2006–2016. *J. Dairy Sci.* **2018**, *101*, 9451–9462. [CrossRef] [PubMed]
135. Heringstad, B.; Klemetsdal, G.; Ruane, J. Selection for mastitis resistance in dairy cattle: A review with focus on the situation in the Nordic countries. *Livest. Prod. Sci.* **2000**, *64*, 95–106. [CrossRef]
136. Gibson, J.P.; Bishop, S.C. Use of molecular markers to enhance resistance of livestock to disease: A global approach. *Rev. Sci. Tech.* **2005**, *24*, 343–353. [CrossRef]
137. Abernethy, D.A.; Upton, P.; Higgins, I.M.; McGrath, G.; Goodchild, A.V.; Rolfe, S.J.; Broughan, J.M.; Downs, S.H.; Clifton-Hadley, R.; Menzies, F.D.; et al. Bovine tuberculosis trends in the UK and the Republic of Ireland, 1995-2010. *Vet. Rec.* **2013**, *172*, 312. [CrossRef]
138. Råberg, L.; Graham, A.L.; Read, A.F. Decomposing health: Tolerance and resistance to parasites in animals. *Philos. Trans. R. Soc. B Biol. Sci.* **2009**, *364*, 37–49. [CrossRef]
139. Bourdon, R.M. *Understanding Animal Breeding*, 2nd ed.; Bourdon, R.M., Ed.; Prentice Hall: Upper Saddler River, NJ, USA, 2014.
140. Hart, B.L. Behavioural defences in animals against pathogens and parasites: Parallels with the pillars of medicine in humans. *Philos. Trans. R. Soc. Lond. B Biol. Sci.* **2011**, *366*, 3406–3417. [CrossRef] [PubMed]
141. Weigel, K.A.; VanRaden, P.M.; Norman, H.D.; Grosu, H. A 100-Year Review: Methods and impact of genetic selection in dairy cattle-From daughter-dam comparisons to deep learning algorithms. *J. Dairy Sci.* **2017**, *100*, 10234–10250. [CrossRef] [PubMed]
142. Rauw, W.M.; Kanis, E.; Noordhuizen-Stassen, E.N.; Grommers, F.J. Undesirable side effects of selection for high production efficiency in farm animals: A review. *Livest. Prod. Sci.* **1998**, *56*, 15–33. [CrossRef]
143. Emmans, G.; Kyriazakis, I. Consequences of genetic change in farm animals on food intake and feeding behaviour. *Proc. Nutr. Soc.* **2001**, *60*, 115–125. [CrossRef] [PubMed]
144. Heringstad, B.; Østerås, O. More than 30 years of health recording in Norway. *ICAR Tech. Ser.* **2013**, *17*, 39–46.
145. Beavers, L.; Van Doormal, B. Improving Existing Traits and Adding Exciting New Ones. Available online: https://www.cdn.ca/Articles/GEBAPR2016/10_Vision%20of%20%20GE%20Services%20-%20ENGLISH.pdf (accessed on 7 July 2020).

146. Miglior, F.; Koeck, A.; Kistemaker, G.; Van Doormaal, B. A New Index for Mastitis Resistance. Available online: https://www.cdn.ca/Articles/GEBMAR2014/DCBGC%20Report_mastitis%20-%20FINAL.pdf (accessed on 7 July 2020).
147. Durmaz, A.A.; Karaca, E.; Demkow, U.; Toruner, G.; Schoumans, J.; Cogulu, O. Evolution of genetic techniques: Past, present, and beyond. *Biomed. Res. Int.* **2015**, *2015*. [CrossRef]
148. Gogolin-Ewens, K.; Meeusen, E.; Scott, P.; Adams, T.; Brandon, M. Genetic selection for disease resistance and traits of economic importance in animal production. *Rev. Sci. Tech.* **1990**, *9*, 865–896. [CrossRef]
149. Andersson, L.; Haley, C.S.; Ellegren, H.; Knott, S.A.; Johansson, M.; Andersson, K.; Andersson-Eklund, L.; Edfors-Lilja, I.; Fredholm, M.; Hansson, I.; et al. Genetic mapping of quantitative trait loci for growth and fatness in pigs. *Science* **1994**, *263*, 1771–1774. [CrossRef]
150. Näslund, J.; Fikse, W.; Pielberg, G.; Lundén, A. Frequency and effect of the bovine acyl-CoA: Diacylglycerol acyltransferase 1 (DGAT1) K232A polymorphism in Swedish dairy cattle. *J. Dairy. Sci.* **2008**, *91*, 2127–2134. [CrossRef]
151. Thaller, G.; Kramer, W.; Winter, A.; Kaupe, B.; Erhardt, G.; Fries, R. Effects of DGAT1 variants on milk production traits in German cattle breeds. *J. Anim. Sci.* **2003**, *81*, 1911–1918. [CrossRef]
152. Do, D.; Schenkel, F.; Miglior, F.; Zhao, X.; Ibeagha-Awemu, E. Targeted genotyping to identify potential functional variants associated with cholesterol content in bovine milk. *Anim. Genet.* **2020**, *51*, 200–209. [CrossRef] [PubMed]
153. Jiang, L.; Liu, J.; Sun, D.; Ma, P.; Ding, X.; Yu, Y.; Zhang, Q. Genome wide association studies for milk production traits in Chinese Holstein population. *PLoS ONE* **2010**, *5*, e13661. [CrossRef] [PubMed]
154. Williams, J.L. The use of marker-assisted selection in animal breeding and biotechnology. *Rev. Sci. Tech.* **2005**, *24*, 379–391. [CrossRef] [PubMed]
155. Wakchaure, R.; Ganguly, S.; Praveen, P.; Kumar, A.; Sharma, S.; Mahajan, T. Marker assisted selection (MAS) in animal breeding: A review. *Drug. Metab. Toxicol.* **2015**, *6*, e127. [CrossRef]
156. Ruane, J.; Colleau, J.J. Marker-assisted selection for a sex-limited character in a nucleus breeding population. *J. Dairy Sci.* **1996**, *79*, 1666–1678. [CrossRef]
157. Wolc, A.; Arango, J.; Jankowski, T.; Settar, P.; Fulton, J.E.; O'Sullivan, N.P.; Fernando, R.; Garrick, D.J.; Dekkers, J.C.J.A.D. Genome-wide association study for Marek's disease mortality in layer chickens. *Avian. Dis.* **2013**, *57*, 395–400. [CrossRef]
158. Meuwissen, T.H.E.; Hayes, B.J.; Goddard, M.E. Prediction of Total Genetic Value Using Genome—Wide Dense Marker Maps. *Genetics* **2001**, *157*, 1819.
159. Piccoli, M.L.; Brito, L.F.; Braccini, J.; Brito, F.V.; Cardoso, F.F.; Cobuci, J.A.; Sargolzaei, M.; Schenkel, F.S. A comprehensive comparison between single-and two-step GBLUP methods in a simulated beef cattle population. *Can. J. Anim. Sci.* **2018**, *98*, 565–575. [CrossRef]
160. Goddard, M.E.; Hayes, B.J.; Meuwissen, T.H. Genomic selection in livestock populations. *Genet. Res.* **2010**, *92*, 413–421. [CrossRef]
161. Miar, Y.; Plastow, G.; Wang, Z. Genomic selection, a new era for pork quality Improvement. *Springer Sci. Rev.* **2015**, *3*, 27–37. [CrossRef]
162. Meuwissen, T.; Hayes, B.; Goddard, M. Accelerating improvement of livestock with genomic selection. *Annu. Rev. Anim. Biosci.* **2013**, *1*, 221–237. [CrossRef]
163. Bishop, S.; Morris, C. Genetics of disease resistance in sheep and goats. *Small. Rumin. Res.* **2007**, *70*, 48–59. [CrossRef]
164. Martin, P.; Barkema, H.W.; Brito, L.F.; Narayana, S.G.; Miglior, F. Symposium review: Novel strategies to genetically improve mastitis resistance in dairy cattle. *J. Dairy. Sci.* **2018**, *101*, 2724–2736. [CrossRef] [PubMed]
165. Weigel, K.A.; Shook, G.E. Genetic Selection for Mastitis Resistance. *Vet. Clin. Food Anim. Pract.* **2018**, *34*, 457–472. [CrossRef] [PubMed]
166. Fang, L.; Sahana, G.; Ma, P.; Su, G.; Yu, Y.; Zhang, S.; Lund, M.S.; Sørensen, P. Exploring the genetic architecture and improving genomic prediction accuracy for mastitis and milk production traits in dairy cattle by mapping variants to hepatic transcriptomic regions responsive to intra-mammary infection. *Genet. Sel. Evol.* **2017**, *49*, 44. [CrossRef]

167. Schneider, M.; Tait Jr, R.G.; Ruble, M.V.; Busby, W.D.; Reecy, J.M. Evaluation of fixed sources of variation and estimation of genetic parameters for incidence of bovine respiratory disease in preweaned calves and feedlot cattle. *J. Anim. Sci.* **2010**, *88*, 1220–1228. [CrossRef]
168. Snowder, G.; Van Vleck, L.D.; Cundiff, L.; Bennett, G. Influence of breed, heterozygosity, and disease incidence on estimates of variance components of respiratory disease in preweaned beef calves. *J. Anim. Sci.* **2005**, *83*, 1247–1261. [CrossRef]
169. Boddicker, N.; Waide, E.H.; Rowland, R.; Lunney, J.K.; Garrick, D.J.; Reecy, J.M.; Dekkers, J. Evidence for a major QTL associated with host response to porcine reproductive and respiratory syndrome virus challenge. *J. Anim. Sci.* **2012**, *90*, 1733–1746. [CrossRef]
170. Cheng, H.; Niikura, M.; Kim, T.; Mao, W.; MacLea, K.S.; Hunt, H.; Dodgson, J.; Burnside, J.; Morgan, R.; Ouyang, M.; et al. Using integrative genomics to elucidate genetic resistance to Marek's disease in chickens. *Dev. Biol.* **2008**, *132*, 365–372. [CrossRef]
171. Heifetz, E.M.; Fulton, J.E.; O'Sullivan, N.P.; Arthur, J.A.; Cheng, H.; Wang, J.; Soller, M.; Dekkers, J.C. Mapping QTL affecting resistance to Marek's disease in an F6 advanced intercross population of commercial layer chickens. *BMC Genom.* **2009**, *10*, 20. [CrossRef]
172. McElroy, J.P.; Dekkers, J.; Fulton, J.; O'Sullivan, N.P.; Soller, M.; Lipkin, E.; Zhang, W.; Koehler, K.J.; Lamont, S.J.; Cheng, H. Microsatellite markers associated with resistance to Marek's disease in commercial layer chickens. *Poult. Sci.* **2005**, *84*, 1678–1688. [CrossRef] [PubMed]
173. Vallejo, R.L.; Bacon, L.D.; Liu, H.-C.; Witter, R.L.; Groenen, M.A.; Hillel, J.; Cheng, H.H. Genetic mapping of quantitative trait loci affecting susceptibility to Marek's disease virus induced tumors in F2 intercross chickens. *Genetics* **1998**, *148*, 349–360. [PubMed]
174. Yonash, N.; Bacon, L.; Witter, R.; Cheng, H. High resolution mapping and identification of new quantitative trait loci (QTL) affecting susceptibility to Marek's disease. *Anim. Genet.* **1999**, *30*, 126–135. [CrossRef]
175. Medzhitov, R.; Schneider, D.S.; Soares, M.P. Disease tolerance as a defense strategy. *Science* **2012**, *335*, 936–941. [CrossRef] [PubMed]
176. Lough, G.; Rashidi, H.; Kyriazakis, I.; Dekkers, J.C.; Hess, A.; Hess, M.; Deeb, N.; Kause, A.; Lunney, J.K.; Rowland, R.R. Use of multi-trait and random regression models to identify genetic variation in tolerance to porcine reproductive and respiratory syndrome virus. *Genet. Sel. Evol.* **2017**, *49*, 37. [CrossRef]
177. Zanella, R.; Settles, M.; McKay, S.; Schnabel, R.; Taylor, J.; Whitlock, R.; Schukken, Y.; Van Kessel, J.; Smith, J.; Neibergs, H. Identification of loci associated with tolerance to Johne's disease in Holstein cattle. *Anim. Genet.* **2011**, *42*, 28–38. [CrossRef] [PubMed]
178. Hanotte, O.; Ronin, Y.; Agaba, M.; Nilsson, P.; Gelhaus, A.; Horstmann, R.; Sugimoto, Y.; Kemp, S.; Gibson, J.; Korol, A.; et al. Mapping of quantitative trait loci controlling trypanotolerance in a cross of tolerant West African N'Dama and susceptible East African Boran cattle. *Proc. Natl. Acad. Sci. USA* **2003**, *100*, 7443–7448. [CrossRef]
179. Phua, S.H.; Hyndman, D.L.; Baird, H.J.; Auvray, B.; McEwan, J.C.; Lee, M.A.; Dodds, K.G. Towards genomic selection for facial eczema disease tolerance in the New Zealand sheep industry. *Anim. Genet.* **2014**, *45*, 559–564. [CrossRef]
180. Restif, O.; Koella, J.C. Concurrent evolution of resistance and tolerance to pathogens. *Am. Nat.* **2004**, *164*, E90–E102. [CrossRef]
181. Roy, B.; Kirchner, J. Evolutionary dynamics of pathogen resistance and tolerance. *Evolution* **2000**, *54*, 51–63. [CrossRef]
182. Drake, J.W.; Holland, J.J. Mutation rates among RNA viruses. *Proc. Natl. Acad. Sci. USA* **1999**, *96*, 13910–13913. [CrossRef]
183. Ayres, J.S.; Schneider, D.S. Tolerance of infections. *Annu. Rev. Immunol.* **2012**, *30*, 271–294. [CrossRef] [PubMed]
184. Raberg, L.; Sim, D.; Read, A.F. Disentangling genetic variation for resistance and tolerance to infectious diseases in animals. *Science* **2007**, *318*, 812–814. [CrossRef]
185. Colditz, I.G.; Hine, B.C. Resilience in farm animals: Biology, management, breeding and implications for animal welfare. *Anim. Prod. Sci.* **2016**, *56*, 1961–1983. [CrossRef]
186. Elgersma, G.G.; de Jong, G.; van der Linde, R.; Mulder, H.A. Fluctuations in milk yield are heritable and can be used as a resilience indicator to breed healthy cows. *J. Dairy Sci.* **2018**, *101*, 1240–1250. [CrossRef] [PubMed]

187. Albers, G.A.; Gray, G.D.; Piper, L.R.; Barker, J.S.; Le Jambre, L.F.; Barger, I.A. The genetics of resistance and resilience to Haemonchus contortus infection in young merino sheep. *Int. J. Parasitol.* **1987**, *17*, 1355–1363. [CrossRef]
188. Bisset, S.A.; Morris, C.A. Feasibility and implications of breeding sheep for resilience to nematode challenge. *Int. J. Parasitol.* **1996**, *26*, 857–868. [CrossRef]
189. Mulder, H.A.; Rashidi, H. Selection on resilience improves disease resistance and tolerance to infections. *J. Anim. Sci.* **2017**, *95*, 3346–3358. [CrossRef]
190. Berghof, T.V.L.; Poppe, M.; Mulder, H.A. Opportunities to Improve Resilience in Animal Breeding Programs. *Front. Genet.* **2018**, *9*, 692. [CrossRef]
191. Abdel-Azim, G.A.; Freeman, A.E.; Kehrli, M.E., Jr.; Kelm, S.C.; Burton, J.L.; Kuck, A.L.; Schnell, S. Genetic basis and risk factors for infectious and noninfectious diseases in US Holsteins. I. Estimation of genetic parameters for single diseases and general health. *J. Dairy Sci.* **2005**, *88*, 1199–1207. [CrossRef]
192. Thompson-Crispi, K.A.; Sewalem, A.; Miglior, F.; Mallard, B.A. Genetic parameters of adaptive immune response traits in Canadian Holsteins. *J. Dairy Sci.* **2012**, *95*, 401–409. [CrossRef] [PubMed]
193. Henryon, M.; Heegaard, P.M.; Nielsen, J.; Berg, P.; Juul-Madsen, H.R. Immunological traits have the potential to improve selection of pigs for resistance to clinical and subclinical disease. *Anim. Sci.* **2006**, *82*, 597–606. [CrossRef]
194. Psifidi, A.; Banos, G.; Matika, O.; Desta, T.T.; Bettridge, J.; Hume, D.A.; Dessie, T.; Christley, R.; Wigley, P.; Hanotte, O. Genome-wide association studies of immune, disease and production traits in indigenous chicken ecotypes. *Genet. Sel. Evol.* **2016**, *48*, 74. [CrossRef]
195. Stear, M.J.; Bishop, S.C.; Mallard, B.A.; Raadsma, H. The sustainability, feasibility and desirability of breeding livestock for disease resistance. *Res. Vet. Sci.* **2001**, *71*, 1–7. [CrossRef]
196. Jie, H.; Liu, Y.-P. Breeding for disease resistance in poultry: Opportunities with challenges. *Worlds Poult. Sci. J.* **2011**, *67*, 687–696. [CrossRef]
197. Schulman, N.F.; Viitala, S.M.; de Koning, D.J.; Virta, J.; Maki-Tanila, A.; Vilkki, J.H. Quantitative trait Loci for health traits in Finnish Ayrshire cattle. *J. Dairy Sci.* **2004**, *87*, 443–449. [CrossRef]
198. Simianer, H.; Solbu, H.; Schaeffer, L. Estimated genetic correlations between disease and yield traits in dairy cattle. *J. Dairy Sci.* **1991**, *74*, 4358–4365. [CrossRef]
199. Van Dorp, T.; Dekkers, J.; Martin, S.; Noordhuizen, J. Genetic parameters of health disorders, and relationships with 305-day milk yield and conformation traits of registered Holstein cows. *J. Dairy Sci.* **1998**, *81*, 2264–2270. [CrossRef]
200. Emanuelson, U. Recording of production diseases in cattle and possibilities for genetic improvements: A review. *Livest. Prod. Sci.* **1988**, *20*, 89–106. [CrossRef]
201. Li, Z.; Nestor, K.E.; Saif, Y.M.; Anderson, J.W.; Patterson, R.A. Effect of selection for increased body weight in turkeys on lymphoid organ weights, phagocytosis, and antibody responses to fowl cholera and Newcastle disease-inactivated vaccines. *Poult. Sci.* **2001**, *80*, 689–694. [CrossRef]
202. van der Most, P.J.; de Jong, B.; Parmentier, H.K.; Verhulst, S. Trade-off between growth and immune function: A meta-analysis of selection experiments. *Funct. Ecol.* **2011**, *25*, 74–80. [CrossRef]
203. Hazel, L.N. The genetic basis for constructing selection indexes. *Genetics* **1943**, *28*, 476–490. [PubMed]
204. Hirooka, H. Economic selection index in the genomic era. *J. Anim. Breed. Genet.* **2019**, *136*, 151–152. [CrossRef] [PubMed]
205. Snowder, G. Genetic selection for disease resistance: Challenges and opportunities. In Proceedings of the Beef Improvement Federation Conference Proceedings, Omaha, NE, USA, 10–13 July 2002; pp. 52–60.
206. Nardone, A.; Ronchi, B.; Lacetera, N.; Ranieri, M.S.; Bernabucci, U. Effects of climate changes on animal production and sustainability of livestock systems. *Livest. Sci.* **2010**, *130*, 57–69. [CrossRef]
207. Meuwissen, T.; Hayes, B.; Goddard, M. Genomic selection: A paradigm shift in animal breeding. *Anim. Front.* **2016**, *6*, 6–14. [CrossRef]
208. Asokan, G.V.; Asokan, V. Leveraging "big data" to enhance the effectiveness of "one health" in an era of health informatics. *J. Epidemiol. Glob. Health* **2015**, *5*, 311–314. [CrossRef]
209. Normandeau, K. Beyond Volume, Variety and velocity Is the Issue of Big Data Veracity. Available online: http://insidebigdata.com/2013/09/12/beyond-volume-variety-velocity-issue-big-data-veracity/ (accessed on 7 July 2020).
210. Berckmans, D. General introduction to precision livestock farming. *Anim. Front.* **2017**, *7*, 6–11. [CrossRef]

211. Ip, R.H.; Ang, L.-M.; Seng, K.P.; Broster, J.; Pratley, J. Big data and machine learning for crop protection. *Comput. Electron. Agric.* **2018**, *151*, 376–383. [CrossRef]
212. Bansal, S.; Chowell, G.; Simonsen, L.; Vespignani, A.; Viboud, C. Big data for infectious disease surveillance and modeling. *J. Infect. Dis.* **2016**, *214*, S375–S379. [CrossRef]
213. Koltes, J.E.; Cole, J.B.; Clemmens, R.; Dilger, R.N.; Kramer, L.M.; Lunney, J.K.; McCue, M.E.; McKay, S.D.; Mateescu, R.G.; Murdoch, B.M. A vision for development and utilization of high-throughput phenotyping and big data analytics in livestock. *Front. Genet.* **2019**, *10*. [CrossRef]
214. Rexroad, C.; Vallet, J.; Matukumalli, L.K.; Reecy, J.; Bickhart, D.; Blackburn, H.; Boggess, M.; Cheng, H.; Clutter, A.; Cockett, N. Genome to phenome: Improving animal health, production, and well-being–a new USDA blueprint for animal genome research 2018–2027. *Front. Genet.* **2019**, *10*, 327. [CrossRef] [PubMed]
215. Halachmi, I.; Guarino, M.; Bewley, J.; Pastell, M. Smart animal agriculture: Application of real-time sensors to improve animal well-being and production. *Annu. Rev. Anim. Biosci.* **2019**, *7*, 403–425. [CrossRef] [PubMed]
216. Khatun, M.; Thomson, P.C.; Clark, C.E.; García, S.C. Prediction of quarter level subclinical mastitis by combining in-line and on-animal sensor data. *Anim. Prod. Sci.* **2020**, *60*, 180–186. [CrossRef]
217. Cole, J.B.; Eaglen, S.A.E.; Maltecca, C.; Mulder, H.A.; Pryce, J.E. The future of phenomics in dairy cattle breeding. *Anim. Front.* **2020**, *10*, 37–44. [CrossRef] [PubMed]
218. Morota, G.; Jarquin, D.; Campbell, M.T.; Iwata, H. Statistical methods for the quantitative genetic analysis of high-throughput phenotyping data. *arXiv* **2019**, arXiv:1904.12341.
219. Morota, G.; Ventura, R.V.; Silva, F.F.; Koyama, M.; Fernando, S.C. Big Data Analytics and Precision Animal Agriculture Symposium: Machine learning and data mining advance predictive big data analysis in precision animal agriculture. *J. Anim. Sci.* **2018**, *96*, 1540–1550. [CrossRef] [PubMed]
220. Ibeagha-Awemu, E.M.; Do, D.N.; Dudemaine, P.-L.; Fomenky, B.E.; Bissonnette, N. Integration of lncRNA and mRNA transcriptome analyses reveals genes and pathways potentially involved in calf intestinal growth and development during the early weeks of life. *Genes* **2018**, *9*, 142. [CrossRef]
221. Suravajhala, P.; Kogelman, L.J.; Kadarmideen, H.N. Multi-omic data integration and analysis using systems genomics approaches: Methods and applications in animal production, health and welfare. *Genet. Sel. Evol.* **2016**, *48*, 38. [CrossRef]
222. Ibeagha-Awemu, E.M.; Peters, S.O.; Bemji, M.N.; Adeleke, M.A.; Do, D.N. Leveraging available resources and stakeholder involvement for improved productivity of African livestock in the era of genomic breeding. *Front. Genet.* **2019**, *10*. [CrossRef]
223. Giuffra, E.; Tuggle, C.K.; Consortium, F. Functional annotation of animal genomes (FAANG): Current achievements and roadmap. *Annu. Rev. Anim. Biosci.* **2019**, *7*, 65–88. [CrossRef]
224. Hayes, B.J.; Daetwyler, H.D. 1000 Bull Genomes Project to Map Simple and Complex Genetic Traits in Cattle: Applications and Outcomes. *Annu. Rev. Anim. Biosci.* **2019**, *7*, 89–102. [CrossRef] [PubMed]

2

Genome-Wide Association Studies Reveal Susceptibility Loci for Digital Dermatitis in Holstein Cattle

Ellen Lai, Alexa L. Danner, Thomas R. Famula and Anita M. Oberbauer *

Department of Animal Science, University of California, Davis, CA 95616, USA; elai@ucdavis.edu (E.L.); aldanner@ucdavis.edu (A.L.D.); trfamula@ucdavis.edu (T.R.F.)

* Correspondence: amoberbauer@ucdavis.edu

Simple Summary: Foot warts (FW), a leading cause of foot problems in dairy cattle, is a welfare concern and causes financial losses due to treatment and reduced milk production. Foot warts, or the technically correct term of digital dermatitis, result from a bacterial infection followed by delayed healing due to both genetic and environmental factors. Dairy farmers are already combatting FW through environmental control, but they do not have genetic selection tools because the genetics influencing FW susceptibility are largely unknown. We sought to identify the genetics associated with FW which can be incorporated into genetic selection tools. Farmers can then use these genetic selection tools to breed cows that are less susceptible to FW. We identified promising genes that play a role in the immune response and wound healing immune functions that, if impaired, could increase a cow's susceptibility to FW. Though these genes were promising, their associated genetic markers had very little influence on FW susceptibility when compared to environmental management. Thus, the findings imply that the best approach for reducing FW prevalence is likely through combining a genetics approach with environmental management.

Abstract: Digital dermatitis (DD) causes lameness in dairy cattle. To detect the quantitative trait loci (QTL) associated with DD, genome-wide association studies (GWAS) were performed using high-density single nucleotide polymorphism (SNP) genotypes and binary case/control, quantitative (average number of FW per hoof trimming record) and recurrent (cases with ≥2 DD episodes vs. controls) phenotypes from cows across four dairies (controls n = 129 vs. FW n = 85). Linear mixed model (LMM) and random forest (RF) approaches identified the top SNPs, which were used as predictors in Bayesian regression models to assess the SNP predictive value. The LMM and RF analyses identified QTL regions containing candidate genes on *Bos taurus* autosome (BTA) 2 for the binary and recurrent phenotypes and BTA7 and 20 for the quantitative phenotype that related to epidermal integrity, immune function, and wound healing. Although larger sample sizes are necessary to reaffirm these small effect loci amidst a strong environmental effect, the sample cohort used in this study was sufficient for estimating SNP effects with a high predictive value.

Keywords: digital dermatitis; foot warts; lameness; genome-wide association study; linear mixed model; random forest; Bayesian estimation; sustainability; animal welfare

---

1. Introduction

Lameness, or abnormal gait, affects 16% of dairy cows in the United States, making lameness the second most prevalent disease in dairy cattle after mastitis [1]. Digital dermatitis (DD) is a common cause of lameness, comprising 70.9% and 36.0% of lameness cases in heifers and cows, respectively [1].

The economic impacts of DD are \$64 to \$153 per episode due to reduced milk production, discarded milk, treatment costs, and additional labor [2,3]. Furthermore, premature culling obligates producers to expand their replacement heifer herd. Because heifers consume inputs without contributing to milk production, a larger replacement heifer herd inflates the economic cost [4] and carbon footprint [5] per unit of milk. Thus, reducing the incidence of DD and associated lameness has great potential to benefit animal welfare, the producer's profit margin, and the environment, bolstering the three pillars of sustainability.

Heritability estimates for DD range from 0.01 to 0.4 [6–8], indicating genetic contributions to DD susceptibility along with a strong environmental influence. Reducing DD incidence, therefore, will likely be achieved through a combination of management and genetic approaches informed by the etiology of DD. Although the etiology of DD has not been completely elucidated, multiple bacterial phylotypes belonging to the genus *Treponema* are consistently found in DD lesions [9]. Accordingly, the main environmental management method for reducing DD incidence is medicated foot baths [10,11], though this treatment is expensive, with estimates of ~\$42 per cow per year [12]. Additionally, the disinfectant compounds commonly used in foot baths raise environmental and health concerns, as the primary ingredients, copper sulfate and formaldehyde, are environmental pollutants [13] and carcinogenic [14], respectively. To alleviate these issues and improve DD prevention, some producers emphasize feet and leg conformation scores or indices that include claw health when selecting sires and, increasingly, rely upon genetic testing for heifers. However, the low genetic correlation between conformation traits and claw health impairs efficient indirect selection against claw lesions when using selection on conformation traits [15].

Currently, no selection index exists specifically for DD susceptibility. Targeted genetic selection against DD and associated lameness requires the identification of genomic regions influencing DD susceptibility. To find the contributing quantitative trait loci (QTL), genome-wide association studies (GWAS) have been undertaken, although the results to date have been discordant. Previous studies found significant and suggestive single nucleotide polymorphisms (SNPs) on *Bos taurus* autosomes (BTAs) 1, 3, 5, 6, 8, 9, 10, 14, and 26 [6,16–19], or no suggestive or significant SNPs [20].

In an effort to improve upon and refine past studies, the present study used strict phenotyping, dairies with similar management practices, and a high-density SNP genotyping array to identify the associations between DD and genomic regions. We hypothesized that certain genetic markers would be associated with DD susceptibility, and that those markers would have small effects. Our results revealed multiple small-effect SNPs were associated with DD and defined QTL that contained candidate genes related to immune function and wound healing, supporting our hypothesis.

2. Materials and Methods

Four commercial dairies in the Central Valley of California, two of which had participated in our previous heritability study [8], provided hoof trimming records and blood samples from which to generate genotypic data. All the procedures were conducted in accordance with the ethical standards set by the University of California, Davis, and approved by the Institutional Animal Care and Use Committee.

2.1. Phenotypic Data

Hoof trimming records were used to generate binary and quantitative phenotypes. Claw lesions and lameness issues were diagnosed by a single hoof trimmer servicing three of the dairies (dairies A, B, and C), and a different hoof trimmer servicing the fourth dairy (dairy D). The hoof trimmer servicing three dairies was trained by Dr. Steven Berry, a veterinarian specializing in claw lesions who offered hoof trimming training workshops to the industry and was a coauthor of our earlier paper [8], and the other trimmer shadowed trained trimmers to standardize the diagnostics. Claw lesions were diagnosed and recorded while the cow was restrained. Claw lesion types and the foot with DD lesions were recorded into the cow's electronic record (dairies A and D) or maintained in a hard copy format (dairies B and C). Each type of claw lesion (e.g., DD, sole ulcer, laminitis, white line disease, foot rot, etc.) and miscellaneous lameness event (e.g., rock, cut, etc.) was tallied for each cow.

Both hoof trimmers utilized similar criteria for defining instances of DD in the cattle to reduce the phenotypic classification variability; specifically, DD was recorded for cows with raised, inflamed lesions on the skin above the heel of the foot or above the interdigital space on the front of the foot. Routine hoof trimming varied by dairy: cows were trimmed at the beginning and middle of lactation, during dry off, and when exhibiting altered gait (dairy A); during dry off and when exhibiting altered gait (dairy B and C); and only when exhibiting altered gait (dairy D). Cases were defined as cows who had exhibited at least one DD lesion, whereas controls had no DD or other lameness records and were 6.5 years of age or older to avoid misphenotyping younger cows who had insufficient time to develop lameness events. Cows may have multiple bouts of DD over their lifetime and, in some cases, the first instance of DD may have occurred before the cows were in milk (i.e., as heifers). Because DD lesions typically last for four to six months [21,22], we defined independent DD lesion episodes as those that were separated by at least six months. Cows with two or more independent DD episodes were considered recurrent cases. Digital dermatitis records that were less than six months apart were considered repeated records of one persistent DD episode. Digital dermatitis was analyzed as a binary phenotype to identify loci influencing general susceptibility to DD and as a quantitative phenotype calculated as the total number of independent DD lesions a cow had divided by the total number of hoof trimming records to standardize the number of lesions by the number of hoof trimming records for each cow. Consequently, the quantitative phenotype for a control cow was zero. Digital dermatitis was also analyzed as a recurrent phenotype (cases with ≥2 DD episodes vs. controls) to identify the loci contributing to reoccurring DD episodes.

2.2. Genome-Wide Association and Linear Mixed Model Analyses

Genomic DNA was extracted from whole blood samples using the QIAGEN QIAamp DNA Blood Mini Kit (QIAGEN Inc., Valencia, CA, USA) and quantified using the NanoDrop (ND-2000 v3.2.1) spectrophotometer (Thermo Scientific, Wilmington, DE, USA). DNA samples were genotyped on the BovineHD BeadChip (777962 SNPs, Illumina Inc., San Diego, CA, USA) by GeneSeek (Lincoln, NE, USA). Raw and processed microarray data were submitted to the NCBI Gene Expression Omnibus database (GEO series record GSE159157). Illumina's GenCall algorithm was used to call genotypes.

GWAS were performed using the binary, quantitative, and recurrent phenotypes using the SNP coordinates from the ARS-UCD1.2 map (accessed August 2020 from the National Animal Genome Research Project's Cattle Genome Analysis Data Repository (https://www.animalgenome.org/repository/cattle/UMC_bovine_coordinates/), version last modified 11 September 2018). The quality filtering of SNP genotypes was performed using PLINK 1.9 [23,24] to remove from further analysis any cows having less than 5% of all SNPs genotyped and SNPs missing genotypes in more than 5% of the cows. SNPs with a minor allele frequency of less than 0.05 were removed to exclude rare variants, and SNPs that deviated significantly from the Hardy–Weinberg equilibrium ($p < 1 \times 10^{-6}$) in controls were removed to exclude systematic genotyping errors.

Family structure is extremely prevalent in the dairy population from breeding elite bulls to hundreds to tens of thousands of cows. To visualize the genetic similarity among cows at this initial dairy, a multi-dimensional scaling (MDS) analysis was performed and the first two dimensions were plotted. The GWA analyses were performed using the genetic analysis program Genome-wide Complex Trait Analysis (GCTA) [25] to fit a linear mixed model (LMM) that tests for the association of SNP genotypes with binary and quantitative DD phenotypes. An LMM was selected for its ability to incorporate a genetic relatedness matrix to correct for familial relatedness and population structure. Linear mixed models are designed for quantitative phenotypes, as LMMs assume that phenotypes are normally distributed; however, LMMs have also been routinely used to analyze binary traits [26,27]. A genetic relatedness matrix was computed and included along with farm as a covariate in the LMM. When fitting the LMM for each SNP, the LMM included the chromosome of the candidate SNP being tested. To reduce false positive associations due to multiple testing across many loci without being overly stringent, the effective number of independent SNPs (M_e) after linkage disequilibrium (LD) pruning was determined using the Genetic Type I error calculator (GEC) and used as the denominator for Bonferroni-corrected thresholds [28]. Significant SNPs were defined as those with $p < 0.05/M_e$, whereas suggestive SNPs were defined as having $p < 1/M_e$ [29]. To calculate the genomic inflation factors (λ_{GC}), chi-squared test statistics were first generated from association *p*-values, and the median of the resulting chi-squared distribution was divided by the median of the expected chi-squared distribution. Quantile-quantile plots (qqplots) and Manhattan plots were plotted in R [30] using the package qqman [31].

2.3. Random Forest Analysis

Random forest (RF) analysis was performed as an additional method for identifying SNPs that appeared to importantly contribute to disease phenotypes. Random forests do not make any assumptions about the inheritance model (additive, dominant, recessive) and are able to test multiple SNPs jointly for association with phenotype. Additionally, the RF approach is unaffected by an uneven farm distribution of cases and controls because RF builds decision trees and estimates the importance of each feature by the frequency it appears in the decision trees, rather than estimating parameters for a model. Consequently, RFs avoid estimating parameters for which there are no data. These properties make RFs well equipped to identify structure within complex genetic architectures like DD susceptibility. Specifically, RF can accommodate data despite uneven sampling across farms, in which contributing SNPs may have different modes of inheritance and where epistasis is likely prevalent.

After converting quality-filtered binary PLINK files into VCF files split by chromosome in PLINK 1.9 [24,32], all the missing genotypes were imputed using BEAGLE 5.1 [33] because the RF analysis cannot handle missing genotypes. The resulting VCF files were converted back to binary PLINK files, which were LD-pruned using a threshold of $R^2 \geq 0.90$ to avoid diluting the importance of SNPs in strong LD during the RF analysis [34] and recoded to additive and dominant component files suitable for importing into R. The additive component (i.e., genotypes coded as 0/1/2 minor alleles) was used as input for the RF analysis in R using the caret package [30,35]. For binary and quantitative phenotypes, RF analysis was implemented with all genome-wide SNPs in one run to estimate the relative importance of explainers, comprised of SNP genotypes and farm. For both runs, the same random sample of two thirds of the cows was used to train the model and calculate variables of importance for each explainer. The RF run for each phenotype built 500 decision trees that included three values of *mtry*, the number of predictors considered at each node of the tree. The value of *mtry* that yielded the most accurate model was used as the final model. The most important explainer was assigned an importance variable of 100, and the other explainers were assigned importance variables relative to the most important explainer (e.g., an explainer with an importance of 50 is 50% as important as the most important explainer). To assess the accuracy of the final model, the remaining third of cows was used as the test population, using the explainers and their relative importance to predict phenotype.

After evaluating the model accuracy using the test population, a threshold of importance was determined by ranking and plotting the SNPs the RF identified as important for each chromosome in a scree plot and finding the rank of the second-order point of inflection using the d2uik option in the inflection package in R [36,37]. SNPs ranking equally as or more important than this threshold were considered important and included in further analyses.

2.4. Bayesian Regression to Assess Model Predictability and Validation

To assess the collective predictive ability of the top SNPs identified in the LMM and RF analyses, the top SNPs from each analysis (i.e., significant and suggestive SNPs from LMM analyses, important SNPs from RF analyses) were tested for association with phenotype using Bayesian regression. Bayesian regression was selected because of its ability to fit multiple SNPs simultaneously while also recognizing that the majority of SNPs have small effects on DD susceptibility [20,38], that some SNPs are likely correlated due to LD, and that not all farms contributed controls to the analyses. Additionally, Bayesian regression enables the thorough evaluation of model fit through leave-one-out (LOO) validation and posterior predictive checking (PPC), the latter of which is a uniquely Bayesian feature.

Suggestive and significant SNPs from the LMM GWAS and important SNPs from the RF analysis were used as predictors along with farm in each Bayesian regression model. Similar to the RF analyses, SNP genotypes were coded as 0/1/2 minor alleles. A Bayesian regression model was fitted for each combination of GWAS method (LMM and RF) and phenotype (binary and quantitative), such that four models were fitted: LMM-binary and RF-binary were fitted using a Bayesian logistic regression model, and LMM-quantitative and RF-quantitative were fitted using a Bayesian generalized linear model for continuous data. Susceptibility to DD appears to be complex and the majority of SNP effects are likely to be small [20,38]. To reflect this distribution of SNP effects, a normal prior with a small-scale N (0,1) was used for the distribution of predictors for all four models. Each of the four models was fitted by sampling from the posterior distribution using the Hamiltonian Monte Carlo algorithm, a Markov chain Monte Carlo (MCMC) algorithm, using the rstanarm package in R [39]. Four parallel chains sampled the posterior distribution, and each chain was run for 10,000 iterations with a warmup of 2500 iterations, keeping every 25th iteration to avoid autocorrelation.

Unlike frequentist regression, which would output a point estimate of each SNP effect, Bayesian regression outputted a distribution of where the true value of each SNP effects fell, defined by the Bayesian uncertainty interval (UI). SNPs with 95% UIs that did not include zero were considered significantly associated with DD susceptibility. For each significant SNP, the probability of disease given a genotype at the significant SNP (coded as 0/1/2 minor alleles) and a 0 genotype at all other SNPs was calculated using the median of SNP effect estimates as point estimates in the inverse logit equation using the R package arm [40]. Diagnostic and Bayesian UI plots for the posterior medians of SNP effects were plotted using the bayesplot package. Leave one out cross validation was performed using the loo package [41,42] in R to predict the phenotype of each cow using the SNP effects estimated from all other cows. The reliability of prediction was assessed using the Pareto *k* diagnostic values outputted from the LOO analysis. Posterior predictive checking (PPC) from the bayesplot package [43] was used to assess the goodness of fit of the model. Posterior predictive checking assessed how well the estimated predictor effects were able to simulate phenotypes with a similar distribution to that of the observed phenotypes.

2.5. *Defining and Annotating QTL Regions*

For the significant and suggestive SNPs identified in the LMM analyses and the important SNPs identified in the RF analyses, the QTL boundaries and regions were defined and annotated. Because SNPs are more likely to be in LD with causal variants than be causal themselves, the linkage disequilibrium in the regions flanking these top SNPs was used to define the boundaries of QTL, per the methods used in previous GWAS studies [44,45]. Specifically, SNPs within 5 Mb of significant and suggestive SNPs that were also in LD ($r^2 \geq 0.5$) were considered as belonging to the same QTL. The SNPs furthest upstream and downstream that were in LD with the target suggestive or significant SNP defined the boundaries of the QTL. Overlapping QTL were combined into one QTL. QTL from the LMM and RF analyses were compared to discern whether the two analyses found the same QTL. QTL regions that were identified in both LMM and RF analyses were explored for candidate genes. Additionally, QTL defined by SNPs that were significant in the Bayesian regression analyses were also explored for candidate genes. Candidate genes were defined as genes falling in QTL regions identified in both LMM and RF analyses or in QTL defined by SNPs that were significant in Bayesian regression and were functionally relevant to DD etiology.

To annotate the QTL regions, the genomic regions search in FAANGMine v1.1 [46] using the ARS_UCD1.2 assembly was implemented to find genes within the QTL regions. The RefSeq identifiers of genes within the QTL were used in a gene ontology and pathway enrichment analysis in FAANGMine to discern whether the genes belonged to higher-order functions and pathways related to DD etiology.

For the gene ontology and pathway enrichment analyses, the Benjamini Hochberg test correction was used to correct for multiple testing, and all the RefSeq genes in *B. taurus* were used as the background population. To identify the functions of individual genes, protein coding genes in QTL defined by SNPs that were significant in two analyses (i.e., LMM, RF, and/or Bayesian regression) were searched in the Mouse Genome Informatics batch query database (http://www.informatics.jax.org/batch) using the mammalian phenotype option [47].

3. Results

3.1. Descriptive Data

Hoof trimming records for 1382 DD-affected cows at dairies A, B, and D from 2002 to 2019 were used to calculate the age of onset statistics. Dairy C did not have hoof trimming records from the beginning of the cows' lives and was thus excluded from calculating the age of onset statistics. The average age of onset for the first episode of DD observed was 3.7 (SD = 1.6) years old and the median was 3.5 years old, indicating a minimum age of 6.5 years old for controls was sufficiently stringent to avoid misphenotyping younger cows. The cases and controls were sampled from 2013 to 2020. Cases were sampled from all four dairies, whereas only dairies A and D had control cows that met our stringent age and soundness requirements (Table 1). In total, 222 cows were genotyped (cases n = 90, controls n = 132), of which six were removed during quality filtering (cases n = 3, controls n = 3), leaving 216 cows for analysis (cases n = 87, controls n = 129). Of the 87 cases, 24 had recurrent FW episodes and were used in the GWAS of controls vs. recurrent FW cases. Forty-seven percent of the DD cases no other claw lesions other than DD during their lifetime. The remaining cases had, in addition to clearly identifiable DD, abscesses, sole fracture, sole ulcers, or bruising. One cow also had foot rot in addition to DD. Of these other claw lesions, only foot rot was considered infectious, whereas the other concomitant lesions were noninfectious and associated with excessive wear of the claw due to hard flooring and/or metabolic issues [48].

Table 1. Distribution of digital dermatitis cases and non-lame controls across the four dairies.

Farm	Case	Control	Total
A	19	112	131
B	22	0	22
C	30	0	30
D	16	17	33
Total	87	129	216

After quality control filtering, 560,277 SNPs remained for the LMM analysis, and 222,060 SNPs (40%) for the RF analyses remained after LD pruning ($r^2 > 0.90$). The MDS analysis indicated no obvious population stratification (Figure S1). The effective number of SNPs (i.e., SNPs that were not in LD) was approximately 158,000 SNPs, yielding a cutoff of significance at 3.2×10^{-7} or 6.5 on the $-\log_{10}(p)$ scale and a suggestive cutoff at 6.3×10^{-6} or 5.2 on the $-\log_{10}(p)$ scale. Manhattan plots for the LMM binary and quantitative analyses are shown in Figure 1 and suggestive and significant SNPs, in Tables 2 and 3. For the recurrent LMM GWAS, the Manhattan plot is depicted in Figure S2 and suggestive and significant SNPs in Table S1. The genomic inflation factors were 0.97 for the binary and quantitative GWASs and 1.0 for the recurrent GWAS; when considered in conjunction with the qqplots, the analyses sufficiently accounted for population structure (Figure S3). In separate analyses, we removed outlier control cows, defined as having a value < −0.10 in the first coordinate and a value < −0.08 in the second coordinate of the MDS plot, and the conclusions of association remained unchanged (Figure S4). Our method of correction for multiple testing (i.e., using the effective number of independent SNPs as the denominator for Bonferroni correction) resulted in more stringent significance thresholds than those based on false discovery rate that are used in other GWASs for DD [6,16,20].

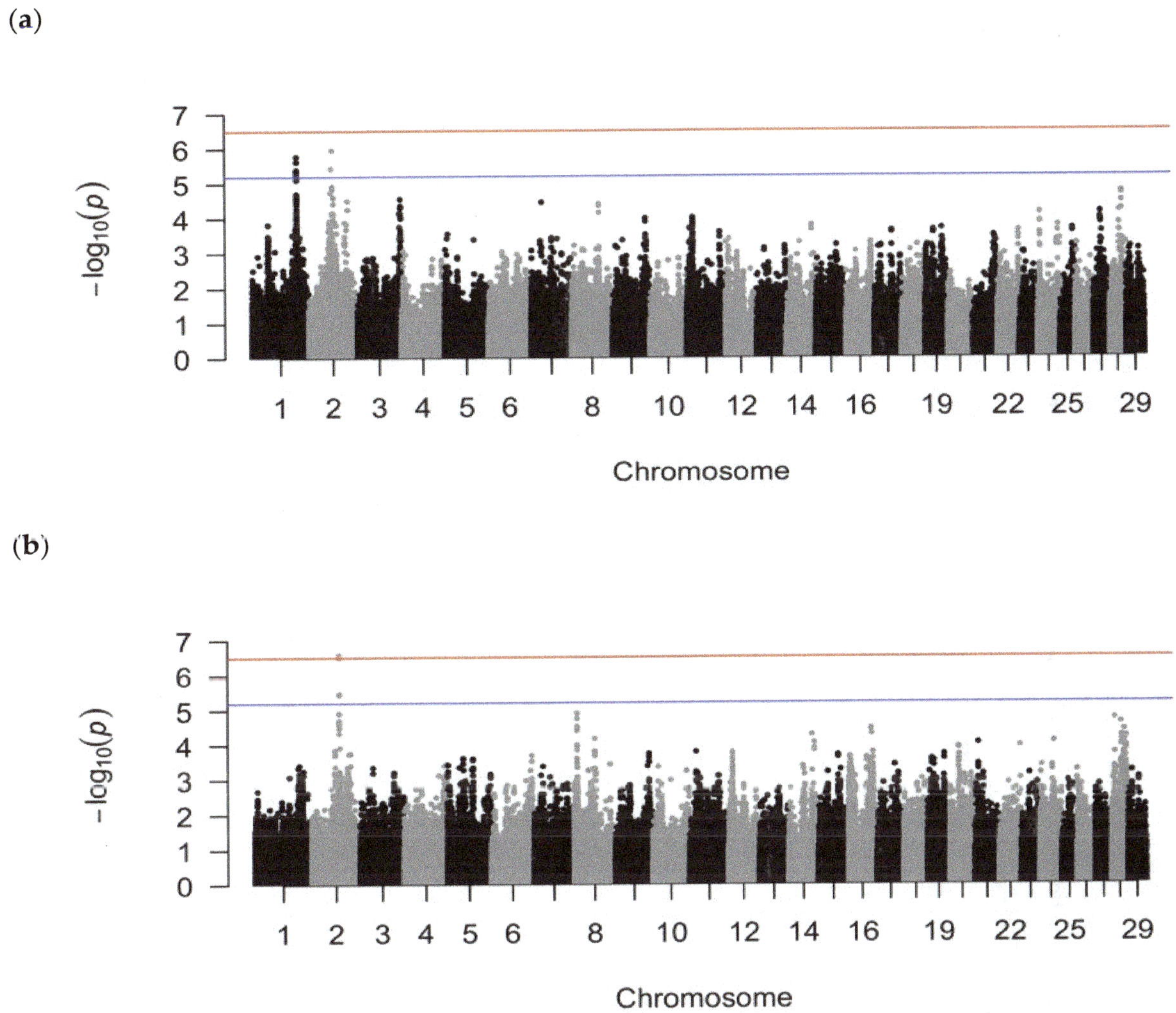

Figure 1. Manhattan plots from the linear mixed model genome-wide association analyses using (**a**) binary phenotypes designating the presence of digital dermatitis (DD) lesions or the absence of any lameness issues and (**b**) quantitative phenotypes calculated by dividing the number of DD episodes by the total number of hoof trimming records. The red line indicates the threshold for genome-wide significance (Bonferroni-corrected using the number of independent SNPs at $p < 0.05$), and the blue line indicates the threshold for suggestive significance (Bonferroni-corrected using the number of independent SNPs at $p < 1$).

Table 2. Suggestive SNPs detected from the linear mixed model genome-wide association analysis using binary phenotypes and their defined QTL.

SNP ID	BTA	SNP Position (bp)	Minor/Major Allele	Minor Allele Count		MAF [a]		Effect Size (SE)	*p*	Significance in Bayesian Regression	QTL Start Position (bp)	QTL End Position (bp)	QTL Size (kb)
				Cases (2n = 174)	Controls (2n = 258)	Cases	Controls						
BovineHD0100035768	1	125563251	A/G	63	54	0.362	0.209	0.178 (0.037)	1.68×10^{-6}	ns	125550933 [b]	125822143 [b]	271.21 [b]
BovineHD0100035771	1	125565548	G/A	63	54	0.362	0.211	0.175 (0.037)	2.31×10^{-6}	ns	125550933 [b]	125822143 [b]	271.21 [b]
BovineHD0100035773	1	125567245	T/C	63	55	0.362	0.213	0.175 (0.037)	2.35×10^{-6}	ns	125550933 [b]	125822143 [b]	271.21 [b]
BovineHD0100035776	1	125570173	G/T	63	55	0.362	0.213	0.175 (0.037)	2.35×10^{-6}	ns	125550933 [b]	125822143 [b]	271.21 [b]
BovineHD0100035780	1	125573042	G/A	63	55	0.362	0.213	0.175 (0.037)	2.35×10^{-6}	ns	125550933 [b]	125822143 [b]	271.21 [b]
BovineHD0100035783	1	125576193	G/A	63	55	0.362	0.213	0.175 (0.037)	2.35×10^{-6}	ns	125550933 [b]	125822143 [b]	271.21 [b]
BovineHD0100035788	1	125598084	G/A	63	57	0.362	0.221	0.164 (0.036)	5.36×10^{-6}	ns	125550933 [b]	125822143 [b]	271.21 [b]
BovineHD4100000712	1	125598643	T/C	63	57	0.362	0.223	0.163 (0.036)	6.31×10^{-6}	ns	125550933 [b]	125822143 [b]	271.21 [b]
BovineHD0100035789	1	125599413	C/T	63	57	0.362	0.221	0.164 (0.036)	5.36×10^{-6}	ns	125550933 [b]	125822143 [b]	271.21 [b]
BovineHD0100035796	1	125608174	A/G	64	56	0.368	0.217	0.163 (0.036)	4.59×10^{-6}	ns	125550933 [b]	125822143 [b]	271.21 [b]
ARS-BFGL-NGS-113021	1	125609019	C/T	64	56	0.368	0.217	0.163 (0.036)	4.59×10^{-6}	ns	125550933 [b]	125822143 [b]	271.21 [b]
BovineHD0100035797	1	125609959	C/T	64	56	0.368	0.217	0.163 (0.036)	4.59×10^{-6}	ns	125550933 [b]	125822143 [b]	271.21 [b]
BovineHD0100035802	1	125627579	C/T	64	56	0.368	0.217	0.163 (0.036)	4.59×10^{-6}	ns	125550933 [b]	125822143 [b]	271.21 [b]
BovineHD0100035803	1	125628401	A/C	64	56	0.368	0.217	0.163 (0.036)	4.59×10^{-6}	ns	125550933 [b]	125822143 [b]	271.21 [b]
BovineHD0100035828	1	125680990	G/A	87	88	0.500	0.341	0.155 (0.034)	4.11×10^{-6}	ns	125550933 [b]	125822143 [b]	271.21 [b]
BovineHD0100035829	1	125681850	C/A	87	88	0.500	0.341	0.155 (0.034)	4.11×10^{-6}	ns	125550933 [b]	125822143 [b]	271.21 [b]
ARS-BFGL-NGS-100109	1	125683184	C/T	87	88	0.500	0.341	0.155 (0.034)	4.11×10^{-6}	ns	125550933 [b]	125822143 [b]	271.21 [b]
BovineHD0100035833	1	125688941	C/T	87	88	0.500	0.341	0.155 (0.034)	4.11×10^{-6}	ns	125550933 [b]	125822143 [b]	271.21 [b]
BovineHD0100035841	1	125700410	A/G	87	89	0.500	0.345	0.152 (0.034)	5.85×10^{-6}	ns	125550933 [b]	125822143 [b]	271.21 [b]
BovineHD0100035842	1	125700857	C/T	87	89	0.500	0.345	0.152 (0.034)	5.85×10^{-6}	ns	125550933 [b]	125822143 [b]	271.21 [b]
BovineHD0100035844	1	125702010	C/T	87	89	0.500	0.345	0.152 (0.034)	5.85×10^{-6}	ns	125550933 [b]	125822143 [b]	271.21 [b]
BovineHD0100035845	1	125702906	G/T	87	89	0.500	0.345	0.152 (0.034)	5.85×10^{-6}	ns	125550933 [b]	125822143 [b]	271.21 [b]
BTA-47853-no-rs	2	63365256	A/G	78	64	0.448	0.248	0.167 (0.036)	3.69×10^{-6}	s	60971364	63389576	2418.2
BovineHD0200019142	2	65836042	G/A	41	32	0.236	0.124	0.224 (0.046)	1.10×10^{-6}	s	65836042	65836042	-

[a] MAF = minor allele frequency. [b] This QTL is defined in both the linear mixed model and random forest analyses for the binary case-control phenotype. s = SNP effect estimated from Bayesian regression was significantly different from zero, as defined by the 95% uncertainty interval. ns = SNP effect estimated from Bayesian regression was not significantly different from zero, as defined by the 95% uncertainty interval.

Table 3. Important SNPs from random forest analysis using binary phenotypes and their defined QTL. Importance variables are expressed as % importance relative to farm (i.e., farm was 100% importance).

SNP ID	BTA	SNP Position (bp)	Minor/Major Allele	Minor Allele Count		MAF [a]		SNP Importance (% Relative to Farm)	Significance in Bayesian Regression	QTL Start Position (bp)	QTL End Position (bp)	QTL Size (kb)
				Cases (2n = 174)	Controls (2n = 258)	Cases	Controls					
BovineHD0100001686	1	5894509	G/A	54	75	0.310	0.291	70.9	ns	5894509	5901795	7.3
BovineHD0100013452	1	47090630	C/T	41	25	0.238	0.098	75.4	ns	43459206	49409839	5950.6
BovineHD0100013140	1	45742004	G/A	35	20	0.201	0.078	75.6	ns	43459206	49409839	5950.6
BovineHD0100013551	1	47618749	T/G	50	27	0.291	0.105	81.5	ns	43459206	49409839	5950.6
BovineHD0100033878	1	118845470	A/G	9	41	0.052	0.159	76.1	ns	114235013	119003717	4768.7
BovineHD0100035876	1	125811728	A/C	70	68	0.402	0.264	79.4	s	125550933 [b]	125822143 [b]	271.21 [b]
BovineHD0200017030	2	59626300	C/T	22	95	0.126	0.368	77.0	s	58016533	59967789	1951.3
BovineHD0200037724	2	129189118	T/C	35	73	0.201	0.283	83.0	ns	128495987	129671807	1175.8
BovineHD0300035231	3	119898047	T/G	52	53	0.299	0.205	76.7	s	119720909	119942789	221.9
BovineHD0400033808	4	115632631	A/G	84	92	0.483	0.357	76.5	ns	115461900	115812750	350.9
ARS-BFGL-NGS-111175	4	119082548	A/C	38	30	0.218	0.116	76.8	ns	116927673	119130213	2202.5
BovineHD0400034694	4	117654227	G/A	53	119	0.305	0.461	76.9	ns	116927673	119130213	2202.5
BovineHD0700005793	7	19675119	C/T	87	102	0.500	0.395	75.5	ns	17910021	19773720	1863.7
BovineHD0700016221	7	54331048	A/G	6	42	0.034	0.163	77.0	ns	49401649	54505899	5104.3
BovineHD1300007641	13	26082265	C/T	69	140	0.397	0.543	76.0	ns	22185154	26101077	3915.9
BovineHD1500016894	15	57724182	A/G	60	59	0.345	0.229	72.9	ns	56807906	58102169	1294.3
BovineHD1600016687	16	58237523	C/T	105	108	0.603	0.419	81.8	ns	56372228	62230342	5858.1
BovineHD1700012893	17	45209840	T/C	62	52	0.356	0.202	80.4	ns	44418753	45224548	805.8
BovineHD1800003369	18	9579005	T/C	100	102	0.575	0.395	79.6	ns	9510127	9582839	72.7
BovineHD1800012376	18	41782168	C/T	27	8	0.155	0.031	88.4	ns	41753915	41863187	109.3
ARS-BFGL-BAC-35025	18	47814171	G/A	32	84	0.184	0.326	79.8	s	47099464	47831459	732.0
BovineHD1900013252	19	46915144	C/T	27	90	0.155	0.349	86.2	ns	46871178	47070613	199.4
BovineHD2200002436	22	8104318	A/G	36	106	0.207	0.411	79.8	ns	7974675	8109630	135.0
BovineHD2200002746	22	9090720	A/G	17	77	0.098	0.298	85.0	ns	9068141	9090720	22.6
BovineHD2600011849	26	42398008	A/G	59	68	0.339	0.264	75.6	ns	40792161	43877138	3085.0
ARS-BFGL-NGS-117055	27	12656552	C/T	86	89	0.494	0.348	75.7	ns	12202138	12834272	632.1

[a] MAF = minor allele frequency. [b] This QTL is defined in both the linear mixed model and random forest analyses for the binary case-control phenotype. s = SNP effect estimated from Bayesian regression was significantly different from zero, as defined by the 95% uncertainty interval. ns = SNP effect estimated from Bayesian regression was not significantly different from zero, as defined by the 95% uncertainty interval.

3.2. SNPs Associated with DD as a Binary Phenotype

The binary LMM GWAS detected 22 suggestive SNPs on BTA1 that fell in the last three introns of *SLC9A9* and two suggestive intergenic SNPs on BTA2 (Table 2). When used to define QTL boundaries, the 22 suggestive SNPs on BTA1 were all in LD and defined one 271.2 kb QTL region at BTA1:125550933–125822143 containing three genes: a long-noncoding RNA gene (LOC112447746), a tRNA-CAU gene, and *SLC9A9*. The BTA2:63365256 (BTA-47853-no-rs) SNP on BTA 2 identified a 2.4 Mb QTL region at BTA2:60971364–63389576 containing 25 genes, whereas the other SNP identified on BTA 2, BTA2:65836042 (BovineHD0200019142), was not in LD with neighboring SNPs ($r^2 < 0.5$). Because the number of genes discovered from the LMM QTL was limited, no gene ontologies or pathways were overrepresented.

When suggestive SNPs from the LMM-binary GWAS were used as predictors in the Bayesian regression models, MCMC sampling was able to efficiently explore the posterior. Though the effects of SNPs on BTA1 were not significantly different from zero at 50% UI, the effects of the two SNPs on BTA2 (BTA-47853-no-rs and BovineHD0200019142) were significantly different from zero at 95% UI (Figure 2, Table 2). Unlike a frequentist 95% confidence interval, which defines the range within which the true value of the SNP effect falls 95% of the time in repeated sampling, a Bayesian 95% uncertainty interval indicates there is a 95% probability that the true value of the SNP effect falls within the range. For example, to give context for the impact of SNP effect size, each minor allele at BTA-47853-no-rs and BovineHD0200019142, respectively, increased the log odds of having DD by 1.3 and 1.5, using the median as the point estimate for SNP effect. A 1.3 increase in the log odds of having DD for each minor allele at BTA-47853-no-rs corresponded to an increase in the probability of having DD by 22% and 54% for heterozygotes and homozygotes of the minor allele relative to homozygotes of the major allele. A 1.5 increase in the log odds of having DD for each minor allele at BovineHD0200019142 corresponded to a 25% and 60% increase in the probability of having DD for the heterozygotes and homozygotes of the minor allele, relative to the homozygotes of the major allele. The relatively large increases in the probability of having DD from each additional minor allele reflects the high minor allele frequency in cases (45%) relative to controls (25%) in this population. Additionally, the magnitude of increase in the probability of DD also depended upon the genotype of the cow at other SNPs. For instance, a cow with a genotype other than homozygous major for all SNPs could have a smaller increase in the probability of DD with each additional minor alelle at BTA-47853-no-rs or BovineHD0200019142.

Using the LMM-binary suggestive SNPs as predictors in the LOO analysis, Pareto k diagnostic values were acceptable ($k \leq 0.7$) for all cows, indicating that the estimated SNP effects were collectively predictive of phenotype within the original population. The LOO analysis indicated that the effective number of predictors in the model was 6.6, considerably lower than the 27 predictors that were actually in the model due to correlated predictors: the SNPs on BTA1 were in LD, and this correlation among predictors reduced the effective number of predictors. The PPC indicated that the observed and simulated data were similar to each other (Figure S5), supporting that the predictor estimates were collectively predictive of phenotype.

Random forest analysis revealed that farm was ranked as the most important explainer, and consequently the importance of SNPs was expressed as the percentage of importance relative to farm. Of the three values of *mtry* that were tested (6, 666, and 222,061), *mtry* = 666 yielded the most accurate model and was selected for further analyses. The accuracy of the selected model (0.69 with 95% CI 0.57–0.80) was not significantly different from the baseline no information rate (in this case, the proportion of controls: 0.64, $p = 0.20$), indicating that the model was unable to call case and control phenotypes more accurately than simply calling the more common phenotype. Random forest analyses found 26 important SNPs from the RF-binary, and using LD to determine the QTL boundaries defined 23 QTL for the RF-binary dataset (Table 3), one of which was the same QTL on BTA1:125550933–125822143 identified from the LMM-binary GWAS. Within the RF-binary QTL, FAANGMine found 566 genes, of which 129 and 188 were used in the pathway and gene ontology enrichment analysis. The Kyoto Encyclopedia of Genes and Genomes (KEGG) pathway herpes simplex virus 1 infection and the Reactome pathways P2Y receptors and nucleotide-like (purinergic) receptors were significantly enriched (Benjamini Hochberg $p = 0.003$, 0.021, and 0.035, respectively).

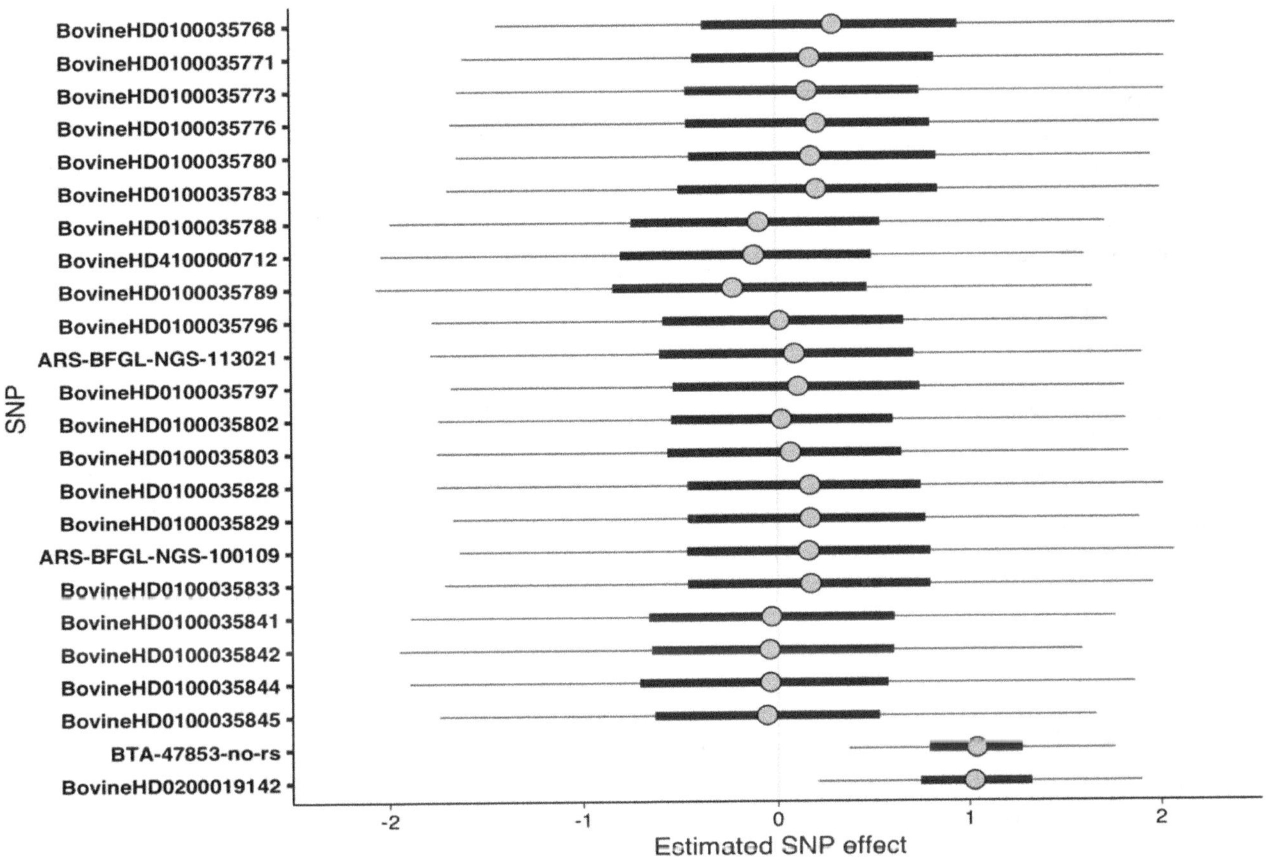

Figure 2. Uncertainty interval (UI) plot for suggestive SNPs on BTA1 (BovineHD0100035768 through BovineHD0100035845) and BTA2 (BTA-47853-no-rs and BovineHD0200019142) from the linear mixed model GWAS using binary phenotypes. Dots represent the median of the SNP effect estimates from Markov chain Monte Carlo draws, thick bars indicate the 50% UI, and the thin lines indicate the 95% UI. SNPs with 95% UI not overlapping zero were considered significant. Positive values of predictor effect estimates indicate a higher risk of DD, whereas negative values indicate a lower risk of DD.

When important SNPs from the RF-binary analyses were used as predictors in the Bayesian logistic regression model, four SNPs had estimated effects that were significantly different from zero, including the SNP defining the QTL at BTA1:125550933–125822143 (Table 3, Figure 3). The important SNPs from the RF-binary analyses were not as predictive of phenotype within the population compared to the suggestive SNPs from the LMM-binary analysis, as evidenced by 13% of cows having high Pareto k diagnostic values ($k > 0.7$) from the LOO analysis. The lower predictability indicates that the RF was able to find small effect SNPs, but also found some noninformative SNPs. Though the PPC indicated that the observed and simulated data were similar to each other (Figure S6), this similarity was likely due to overfitting.

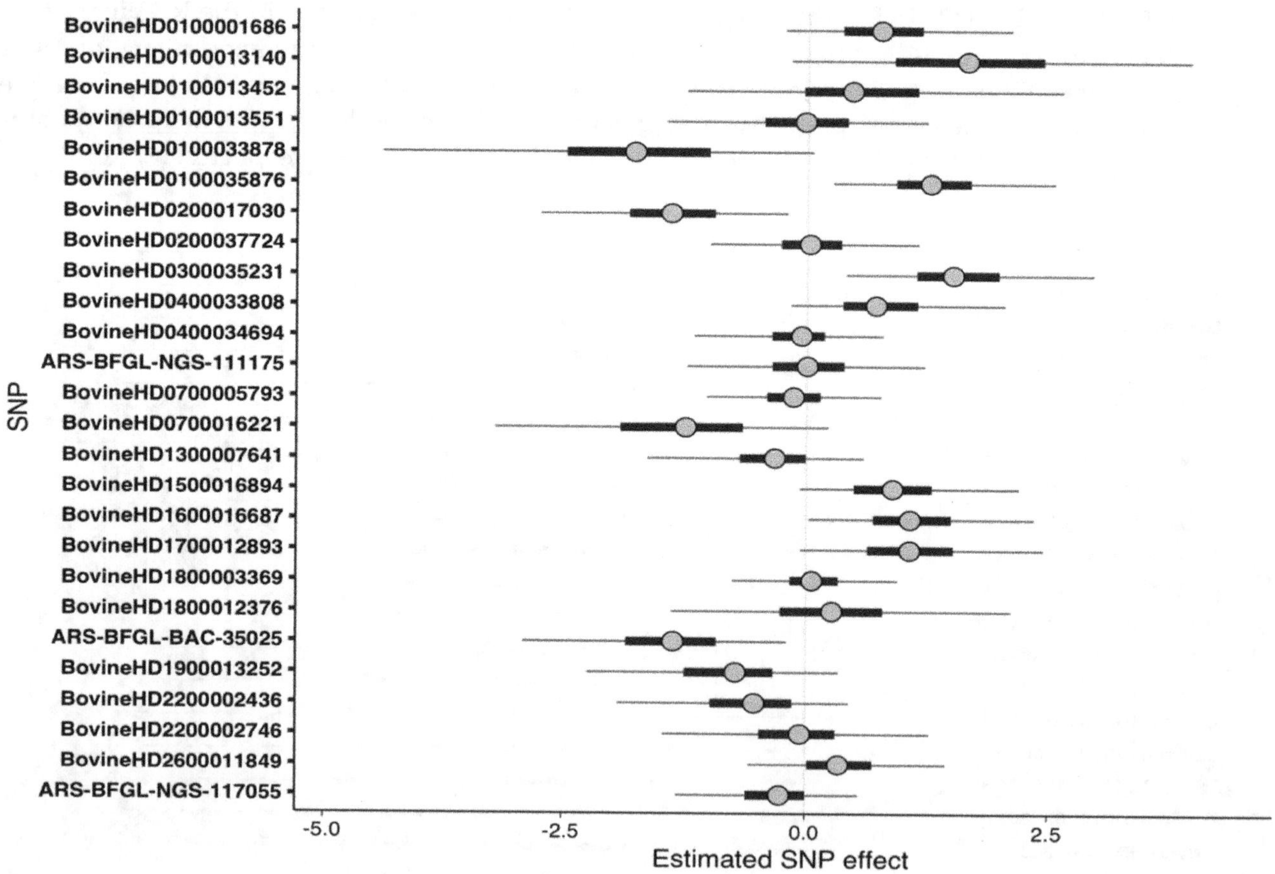

Figure 3. Uncertainty interval (UI) plot for important SNPs from the random forest analysis using binary phenotypes. Dots represent the median of the SNP effect estimates from the Markov chain Monte Carlo draws, thick bars indicate the 50% UI, and the thin lines indicate the 95% UI. SNPs with 95% UI not overlapping zero were considered significant. Positive values of predictor effect estimates indicate a higher risk of DD, whereas negative values indicate a lower risk of DD.

3.3. SNPs Associated with DD as a Quantitative Phenotype

The quantitative LMM GWAS identified seven significant and two suggestive SNPs, all of which were intergenic (Table 4). The gene nearest to these nine SNPs was a suppressor of cytokine-signaling 6-like pseudogene (LOC615204) falling between the seven significant and two suggestive SNPs. When these nine SNPs were used to determine the QTL boundaries, all nine SNPs were in LD ($r^2 > 0.5$) and defined a 2 Mb QTL region at BTA2:77930065–79925981 (Table 4). This 2 Mb QTL region included nine genes, including LOC615204. The recurrent DD cases vs. controls placed more emphasis on finding genetic differences between controls and cases with more DD cases, similar to the LMM-quantitative GWAS; however, the LMM GWAS using recurrent DD cases vs. controls identified QTL regions in common with the LMM-binary and not the LMM-quantitative GWAS. In the recurrent GWAS, the same SNPs observed on BTA1 from the LMM-binary analyses formed a peak of association but did not reach suggestive significance, whereas three SNPs on BTA2 in addition to the two detected in the LMM-binary GWAS reached suggestive significance (Figure S2, Table S1). The three additional suggestive SNPs on BTA2 revealed by the recurrent analysis defined a 328 kb QTL at BTA2:65836042–66217730 that was not in LD with the QTL at BTA2:60971364–63389576 defined by BTA-47853-no-rs at BTA2:63365256 in both the binary and recurrent LMM GWASs (Table S1).

Table 4. Significant and suggestive SNPs detected from the linear mixed model genome-wide association analysis using quantitative phenotypes and their defined QTL.

SNP ID	BTA	SNP Position (bp)	MAF [a]	Effect Size (SE)	p	QTL Start Position (bp)	QTL End Position (bp)	QTL Size (kb)
BovineHD0200022555	2	78069923	0.231	0.127 (0.025)	3.14×10^{-7} *	77930065	79925981	1995.9
BovineHD0200022557	2	78080217	0.231	0.127 (0.025)	3.14×10^{-7} *	77930065	79925981	1995.9
Hapmap43777-BTA-115985	2	78080944	0.233	0.128 (0.025)	2.66×10^{-7} *	77930065	79925981	1995.9
BovineHD0200022559	2	78092854	0.231	0.127 (0.025)	3.14×10^{-7} *	77930065	79925981	1995.9
BovineHD0200022560	2	78100071	0.231	0.127 (0.025)	3.14×10^{-7} *	77930065	79925981	1995.9
BovineHD0200022562	2	78110140	0.231	0.127 (0.025)	3.14×10^{-7} *	77930065	79925981	1995.9
BovineHD0200022563	2	78111523	0.231	0.127 (0.025)	3.14×10^{-7} *	77930065	79925981	1995.9
BovineHD0200022605	2	78307821	0.28	0.107 (0.023)	3.68×10^{-7} †	77930065	79925981	1995.9
BovineHD0200022737	2	78767889	0.278	0.108 (0.023)	3.43×10^{-7} †	77930065	79925981	1995.9

[a] MAF = minor allele frequency. * = genome-wide significant. † = genome-wide suggestive significance.

When the significant and suggestive SNPs from the LMM-quantitative analysis were used as predictors in Bayesian regression, MCMC sampling to fit the model was unable to efficiently explore the posterior likely because the phenotypes did not follow a normal distribution as expected by the model. This resulted in unreliable results and thereby prevented further analyses. The limited number of genes within the LMM-quantitative QTL on BTA 2:77930065–79925981 prevented the detection of overrepresented gene ontologies or pathways.

Random forest analysis using quantitative phenotypes revealed that, similar to the RF-binary rankings, farm was ranked as the most important explainer. The 15 important SNPs identified from the RF-quantitative analysis defined 13 QTL distinct from those defined in the LMM-quantitative analysis (Table 5). The RF-quantitative QTL contained 124 genes. The 28 and 13 genes that were used in pathway analysis using KEGG and Reactome pathways did not find enriched pathways. The 37 genes used in gene ontology enrichment analysis did not have significantly overrepresented gene ontologies after multiple testing correction.

Although no pathways or gene ontologies were enriched from the RF-quantitative dataset, the important SNPs detected were nonetheless predictive of phenotype when used as predictors in Bayesian regression. MCMC sampling to fit the Bayesian model was able to explore the posterior sufficiently, resulting in convergence. Three of the important SNPs had effect sizes significantly greater than zero at 95% UI (Figure 4, Table 5). The LOO analysis indicated that the 15 SNPs were predictive of quantitative phenotype, as all the cows had Pareto k diagnostic values that were acceptable ($k \leq 0.7$). The PPC demonstrated that the simulated data followed a similar distribution to the original data, though the frequency of more extreme phenotypes was dampened (Figure S7).

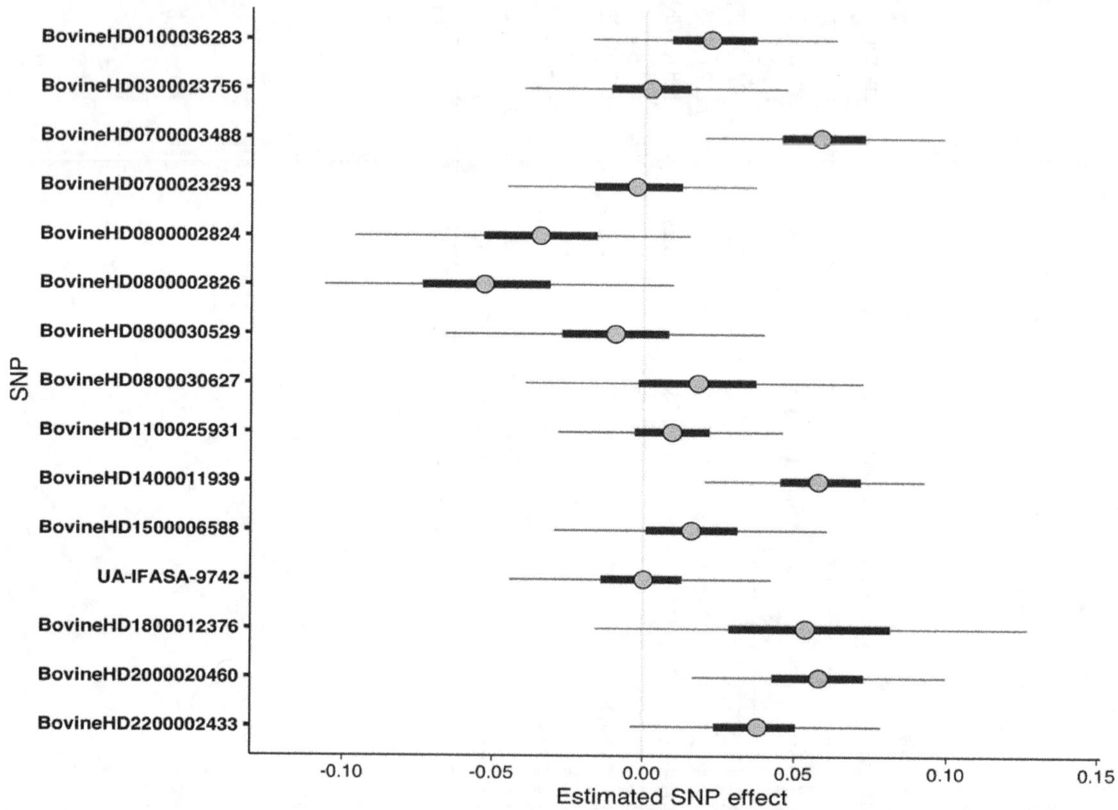

Figure 4. Uncertainty interval (UI) plot for important SNPs from the random forest analysis using quantitative phenotypes. Dots represent the median of the SNP effect estimates from the Markov chain Monte Carlo draws, thick bars indicate the 50% UI, and the thin lines indicate the 95% UI. SNPs with 95% UI not overlapping zero were considered significant. Positive values of the predictor effect estimates indicate a phenotypic value for DD, whereas negative values indicate a phenotypic value for DD.

Table 5. Important SNPs from random forest analysis using quantitative phenotypes and their defined QTL. Importance variables are expressed as % importance relative to farm (i.e., farm had 100% importance).

SNP ID	BTA	SNP Position (bp)	Minor/ Major Allele	MAF [a]	SNP Importance (% Relative to Farm)	Significance in Bayesian Regression	QTL Start Position (bp)	QTL End Position (bp)	QTL Size (kb)
BovineHD0100036283	1	127408427	A/G	0.350	8.9	ns	127389567	127408427	18.9
BovineHD0300023756	3	82473975	A/G	0.391	8.5	ns	82468446	82480613	12.2
BovineHD0700003488	7	12238249	T/G	0.354	17.1	s	11979738	12261707	282.0
BovineHD0700023293	7	77533459	T/C	0.220	8.7	ns	77242189	78032023	789.8
BovineHD0800002826	8	8983282	C/T	0.463	8.7	ns	8671707	9806692	1135.0
BovineHD0800002824	8	8979816	G/A	0.373	10.6	ns	8671707	9806692	1135.0
BovineHD0800030529	8	100994105	C/T	0.402	10.5	ns	100412296	102353854	1941.6
BovineHD0800030627	8	101328029	G/A	0.350	9.5	ns	100412296	102353854	1941.6
BovineHD1100025931	11	89788438	C/A	0.387	9.9	ns	89375874	89788438	412.6
BovineHD1400011939	14	39785964	T/C	0.448	10.0	s	39785964	39818361	32.4
BovineHD1500006588	15	24668401	A/G	0.250	11.2	ns	24668401	24771237	102.8
UA-IFASA-9742	15	42081374	G/T	0.250	8.6	ns	42081374	42092689	11.3
BovineHD1800012376	18	41782168	C/T	0.081	9.6	ns	41753915	41863187	109.3
BovineHD2000020460	20	69870827	T/C	0.308	8.3	s	69696705	71850045	2153.3
BovineHD2200002433	22	8091674	T/C	0.205	9.1	ns	6375507	8317371	1941.9

[a] MAF = minor allele frequency. s = SNP effect estimated from Bayesian regression was significantly different from zero, as defined by the 95% uncertainty interval. ns = SNP effect estimated from Bayesian regression was not significantly different from zero, as defined by the 95% uncertainty interval.

4. Discussion

The genetic component of DD susceptibility is highly complex and heterogeneous [20,38], as demonstrated by the numerous and varied QTL detected in previous studies [6,16–20]. We sought to further identify the QTL contributing to DD susceptibility using a high-density SNP array and LMM and RF analytical approaches on well-phenotyped DD cases and controls. The LMM GWAS and RF analyses revealed suggestive, significant, and important SNPs that defined QTL regions in binary, quantitative, and recurrent DD phenotypes. The LMM GWAS using recurrent DD cases vs. controls indicated that the recurrent DD cases were contributing to the significance of association in the LMM-binary GWAS on BTA1 and BTA2, but not in the LMM-quantitative GWAS. Bayesian regression allowed for an intuitive estimate of SNP effects and the robust evaluation of model fit through the LOO and PPC analyses, providing additional distinctions of informative and noninformative SNPs among the top SNPs. QTL regions were explored for candidate genes if the QTL was defined by the top SNPs (i.e., significant or suggestive SNPs from LMM analyses or important SNPs in RF analyses) that were also significant in Bayesian regression or were top SNPs in both LMM and RF analyses. That is, nine QTL were investigated further (Table 6).

Within these QTL regions, we identified likely candidate genes based on their relevance to DD etiology. DD is associated with Treponema bacteria invading the dermis and epidermis, likely through hair follicles, and results in a raised erosive lesion [21,49]. The infection elicits a strong initial activation of the innate immune response [50] that is then attenuated by the treponemes [51], leading to prolonged inflammation and a delayed adaptive immune response [52]. Within the adaptive immune response, the antibody-mediated immune response is mainly responsible for defending the host against extracellular pathogens [53], such as treponemes. After the immune response, the skin then attempts to heal the wound, a process that is also impaired by treponemes [51]. As such, changes in the sequence or expression of genes related to maintaining epidermal integrity, immune response, or wound repair could affect a cow's DD susceptibility and the persistence of a DD lesion. Previous work has indicated that genes related to these three functions were dysregulated in DD lesions [18,51]. Therefore, we considered candidate genes as those with associated phenotypes, as determined by MGI, that pertained to these functions and fell within the six QTL regions, resulting in six candidate genes: *CXCR4*, *MGAT5*, *CACNA1A*, *TERT*, *SLC9A3*, and *AHRR* (Table 6, Table S2). All six candidate genes were related to immune function, and *TERT* was also associated with skin hyperplasia and wound healing (Table S2). Similarly, we defined functionally relevant gene ontologies and pathways as those related to these three functions. The QTL on BTA18 contained 16 zinc finger genes that were part of the herpes simplex virus 1 infection pathway, implying an immune function of these genes that could also play a role in DD infection (Table 6).

A limitation of the study is the small sample size. Minimizing phenotypic variation and increasing sample size are both methods to improve the detection of small-effect SNPs, but often pursuing one of these approaches comes at the expense of the other—for example, in this study, large sample size. Our strict phenotypic criteria also caused the controls to be from only two dairies, which was partially accounted for in the LMM analyses by including a covariate term. While the uneven sampling of dairies can be problematic in frequentist methods such as LMM, those issues were avoided in RF analyses and Bayesian estimation because these models account for parameters that did not exist (e.g., a control cow from Farm B or C). Furthermore, the SNPs that defined the QTL regions containing promising candidate genes were significant, suggestive, or important in the LMM and RF analyses, some of which also had nonzero effect sizes estimated from Bayesian regression despite the small sample size. For the quantitative phenotypes, a larger sample size might have more normally distributed phenotypes that the model expects, thereby improving the efficiency of MCMC sampling and more accurate SNP effect estimates. Although the sample size of this study was limited due to our intentionally reducing phenotypic variation, which may have prevented the detection of additional small SNP effects, the sample size was sufficient to very accurately predict the phenotype within the original population. Future replication studies are necessary to determine how well the SNP effects estimated in this study population can be extrapolated to larger populations in different geographical regions and other dairies.

Table 6. Quantitative trait loci (QTL) defined by SNPs that were significant in at least two analyses: linear mixed model (LMM), random forest (RF), or Bayesian regression of top SNPs from linear mixed model (LMM-B) or random forest (RF-B) containing functionally relevant pathways or genes.

Phenotype	BTA	QTL Start Position (bp)	QTL End Position (bp)	QTL Size (kb)	Methodology Used in Defining the QTL	Relevant Pathways	Candidate Genes in QTL
Binary	1	125550933	125822143	271.2	LMM, LMM-B, RF, RF-B		
	2	60971364	63389576	2418.2	LMM, LMM-B		*CXCR, MGAT5*
	2	58016533	59967789	1951.3	RF, RF-B		
	2	65836042	65836042	-	LMM, LMM-B		
	3	119720909	119942789	221.9	RF, RF-B		
	18	47099464	47831459	732.0	RF, RF-B	Herpes simplex virus 1 infection	
Quantitative	7	11979738	12261707	282.0	RF, RF-B		*CACNA1A*
	14	39785964	39818361	32.4	RF, RF-B		
	20	69696705	71850045	2153.3	RF, RF-B		*TERT, SLC9A3, AHRR*

In addition to minimizing phenotyping variation, our GWAS used high-density SNP genotyping to increase the resolution of QTL detection. Previous studies [16,17,20,38,54] had larger sample sizes than our study, achieved by using dairies across multiple geographic regions and various lower-density SNP panels (maximum 76 K SNPs). The lower-resolution SNP panels in those studies may have prevented the detection of smaller linkage disequilibrium blocks (<20 kb) in Holstein cattle [55] and contributed to the inconsistency of genomic regions detected. Although two previous studies found associated loci on BTA1, for one study the suggestive SNPs were in a different region [6], while the other study did not provide SNP coordinates to permit comparisons [16]. Similarly, other GWASs also detected the associated SNPs on BTA3 [17,19] and BTA14 [6], but in different regions. Other GWASs did not detect SNPs on the same chromosomes as our GWAS [54] or did not detect any suggestive or significant SNPs [20]. The published GWASs with smaller sample sizes using the high-density SNP array were able to find SNPs associated for other traits in Holstein cattle, including digital cushion thickness [56], mastitis resistance [57], and fat deposition [58]. Our study using tightly controlled cases and controls was the first to use high-density SNP genotypes in a GWAS for DD susceptibility for improved resolution and the first to find significant and suggestive SNPs on BTA2, 7, 18, and 20 in regions containing likely candidate genes or genes in relevant pathways. The multiplicity of associated chromosomal regions supports that the genetic component of DD susceptibility is heterogeneous and highly complex, such that different combinations of loci with small effects contribute to DD susceptibility, as suggested by previous authors [20,38]. The complex genetic architecture of DD susceptibility likely reflects multiple physiological systems (e.g., immune system, hair morphology, skin matrix remodeling) interacting in the etiology of DD.

The lack of congruence in the genomic regions associated with DD across published studies and the small effect sizes of those QTLs identified further supports that, in addition to many low-impact loci, non-genetic factors strongly influence DD susceptibility. The ranking of farm as the most important predictor in the RF analyses supports the concept that farm management (e.g., hoof trimming regimen, methods of preventing and treating DD) plays a significant role in reducing DD prevalence. Employing genetic selection in combination with environmental management will likely further reduce DD prevalence.

5. Conclusions

GWAS using LMM and RF approaches identified loci containing six genes on BTA1, 7, and 20 that regulate skin integrity, immune function, and wound repair: *CXCR4*, *MGAT5*, *CACNA1A*, *TERT*, *SLC9A3*, and *AHRR*. Bayesian estimation of SNP effects was used to additionally distinguish between informative and noninformative SNPs and indicated that the top SNPs from LMM-binary and RF-quantitative were collectively predictive of binary and quantitative phenotypes. Despite our identifying significant QTL, the absence of the congruency of associated SNPs in this study compared to other studies and the consistent ranking of the farm as the most important predictor in the RF analyses support the notion that DD susceptibility is heavily influenced by management, and the remaining genetic component is heterogeneous and highly complex. Thus, although farm management may be the most effective short-term method for reducing DD prevalence, combining genetic selection with management will likely be the most effective and sustainable long-term solution.

Supplementary Materials:
Table S1. Suggestive SNPs detected from the linear mixed model genome-wide association analysis using recurrent phenotypes and their defined QTL. Table S2. Candidate genes found within the nine QTL defined by SNPs that were significant/important in at least two of the following analyses: linear mixed model, random forest, and/or Bayesian regression. Figure S1. Multidimensional scaling plot depicting the first two dimensions. Each dot represents a cow, status is indicated by point shape, and farm is indicated by point color. Figure S2. Manhattan plot for the linear mixed model genome-wide association analysis using binary phenotypes from recurrent cases vs. controls. Figure S3. Quantile-quantile plots depicting observed and expected p-values from linear mixed model genome-wide association analyses using (a) binary, (b) quantitative, and (c) binary recurrent phenotypes in the full dataset of 261 cows; and (d) binary and (e) quantitative phenotypes in the subset of 188 cows after removing outlier cows. The red line indicates when observed and expected *p*-values are equivalent. Figure S4.

Manhattan plots from linear mixed model genome-wide association analyses excluding the outlier control cows using (a) binary phenotypes designating the presence of digital dermatitis (DD) lesions or absence of any lameness issues and (b) quantitative phenotypes calculated by dividing the number of DD episodes by the total number of hoof trimming records. The red line indicates the threshold for genome-wide significance (Bonferroni-corrected using the number of independent SNPs at $p < 0.05$), and the blue line indicates the threshold for suggestive significance (Bonferroni-corrected using the number of independent SNPs at $p < 1$). Genomic inflation factors (lambda) are indicated in figure titles. Figure S5. Posterior predictive check bar plot for Bayesian regression estimating effects of suggestive SNPs detected in the linear mixed model genome-wide association study using binary phenotypes. Gray bars represent the actual phenotypes and black dots with intervals represent the median and uncertainty intervals of the phenotypes of replicates (y_{rep}), which were simulated from estimated effects of predictors. Figure S6. Posterior predictive check bar plot for Bayesian regression estimating effects of suggestive SNPs detected in the random forest using binary phenotypes. Gray bars represent the actual phenotypes and black dots with intervals represent the median and uncertainty intervals of the phenotypes of replicates (y_{rep}), which were simulated from estimated effects of predictors. Figure S7. Posterior predictive check distribution plot for Bayesian regression estimating effects of suggestive SNPs detected in the random forest using quantitative phenotypes. The black line represents the actual phenotypic distribution and grey lines dots represent the phenotypic distribution of replicates (y_{rep}), which were simulated from estimated effects of predictors.

Author Contributions: Conceptualization, A.M.O., T.R.F., E.L. and A.L.D.; methodology, A.M.O., T.R.F. and E.L.; software, T.R.F., E.L.; validation, A.M.O., T.R.F. and E.L.; formal analysis, T.R.F. and E.L.; investigation, E.L. and A.L.D.; resources, A.M.O.; data curation, E.L. and A.L.D.; writing—original draft preparation, A.M.O., T.R.F., E.L. and A.L.D.; writing—review and editing, A.M.O., T.R.F., E.L. and A.L.D.; visualization, E.L.; supervision, A.M.O. and T.R.F.; project administration, A.M.O. and E.L.; funding acquisition, A.M.O. All authors have read and agreed to the published version of the manuscript.

Acknowledgments: We thank the producers for their participation and the hoof trimmers for lending their expertise. We gratefully acknowledge the infrastructure support of the Department of Animal Science, College of Agricultural and Environmental Sciences, and the California Agricultural Experiment Station of the University of California, Davis.

References

1. USDA. *Dairy 2014, Dairy Cattle Management Practices in the United States*; USDA–APHIS–VS–CEAH–NAHMS: Fort Collins, CO, USA, 2018.
2. Dolecheck, K.A.; Overton, M.W.; Mark, T.B.; Bewley, J.M. Use of a stochastic simulation model to estimate the cost per case of digital dermatitis, sole ulcer, and white line disease by parity group and incidence timing. *J. Dairy Sci.* **2019**, *102*, 715–730. [CrossRef]
3. Cha, E.; Hertl, J.A.; Bar, D.; Gröhn, Y.T.; Grohn, Y.T. The cost of different types of lameness in dairy cows calculated by dynamic programming. *Prev. Vet. Med. J.* **2010**, *97*, 1–8. [CrossRef] [PubMed]
4. Hadley, G.L.; Wolf, C.A.; Harsh, S.B. Dairy cattle culling patterns, explanations, and implications. *J. Dairy Sci.* **2006**, *89*, 2286–2296. [CrossRef]
5. Ratwan, P.; Mandal, A.; Kumar, M.; Karunakaran, M.; Dutta, T.K. Carbon footprints of dairy animals: Causes and its mitigation. *Res. Rev. J. Dairy Sci. Technol.* **2015**, *4*, 6–11.
6. Biemans, F.; de Jong, M.C.M.; Bijma, P. A genome-wide association study for susceptibility and infectivity of Holstein Friesian dairy cattle to digital dermatitis. *J. Dairy Sci.* **2019**, *102*, 6248–6262. [CrossRef] [PubMed]
7. Onyiro, O.M.; Andrews, L.J.; Brotherstone, S. Genetic parameters for digital dermatitis and correlations with locomotion, production, fertility traits, and longevity in holstein-friesian dairy cows. *J. Dairy Sci.* **2008**, *91*, 4037–4046. [CrossRef] [PubMed]
8. Oberbauer, A.M.; Berry, S.L.; Belanger, J.M.; McGoldrick, R.M.; Pinos-Rodriquez, J.M.; Famula, T.R. Determining the heritable component of dairy cattle foot lesions. *J. Dairy Sci.* **2013**, *96*, 605–613. [CrossRef]
9. Brandt, S.; Apprich, V.; Hackl, V.; Tober, R.; Danzer, M.; Kainzbauer, C.; Gabriel, C.; Stanek, C.; Kofler, J. Prevalence of bovine papillomavirus and Treponema DNA in bovine digital dermatitis lesions. *Vet. Microbiol. J.* **2011**, *148*, 161–167. [CrossRef]
10. Holzhauer, M. Foot bathing dairy cows with antibiotics. *Vet. Rec.* **2017**, *181*, 270. [CrossRef]
11. Holzhauer, M.; Bartels, C.J.; Bergsten, C.; van Riet, M.M.J.; Frankena, K.; Lam, T.J.G.M. The effect of an acidified, ionized copper sulphate solution on digital dermatitis in dairy cows. *Vet. J.* **2012**, *193*, 659–663. [CrossRef]

12. Cook, N.B. A Review of the design and management of footbaths for dairy cattle. *Vet. Clin. North Am. Food Anim. Pract.* **2017**, *33*, 195–225. [CrossRef] [PubMed]
13. Epperson, B.; Midla, L. Copper sulfate for footbaths—Issues and alternatives. In Proceedings of the Tri-State Dairy Nutrition Conference, Fort Wayne, IN, USA, 24 April 2007; pp. 51–54.
14. NTP (National Toxicology Program). *Report on Carcinogens*; Research Triangle Park: Durham, NC, USA, 2016.
15. van der Linde, C.; de Jong, G.; Koenen, E.P.C.; Eding, H. Claw health index for Dutch dairy cattle based on claw trimming and conformation data. *J. Dairy Sci.* **2010**, *93*, 4883–4891. [CrossRef] [PubMed]
16. Malchiodi, F.; Koeck, A.; Christen, A.M.; Schenkel, F.S.; Kelton, D.F.; Miglior, F. *Genetic Parameters and Genome Wide Association Study of Individual Hoof Lesions in Canadian Holsteins Using Different Contemporary Groups*; Canadian Dairy Network: Guelph, ON, Canada, 2015.
17. Sánchez-Molano, E.; Bay, V.; Smith, R.F.; Oikonomou, G.; Banos, G. Quantitative trait loci mapping for lameness associated phenotypes in holstein–friesian dairy cattle. *Front. Genet.* **2019**, *10*. [CrossRef]
18. Scholey, R.A.; Evans, N.J.; Blowey, R.W.; Massey, J.P.; Murray, R.D.; Smith, R.F.; Ollier, W.E.; Carter, S.D. Identifying host pathogenic pathways in bovine digital dermatitis by RNA-Seq analysis. *Vet. J.* **2013**, *197*, 699–706. [CrossRef]
19. Naderi, S.; Bohlouli, M.; Yin, T.; Konig, S.; König, S. Genomic breeding values, SNP effects and gene identification for disease traits in cow training sets. *Anim. Genet.* **2018**, *49*, 178–192. [CrossRef] [PubMed]
20. van der Spek, D.; van Arendonk, J.A.; Bovenhuis, H. Genome-wide association study for claw disorders and trimming status in dairy cattle. *J. Dairy Sci.* **2015**, *98*, 1286–1295. [CrossRef]
21. Read, D.H.; Walker, R.L. Papillomatous digital dermatitis (footwarts) in California dairy cattle: Clinical and gross pathologic findings. *J. Vet. Diagn. Investig.* **1998**, *10*, 67–76. [CrossRef]
22. Krull, A.C.; Shearer, J.K.; Gorden, P.J.; Scott, H.M.; Plummer, P.J. Digital dermatitis: Natural lesion progression and regression in Holstein dairy cattle over 3 years. *J. Dairy Sci.* **2016**, *99*, 3718–3731. [CrossRef]
23. Purcell, S.M.; Chang, C.C. PLINK 1.9. Available online: https://www.cog-genomics.org/plink/1.9/ (accessed on 19 February 2020).
24. Chang, C.C.; Chow, C.C.; Tellier, L.C.; Vattikuti, S.; Purcell, S.M.; Lee, J.J. Second-generation PLINK: Rising to the challenge of larger and richer datasets. *Gigascience* **2015**, *4*, 7. [CrossRef]
25. Yang, J.; Lee, S.H.; Goddard, M.E.; Visscher, P.M. GCTA: A tool for genome-wide complex trait analysis. *Am. J. Hum. Genet.* **2011**, *88*, 76–82. [CrossRef]
26. Lippert, C.; Listgarten, J.; Liu, Y.; Kadie, C.M.; Davidson, R.I.; Heckerman, D. FaST linear mixed models for genome-wide association studies. *Nat. Methods* **2011**, *8*, 833–835. [CrossRef]
27. Zhou, X.; Stephens, M. Genome-wide efficient mixed-model analysis for association studies. *Nat. Genet.* **2012**, *44*, 821–824. [CrossRef] [PubMed]
28. Li, M.-X.; Yeung, J.M.Y.; Cherny, S.S.; Sham, P.C. Evaluating the effective numbers of independent tests and significant p-value thresholds in commercial genotyping arrays and public imputation reference datasets. *Hum. Genet.* **2012**, *131*, 747–756. [CrossRef] [PubMed]
29. Lander, E.; Kruglyak, L. Genetic dissection of complex traits: Guidelines for interpreting and reporting linkage results. *Nat. Genet.* **1995**, *11*, 241–247. [CrossRef] [PubMed]
30. R Development Core Team. R: A language and Environment for Statistical Computing. Available online: https://www.r-project.org/ (accessed on 10 August 2020).
31. Turner, S.D. qqman: An R package for visualizing GWAS results using QQ and manhattan plots. *bioRxiv* **2014**, 5165. [CrossRef]
32. Purcell, S.; Neale, B.; Todd-Brown, K.; Thomas, L.; Ferreira, M.A.R.; Bender, D.; Maller, J.; Sklar, P.; De Bakker, P.I.W.; Daly, M.J. PLINK: A tool set for whole-genome association and population-based linkage analyses. *Am. J. Hum. Genet.* **2007**, *81*, 559–575. [CrossRef]
33. Browning, B.L.; Zhou, Y.; Browning, S.R. A one-penny imputed genome from next-generation reference panels. *Am. J. Hum. Genet.* **2018**, *103*, 338–348. [CrossRef]
34. Goldstein, B.A.; Hubbard, A.E.; Cutler, A.; Barcellos, L.F. An application of Random Forests to a genome-wide association dataset: Methodological considerations and new findings. *BMC Genet.* **2010**, *11*, 49. [CrossRef]
35. Kuhn, M. Building predictive models in R using the caret package. *J. Stat. Softw.* **2008**, *28*, 1–26. [CrossRef]
36. Christopoulos, D.T. On the efficient identification of an inflection point on the efficient identification of an inflection point. *Int. J. Math. Sci. Comput.* **2016**, *6*, 13–20.

37. Christopoulos, D.T. Introducing Unit Invariant Knee (UIK) As an objective choice for elbow point in multivariate data analysis techniques. *SSRN Electron. J.* **2017**, 1–7. [CrossRef]
38. Biemans, F.; Bijma, P.; Boots, N.M.; de Jong, M.C.M. Digital dermatitis in dairy cattle: The contribution of different disease classes to transmission. *Epidemics* **2018**, *23*, 76–84. [CrossRef] [PubMed]
39. Goodrich, B.; Gabry, J.; Ali, I.; Brilleman, S. Rstanarm: Bayesian Applied Regression Modeling via Stan. Available online: https://mc-stan.org/rstanarm/ (accessed on 7 August 2020).
40. Gelman, A.; Su, Y.-S.; Yajima, M.; Hill, J.; Pittau, M.G.; Kerman, J.; Zheng, T.; Dorie, V. *R Package ARM: Data Analysis Using Regression and Multilevel/Hierarchical Models*; Cambridge University Press: Cambridge, UK, 2007.
41. Vehtari, A.; Gabry, J.; Magnusson, M.; Yao, Y.; Andrew, Y.; Bürkner, P.-C.; Paananen, T.; Gelman, A. Loo: Efficient Leave-one-out Cross-Validation and WAIC for Bayesian Models. Available online: https://mc-stan.org/loo/ (accessed on 30 September 2020).
42. Vehtari, A.; Gelman, A.; Gabry, J. Practical Bayesian model evaluation using leave-one-out cross-validation and WAIC. *Stat. Comput.* **2017**, *27*, 1413–1432. [CrossRef]
43. Gabry, J.; Simpson, D.; Vehtari, A.; Betancourt, M.; Gelman, A. Visualization in Bayesian workflow Jonah. *J. R. Stat. Soc.* **2019**, *182*, 389–402. [CrossRef]
44. Richardson, I.W.; Berry, D.P.; Wiencko, H.L.; Higgins, I.M.; More, S.J.; McClure, J.; Lynn, D.J.; Bradley, D.G. A genome-wide association study for genetic susceptibility to Mycobacterium bovis infection in dairy cattle identifies a susceptibility QTL on chromosome 23. *Genet. Sel. Evol.* **2016**, *48*, 19. [CrossRef]
45. Twomey, A.J.; Berry, D.P.; Evans, R.D.; Doherty, M.L.; Graham, D.A.; Purfield, D.C. Genome-wide association study of endo-parasite phenotypes using imputed whole-genome sequence data in dairy and beef cattle. *Genet. Sel. Evol.* **2019**, *51*, 1–17. [CrossRef] [PubMed]
46. Functional Annotation of Animal Genomes (FAANG) Consortium FAANGMine. Available online: http://128.206.116.18:8080/faangmine/begin.do (accessed on 3 August 2020).
47. Smith, C.L.; Eppig, J.T. The mammalian phenotype ontology: Enabling robust annotation and comparative analysis. *Wiley Interdiscip. Rev. Syst. Biol. Med.* **2009**, *1*, 390–399. [CrossRef]
48. Shearer, J.K.; van Amstel, S.R. Pathogenesis and treatment of sole ulcers and white line disease. *Vet. Clin. North Am. Food Anim. Pr.* **2017**, *33*, 283–300. [CrossRef]
49. Evans, N.J.; Brown, J.M.; Demirkan, I.; Singh, P.; Getty, B.; Timofte, D.; Vink, W.D.; Murray, R.D.; Blowey, R.W.; Birtles, R.J.; et al. Association of unique, isolated treponemes with bovine digital dermatitis lesions. *J. Clin. Microbiol.* **2009**, *47*, 689–696. [CrossRef]
50. Watts, K.M.; Fodor, C.; Beninger, C.; Lahiri, P.; Arrazuria, R.; De Buck, J.; Knight, C.G.; Orsel, K.; Barkema, H.W.; Cobo, E.R.; et al. A differential innate immune response in active and chronic stages of bovine infectious digital dermatitis. *Front. Microbiol.* **2018**, *9*, 1586. [CrossRef]
51. Zuerner, R.L.; Heidari, M.; Elliott, M.K.; Alt, D.P.; Neill, J.D. Papillomatous digital dermatitis spirochetes suppress the bovine macrophage innate immune response. *Vet. Microbiol.* **2007**, *125*, 256–264. [CrossRef]
52. Refaai, W.; Ducatelle, R.; Geldhof, P.; Mihi, B.; El-shair, M.; Opsomer, G. Digital dermatitis in cattle is associated with an excessive innate immune response triggered by the keratinocytes. *BMC Vet. Res.* **2013**, *9*, 193. [CrossRef] [PubMed]
53. Murphy, K.; Weaver, C. *Janeway's Immunobiology*, 9th ed.; Garland Science: New York, NY, USA, 2016; ISBN 978-0-8153-4243-4.
54. Scholey, R.A.; Blowey, R.W.; Murray, R.D.; Smith, R.F.; Cameron, J.; Massey, J.P.; Ollier, W.E.; Carter, S.D. Investigating host genetic factors in bovine digital dermatitis. *Vet. Rec.* **2012**, *171*, 624. [CrossRef] [PubMed]
55. Pérez O'Brien, A.M.; Mészáros, G.; Utsunomiya, Y.T.; Sonstegard, T.S.; Garcia, J.F.; Van Tassell, C.P.; Carvalheiro, R.; da Silva, M.V.B.; Sölkner, J. Linkage disequilibrium levels in Bos indicus and Bos taurus cattle using medium and high density SNP chip data and different minor allele frequency distributions. *Livest. Sci.* **2014**, *166*, 121–132. [CrossRef]
56. Stambuk, C.R.; Staiger, E.A.; Nazari-Ghadikolaei, A.; Heins, B.J.; Huson, H.J. Phenotypic characterization and genome-wide association studies of digital cushion thickness in Holstein cows. *J. Dairy Sci.* **2020**, *103*, 3289–3303. [CrossRef]

57. Kurz, J.P.; Yang, Z.; Weiss, R.B.; Wilson, D.J.; Rood, K.A.; Liu, G.E.; Wang, Z. A genome-wide association study for mastitis resistance in phenotypically well-characterized Holstein dairy cattle using a selective genotyping approach. *Immunogenetics* **2019**, *71*, 35–47. [CrossRef]
58. Lehner, S.; Zerbin, I.; Doll, K.; Rehage, J.; Distl, O. A genome-wide association study for left-sided displacement of the abomasum using a high-density single nucleotide polymorphism array. *J. Dairy Sci.* **2018**, *101*, 1258–1266. [CrossRef]

3

Genome-Wide Association Study in Mexican Holstein Cattle Reveals Novel Quantitative Trait Loci Regions and Confirms Mapped Loci for Resistance to Bovine Tuberculosis

Sara González-Ruiz [1], Maria G. Strillacci [2,*], Marina Durán-Aguilar [3], Germinal J. Cantó-Alarcón [3], Sara E. Herrera-Rodríguez [4], Alessandro Bagnato [2], Luis F. Guzmán [5], Feliciano Milián-Suazo [3] and Sergio I. Román-Ponce [6,*]

1 Doctorado en Ciencias Biológicas, Universidad Autónoma de Querétaro, Avenida de las Ciencias S/N Juriquilla, Delegación Santa Rosa Jáuregui, Querétaro C.P. 76230, Mexico
2 Department of Veterinary Medicine, Università degli Studi di Milano, Via Trentacoste, 2, 20134 Milano, Italy
3 Facultad de Ciencias Naturales, Universidad Autónoma de Querétaro, Avenida de las Ciencias S/N Juriquilla, Delegación Santa Rosa Jáuregui, Querétaro C.P. 76230, Mexico
4 Centro de Investigación y Asistencia en Tecnología y Diseño del Estado de Jalisco A.C., Guadalajara C.P. 44270, Mexico
5 Centro Nacional de Recursos Genéticos, INIFAP, Tepatitlán de Morelos 47600, Mexico
6 Centro Nacional de Investigación Disciplinaria en Fisiología y Mejoramiento animal, INIFAP, SAGARPA, Km. 1 Carretera a Colón, Ajuchitlán, Colón, Querétaro C.P. 76280, Mexico
* Correspondence: maria.strillacci@unimi.it (M.G.S.); roman.sergio@inifap.gob.mx (S.I.R.-P.)

Simple Summary: Bovine tuberculosis is an infectious disease of cattle caused by *Mycobacterium bovis* characterized by the formation of tubercles in any organ or tissue. Bovine tuberculosis represents a significant veterinary and public health problem in many parts of the world. It is zoonotic, transmitted to humans through consumption of infected milk and other cattle products. Although many factors influence infection and progression of the disease, there must be an important host genetic component that explains why some animals get sick and others remain healty. We present evidence of genetic variants associated with resistance to tuberculosis in Mexican Holstein dairy cattle using a case-control approach with a selective DNA pooling. Here, we identified novel quantitative trait loci regions harboring genes involved in *Mycobacterium* spp. immune response. This is a first screening about resistance to tuberculosis infection on Mexican Holstein cattle based on a dense single nucleotide polymorphism chip. The identified genes belong to both, the already known, and the undisclosed quantitative trait loci regions.

Abstract: Bovine tuberculosis (bTB) is a disease of cattle that represents a risk to public health and causes severe economic losses to the livestock industry. Recently, genetic studies, like genome-wide association studies (GWAS) have greatly improved the investigation of complex diseases identifying thousands of disease-associated genomic variants. Here, we present evidence of genetic variants associated with resistance to TB in Mexican dairy cattle using a case-control approach with a selective DNA pooling experimental design. A total of 154 QTLRs (quantitative trait loci regions) at 10% PFP (proportion of false positives), 42 at 5% PFP and 5 at 1% PFP have been identified, which harbored 172 annotated genes. On BTA13, five new QTLRs were identified in the *MACROD2* and *KIF16B* genes, supporting their involvement in resistance to bTB. Six QTLRs harbor seven annotated genes that have been previously reported as involved in immune response against *Mycobacterium* spp: BTA (*Bos taurus* autosome) 1 (*CD80*), BTA3 (*CTSS*), BTA 3 (*FCGR1A*), BTA 23 (*HFE*), BTA 25 (*IL21R*), and BTA 29 (*ANO9* and *SIGIRR*). We identified novel QTLRs harboring genes involved in *Mycobacterium* spp.

immune response. This is a first screening for resistance to TB infection on Mexican dairy cattle based on a dense SNP (Single Nucleotide Polymorphism) chip.

Keywords: bovine tuberculosis resistance; DNA pooling; SNP; QTL; genome-wide association study

---

1. Introduction

Bovine tuberculosis (bTB), caused by *Mycobacterium bovis* is a chronic infectious disease characterized by granulomas in affected tissues [1,2]. *M. bovis* infects a wide range of mammalian hosts, domestic and wildlife species, and humans; therefore, it is a risk to public health [3]. It has been estimated that nearly 10 million people are affected by tuberculosis worldwide every year, and that the proportion of cases due to *M. bovis* in humans during the last two decades was from 0.5% to 13%, depending on the study population [4–6]. Additionally, bTB causes economic losses to the livestock industry: infected animals have poor production performance, die or are disposed of prematurely [7,8]. Cattle TB is considered the fourth most significant livestock disease in terms of impact on human health in developing countries, including risks to species other than cattle and the wildlife species [9]. The disease persists in livestock in spite of the on-going eradication program that has been established. The program relies on a test-and-slaughter strategy in herds of cattle, and carcass inspection at abattoirs [10].

Recently, genetic studies like genome-wide association studies (GWASs) have greatly improved the understanding of complex diseases identifying thousands of disease-associated genomic variants [11]. Evidence suggests that genetic variation and resistance to bTB exists in many species, including humans, mice, deer and cattle [12,13]. Heritability values estimated on UK and Irish cattle populations have shown that individual variability for host resistance to TB has a genetic basis [14,15]. Other studies have also shown genetic variation for resistance of cattle to TB [15]; higher resistance has been reported in *Bos taurus indicus* compared to *Bos taurus* [16,17].

In Mexico, bTB is still an endemic disease, and the availability of genomic tools, such as high-density SNP (Single Nucleotide Polymorphism), allow disclosing QTL (quantitative trait loci) regions harboring genes involved in the immune response against TB, as previously reported in different cattle populations. Several studies have in fact identified genetic loci associated with bTB resistance. They included polymorphisms in candidate genes like *SLC11A1* in African Zebu cattle [18], *TLR1* in Chinese Holsteins [19], SNP on BTA23 in Irish dairy herds [20], and three other genetic loci on BTA2 and 13 were also associated [21]. A GWAS involving Irish Holsteins identified a genomic region in BTA22 containing the taurine transporter gene *SLC6A6*, which was suggestively associated with resistance [22]. In a case-control study, GWAS used in *Mycobacterium avium* subsp. paratuberculosis (MAP) identified chromosomal regions (BTA9, BTA11 and BTA12) associated with this disease; and provides evidence of genetic loci involvement in humoral response to MAP [23].

Therefore, the aim of this study was to identify QTL regions involved in resistance to TB in Mexican dairy cattle using a GWAS case-control approach with a selective DNA pooling experimental design.

2. Materials and Methods

This project was approved by the Bioethics Committee of the Natural Sciences Department of the Autonomous University of Queretaro under registry number 29FCN2016.

2.1. Tissue Samples

Tissue samples were collected from carcasses at slaughterhouses in the States of Jalisco and Aguascalientes. These two states are located in central Mexico where the within-herd prevalence of tuberculosis in dairy cattle is about 16% [24,25]. Animals slaughtered were Holstein cows from small family-run herds with an average size of 70 head.

Even when all lymph nodes and internal organs were checked for the presence of lesions, tissue samples selected were taken only from lymph nodes in head (retropharyngeal), thorax (tracheobronchial and mediastinal), abdomen (mesenteric), and lungs. Tissue samples were collected both from animals with visible lesions and from animals with no visible lesions at carcass inspection. After collection, tissue samples were immediately placed in a cooler with ice and taken to the laboratory where they were kept at −20 °C until analysis. Hair samples were taken from the ear in the same animals as a source of DNA for SNP genotyping. Epidemiological data for each animal included herd and States of sampling, sex, age, and the organ affected, and was used to evaluate homogeneity of prevalence of bTB across different geographical areas of sample collection.

2.2. Bacteriological Analysis

All tissue samples were cultured in Stonebrink and Lowenstein-Jensen media with pyruvate for the isolation of *M. bovis* (Figure 1). Briefly, tissue samples were first surface-sterilized with 1:1000 solution of sodium hypochlorite, and then macerated and decontaminated with a 10% solution of hydrochloric acid as previously reported [25,26].

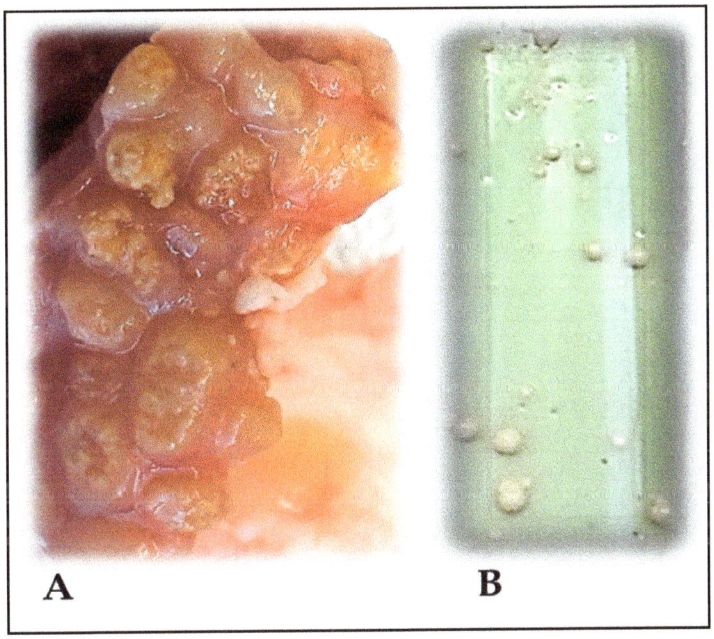

Figure 1. Tracheobronchial lymph nodes with visible lesions of Bovine tuberculosis (bTB) (**A**). Colonies of *M. bovis* in Stonebrink media (**B**).

2.3. Experimental Design, DNA Extraction, Pooling and Genotyping

A total of 375 biological samples were included in the study, 150 cases (tissue samples with visible lesions and culture positive) and 225 controls (tissue samples with no visible lesions and culture negative), collected from carcasses. All samples were from the same geographic area and, in some cases, from the same herd, to ensure similar level of exposure to the pathogen as previously described [24,25].

A selective DNA pooling design [27] was used in this study to identify QTL regions associated with resistance to bTB in a case control study. This experimental design has been shown to be effective, appropriate, powerful to perform association studies, and highly accurate compared with experimental designs using individual-sample genotyping [28,29]. Selective DNA pooling has been extensively used in GWAS mapping studies in livestock for mapping QTL in quantitative traits [29,30], and in case control studies in cattle [31,32].

With the advent of dense SNP chip arrays, the source of variation related to the experimental design and the methodology to control and accurately account for it has been discussed and established [33,34].

DNA extraction was performed using a commercial kit (Wizard® Genomic DNA Purification Kit, Thermo Fisher Scientific, Waltham, MA, USA) following the manufacturer recommendations. Quantity and quality control on each DNA sample was performed by spectrophotometry with NanoDrop™ 2000 equipment (Thermo Fisher Scientific). Integrity of the DNA was determined by electrophoresis on a 1% agarose gel pre-stained with GelRed® Nucleic Acid Gel Stain (Biotium, Fremont, CA, USA).

All DNA samples were normalized at a concentration of 50 ng/μL. DNA pools were then built by taking equivalent amounts of volume from each DNA sample, thus the final concentration for each pool was 50 ng/μL according to Illumina array requirements.

A total of 75 DNA samples were used in building each pool, and biological, technical and array replicates were designed as suggested [33,34]. Pools for cases were composed of two independent groups of 75 animals (average age of 47 ± 1.8 months and the proportion was 75% females and 25% males) positive for visible lesions at carcass inspection and positive for *M. bovis* isolation by culture (Figure 1). These two pools represent two independent biological replicates. The pools for controls were composed of three independent groups of 75 animals (average age of 43 ± 2.8 months and the proportion was 62% females and 38% males) with no visible lesions and negative for *M. bovis* isolation by culture. Each of the pools was produced in two replicates to account for possible errors in pooling the individuals (technical pooling replicates, i.e., Pool_Rep "_A" and "_B" in Table 1) and respectively genotyped three times to account for array technical error (technical array replicates, i.e., Array_Rep "_1", "_2", and "_3" in Table 1).

Table 1. Scheme of case (CA) and controls (CT) pool definitions, and of genotyping.

CASES			CONTROLS		
Biological	**Technical**		**Biological**	**Technical**	
Bio_rep [a]	**Pool_Rep** [b]	**Array_Rep** [c]	**Bio_rep** [a]	**Pool_Rep** [b]	**Array_Rep** [c]
CA_1	CA1_A	CA_1A_1	CT_1	CT1_A	CT_1A_1
		CA_1A_2			CT_1A_2
		CA_1A_3			CT_1A_3
	CA1_B	CA_1B_1		CT1_B	CT_1B_1
		CA_1B_2			CT_1B_2
		CA_1B_3			CT_1B_3
CA_2	CA2_A	CA_2A_1	CT_2	CT2_A	CT_2A_1
		CA_2A_2			CT_2A_2
		CA_2A_3			CT_2A_3
	CA2_B	CA_2B_1		CT2_B	CT_2B_1
		CA_2B_2			CT_2B_2
		CA_2B_3			CT_2B_3
			CT_3	CT3_A	CT_3A_1
					CT_3A_3
					CT_3A_3
				CT3_B	CT_3B_1
					CT_3B_3
					CT_3B_3

[a] Bio_rep = biological replicate; [b] Pool_Rep = technical pooling replicate; [c] Array_Rep = technical array replicate.

The 10 pools (biological and technical replicates) were processed in three array replicates each, on the Illumina BovineHD BeadChips (777,962 SNP), following the Infinium protocol obtaining a total of 30 sets of B-allele frequency for each SNP. SNPs position was determined according to the UMD 3.1 bovine assembly.

2.4. *Statistical Analysis of Pool*

The B-allele frequencies (BAF) values for each SNP were obtained from the self-normalization algorithm of Illumina BeadStudio software® for each of the three arrays technical replicates of the 10 pools. The BAF is a very accurate measure of the frequency of the alleles in all individuals together in a pool as previously reported [29].

First, a quality control was performed at array technical replicate comparing the standard deviation (SD) distribution of B-allele frequencies among each triplet of array technical replicates. Two array-replicates, one case and one control, were eliminated from the analysis because the value of their B-allele frequency diverged from the other two technical array-replicates. Second, a quality control on the BAF estimation was performed at SNP level as follows: the SD among BAF from the replicate assays (biological, pool and array technical replicates) within cases and controls was calculated, and the markers showing the largest 10% SD were excluded from the analysis. Finally, only SNPs with minor allele frequency (MAF) ≥0.05 were retained. After editing, a total of 438,555 SNPs (of which 10,034 were on BTX (*Bos taurus* X autosome) were used in the association analysis.

GWAS was performed comparing at each marker the allele frequencies obtained for the cases pools with those obtained in the control pools for each marker (averaged over replicates within case and within control) according to the selective DNA pooling (SDP) design and methods as described in detail [31,32]. GWAS was performed after excluding monomorphic SNPs, SNPs mapped on BTY, mitochondrial SNPs, and SNPs without chromosome position.

A single-marker test for marker-trait association was used, and the *p*-value for each marker calculated as:

$$\text{Ztest} = \text{Dtest}/\text{SD (Dnull)} \tag{1}$$

where: Dtest is the difference of the B-allele frequencies means among tails, and Dnull is the difference of the B-allele frequencies means within tails.

2.5. *Quantitative Trait Loci Region Definition*

The nominal P values at different PFP (proportion of false positives) thresholds, i.e., 1%, 5% and 10%, have been identified according to Fernando et al. [34,35], and the corresponding −log10 (*p*-value) calculated, resulting: (i) for PFP at 1%, 4.58; (ii) for PFP at 5%, 3.17; (iii) for PFP at 10%, 2.53. As in Lipkin et al. [31], moving averages of −log10 (*p*-values) were calculated considering a window of 16 SNP markers, corresponding to an average-window-size of about 100 Kb. As shown in Lipkin et al. [31], PFP is the appropriate approach to correct for multiple testing when the moving averages approach proposed by the same authors is used to identify QTL regions. As such the window average values above the PFP thresholds of 1%, 5% and 10% have been considered as leading QTL average. A 1 log drop in flanking average values defined the boundaries of the QTL region (QTLR). The leading SNP is the one showing the largest −log10 (*p*-value) among those in each QTLR.

2.6. *Functional Annotation of the QTLR*

The SNPchiMp online database [36] was utilized to match the Illumina SNP name with the SNP rsID (Reference SNP cluster ID). The European Variation Archive (EVA) variant browser of EMBL-EBI [37] allowed annotating all the leading SNPs through the rsID. The full genes set (*Bos taurus*: Ensemble Gene 92) was used [38]. Gene ontology (GO) functional annotation and KEGG pathway analyses using the Gene ontology (GO) and pathway analyses were performed using the DAVID Bioinformatics Resources software, version 6.8 [39]. In addition, bovine QTL available from Animal Genome Database [40] were catalogued into our QTLRs by overlapping.

STRING (Search Tool for the Retrieval of Interacting Genes/Proteins) was used to investigate the existence of gene networks in cattle among ones in QTLRs identified with PFP at 10%. Those found in the gene network were annotated by STRING using both bovine and human databases.

3. Results

From the 375 animals included in the study, 34% were males, and 65% females, ages 12 to 108 months; 44 months was the most frequent age (22%). From the cases group, lesions were found mainly in lymph nodes of head (retropharyngeal 51%) and thorax (mediastinal and tracheobronchial, 61%), some animals had lesions in more than one lymph node.

QTLRs Associated with Resistance/Susceptibility to bTB

A total 154 QTLRs at 10% PFP were identified (Figure 2, Table S1). In general, all these regions were distributed homogeneously over all autosomes (with the exception that none were found on BTA15 and BTA17), and on chromosome X (n. 2), defined by 3296 SNPs. The average length of the QTLRs was 93,446 bp. Table S1 also includes information about the position of the leading SNP for each QTLR on the chromosome, the number of SNPs defining the regions, and its location in the genes annotated within the QTLR, and the number of SNPs pertaining to the regions above each of the three PFP thresholds.

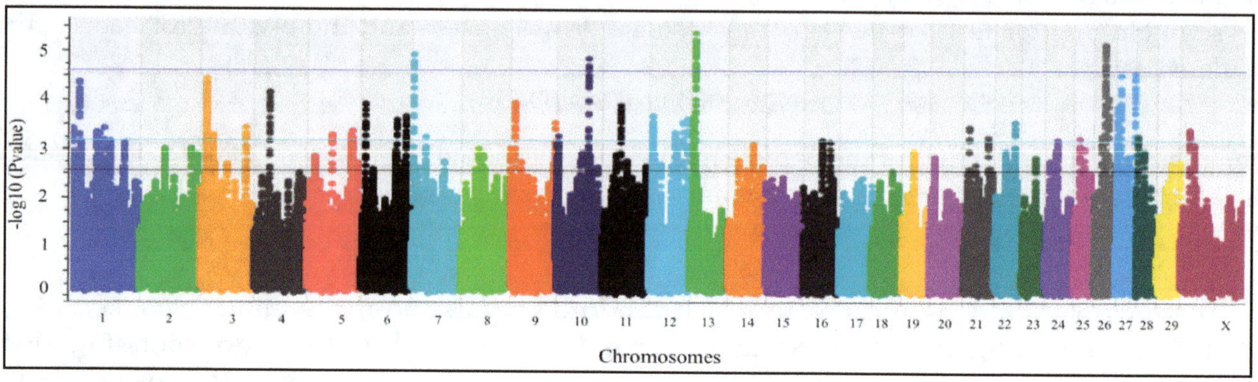

Figure 2. Manhattan plots of QTLR (Quantitative Trait Loci Regions) for all chromosomes. Horizontal lines represent the 1% PFP (proportion of false positives) (blue), the 5% PFP (light blue), and the 10% PFP (black) thresholds.

One hundred and seventy-two genes (including 2 miRNA and 5 tRNA) were catalogued in the QTLRs using the *Bos taurus* Ensembl Gene annotation release 92 (Table S2). The DAVID (The Database for Annotation, Visualization and Integrated Discovery) Database recognized all these genes (excluding miRNA and tRNA), but not for all of them provided the annotated information according to the GO (Gene Ontology) and the KEGG (Kyoto Encyclopedia of Genes and Genomes) pathways terms as in Table 2 (reporting only gene function classifications resulted with a nominal p value ≤ 0.05). As shown in Table 2, most genes refer to the immune response and structural terms. Table S2 reports: (i) the list of genes annotated in the QTLRs (list of genes); (ii) the gene annotation according to the DAVID database classification reported as clustered and not clustered genes including those with a nominal p value ≥ 0.05.

Table 2. Results of the gene annotation: DAVID GO and pathway analysis (KEGG).

Term	Count	*p*-Value	Genes
Biological process			
GO:0006334: nucleosome assembly	6	9.42×10^{5}	*HIST1H2BB, HIST1H1C, HIST1H1A, H2B, HIST1H3G,* HIST1H3I
GO:0006335: DNA replication-dependent nucleosome assembly	3	6.12×10^{3}	*H4, HIST1H3G, HIST1H3I*
GO:0051290: protein heterotetramerization	3	6.81×10^{3}	*H4, HIST1H3G, HIST1H3I*
GO:0098792: xenophagy	5	2.27×10^{3}	*TMEM39A, SNRPB2, CPA3, HIST1H3G, HIST1H3I*
GO:0002230: positive regulation of defense response to virus by host	5	3.68×10^{3}	*TMEM39A, SNRPB2, CPA3, HIST1H3G, HIST1H3I*
GO:0046627: negative regulation of insulin receptor signaling pathway	3	9.09×10^{3}	*PRKCD, KANK1, PRKCB*
GO:0042742: defense response to bacterium	4	1.63×10^{2}	*STAB1, FCGR1A, PRKCD, TMF1*
Cellular Components			
GO:0000786: nucleosome	7	1.60×10^{5}	*H4, HIST1H1C, HIST1H1A, H2B, HIST1H2AK, HIST1H3G, HIST1H3I*
GO:0000788: nuclear nucleosome	5	2.47×10^{4}	*HIST1H2BB, H2B, HIST1H3G, HIST1H3I*
GO:0000784: nuclear chromosome, telomeric region	4	2.3×10^{2}	*H4, TNKS, HIST1H3G, HIST1H3I*
GO:0030176: integral component of endoplasmic reticulum membrane	4	1.50×10^{2}	*PIGG, SARAF, MBOAT4, SLC27A2*
GO:0005615: extracellular space	13	3.32×10^{2}	*A2M, H2B, HFE, FSTL1, CTSS, OVOS2, ESF1, VEGFC, GPI, CTSK, CPA3, CPB1, SMARCA4*
GO:0005788: endoplasmic reticulum lumen	3	4.77×10^{2}	*EOGT, SLC27A2, POGLUT1*
Molecular Functions			
GO:0046982: protein heterodimerization activity	5	7.15×10^{3}	*AGTR1, HIST1H2BB, H4, H2B, FOXP1*
GO:0042393: histone binding	3	3.67×10^{2}	*H4, PRKCB, SMARCA4*
KEGG Pathways			
bta05322: Systemic lupus erythematosus	9	7.64×10^{8}	*HIST1H2BB, H4, CD80, FCGR1A, HIST2H2BF, H2B, HIST1H2AK, HIST1H3G, HIST1H3I*
bta05034: Alcoholism	8	4.32×10^{6}	*HIST1H2BB, HRAS, H4, HIST2H2BF, H2B, HIST1H2AK, HIST1H3G, HIST1H3I*
bta05203: Viral carcinogenesis	5	1.92×10^{3}	*HIST1H2BB, HRAS, H4, HIST2H2BF, H2B*
bta00514: Other types of O-glycan biosynthesis	3	2.18×10^{2}	*ST6GAL2, EOGT, POGLUT1*

In Figure 3, the gene network obtained for genes annotated with STRING is shown for *Bos taurus* and *Homo sapiens* proteins. The genes shown are only the ones in QTLRs that were part of a network. Table S3 reports the GO and pathway analysis for the genes included in the networks of Figure 3.

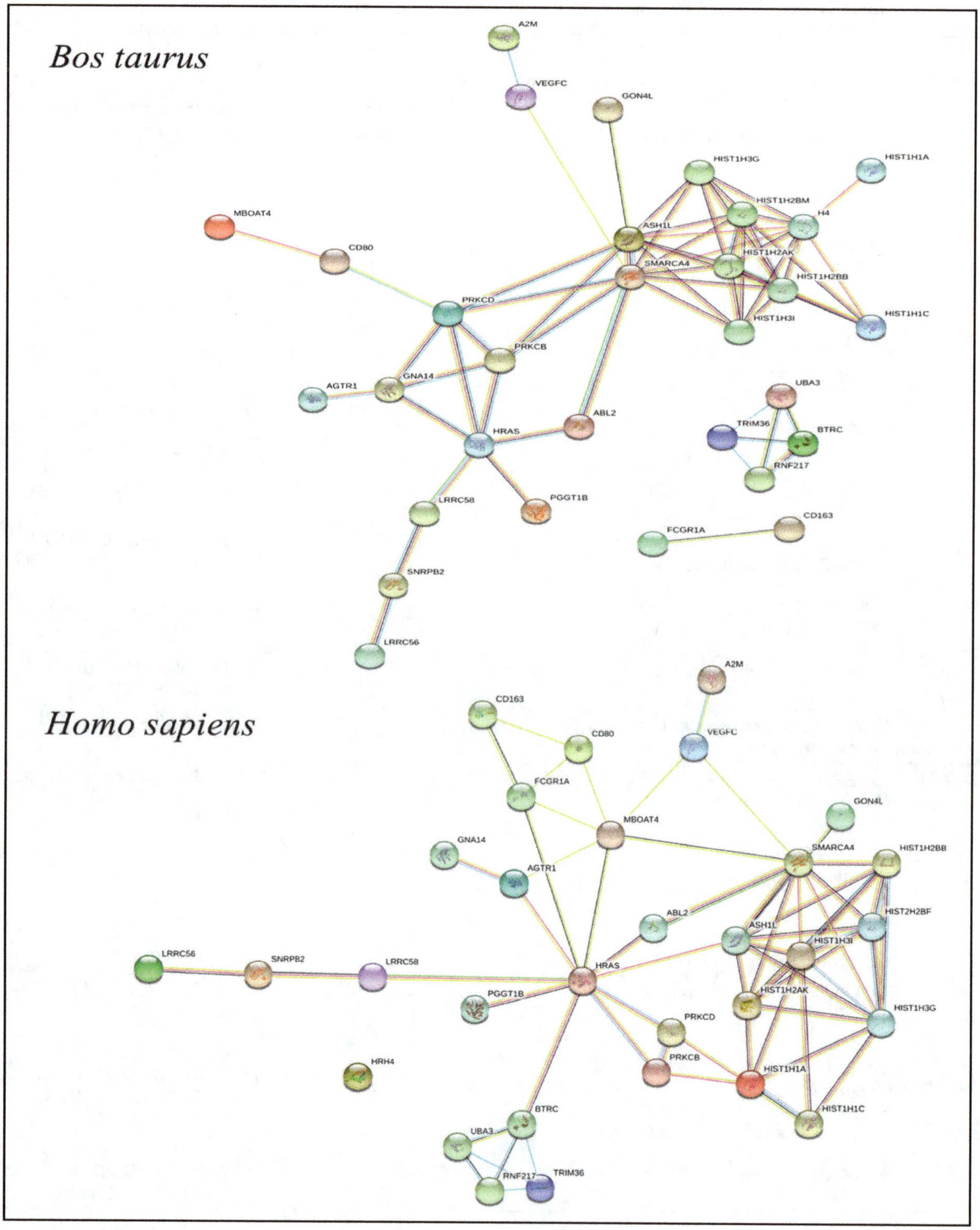

Figure 3. Gene networks in cattle among the ones in QTLRs identified with PFP at 10% (Bovine and Human databases).

4. Discussion

Bovine TB is one of the most prevalent and important diseases in the livestock industry, as well as in wildlife and human population [3]; its eradication is still a priority for many countries. Current strategies to reduce the prevalence in the herds of livestock focus primarily on test-and-disposal of reactors, and abattoir surveillance. In developing countries, however, the success of these programs has been partial because of the poor sensitivity of the tuberculin test and the difficulties tracing back infected animals identified at slaughterhouses. New strategies have been recommended, such as vaccination, in either cattle or the wildlife species [41], estimation of direct genomic estimated breeding values (EBVs) in UK dairy cattle [42], or to increase host resistance through breeding practices [43]. Recent studies in fact have disclosed genetic variability affecting resistance to bTB [20,41,43–48] suggesting the possibility of implementing genomic selection for that feature in cattle.

The genes present in the novel QTLRs according to the PFP, 1%, 5% and 10% *p* values threshold were:

4.1. QTLR_1%_PFP

Five QTLRs distributed on different BTA (7, 10, 13, 30 and 31) were identified, but the three genes mapping within these regions are not involved in metabolic pathways associated with bTB.

4.2. QTLR_5%_PFP

4.2.1. BTA 1

The QTLR_10 and QTLR_16 include genes involved in immune response to disease. In detail, the first region harbors the TIGIT gene (T cell immunoreceptor with Ig and ITIM (Immunoreceptor tyrosine-based inhibitory motif) domain), an inhibitor of the T cell proliferation, the cytokine production in CD4+ T cells, and of the NK cells cytolytic activity [49]. As reported by Joller et al. [50], the altered balance between activation and inhibitory immune signals can result in increased susceptibility to infection or to induction of autoimmunity.

The *NAALADL2* gene (N-acetylated alpha-linked acidic dipeptidase-like 2), whose function is not well known, is located within the QTLR_16. This gene promotes a pro-migratory and pro-metastatic phenotype in cancer [51], and was recently associated with bovine respiratory disease susceptibility [31].

4.2.2. BTA 3

The *TRIM33* gene (Tripartite motif containing 33), located in QTLR_27 on BTA 3, is involved in migration of macrophages and neutrophils towards inflammatory stimulus in vertebrate tissues [52]. Weng et al. [53] reported *TRIM33* roles in transcriptional regulation during hematopoiesis, tumor suppressor activity in multiple tissues, erythropoiesis, and DNA repair.

4.2.3. BTA 5

On this chromosome, the QTLR_37 harbors the *CD163* gene (CD163 molecule). This gene, expressed on monocytes, macrophages and subpopulations of hematopoietic progenitor is involved in the clearance of haptoglobin–hemoglobin complexes by mediating endocytosis, and prevents the toxic and oxidative effects of free hemoglobin. Different mediators regulate the *CD163* gene expression: up-regulation by glucocorticoids and IL10, and down-regulation by lipopolysaccharide, gamma-interferon, and tumor necrosis factor alpha [54].

4.2.4. BTA 13

Interestingly, from 8.1 Mb to 10.2 Mb, five QTLRs (QTLR_95, QTLR_96, QTLR_97, QTLR_98 and QTLR_99) are found: the first four located within the gene *MACROD2* (MACRO domain containing 2), and the fifth one is in between the end of the gene *MACROD2* and a second gene *KIF16B* (Kinesin Family Member 16 B) (Figure 4). The individual −log10 *p* values show very clear peaks supporting the indication that in this 2 Mb region the *MACROD2* gene and the *KIF16B* gene may play a role in resistance to TB. According to Figure 4 showing the introns and exons of *MACROD2* gene (NCBI refseq gene 105) and the GWAS results for this chromosomal region, the QTLR_98 includes three exons (blue vertical lines). Nevertheless, the *MACROD2* gene is very long and its annotation still needs additional validation [55].

The *KIF16B* gene encodes a kinesin-like protein that could be involved in intracellular trafficking [56].

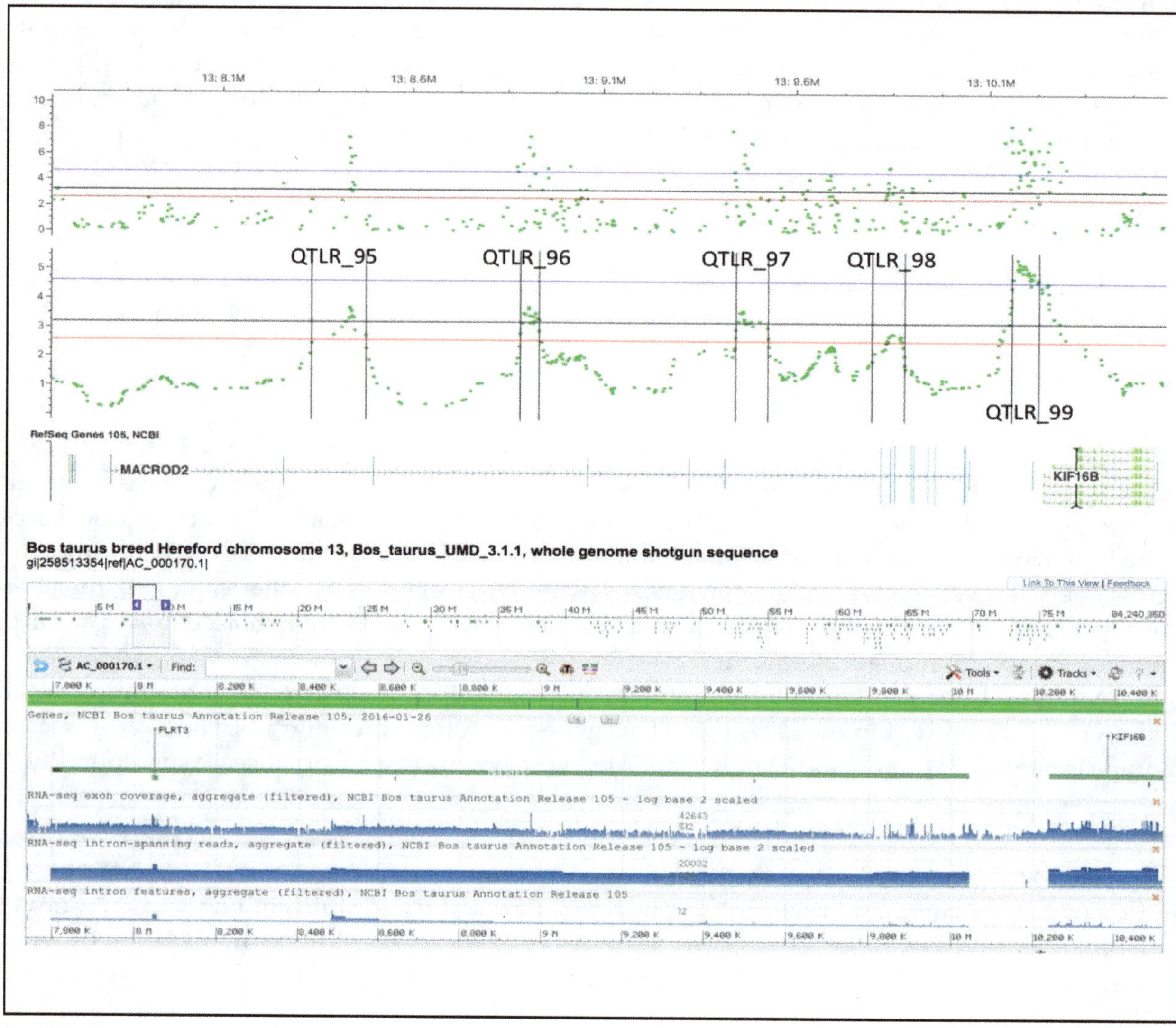

Figure 4. The location of MACROD2 gene is spread over the QTLRs 95–98 (NCBI refseq gene 105).

4.3. *QTLR_10%_PFP*

BTA 2

The *DNER* gene (delta/notch-like EGF repeat containing) within the QTLR_21 on BTA 2, is among those differentially expressed for inflammatory diseases, connective tissue disorders and immunological diseases in cattle [57]. In addition, the *DNER* gene expression level has been shown to decrease in highly marbled beef cattle [58].

Six QTLRs harbor seven genes that have been already associated with susceptibility/resistance to TB: QTLR_12 on BTA 1 (*CD80*), QTLR_25 on BTA3 (*CTSS*), QTLR_26 on BTA 3 (*FCGR1A*), QTLR_127 on BTA 23 (*HFE*), QTLR_133 on BTA 25 (*IL21R*), and QTLR_152 on BTA 29 (*ANO9* and *SIGIRR*). These genes are all involved in immune response against *Mycobacterium* spp.

- Cathepsins, including Cathepsin S (*CTSS*) are proteolytic enzymes that function mainly in lysosomes, where they contribute to pathogen killing by their involvement in antigen presentation pathways. Pires et al. [59] demonstrated the role of this class of proteins in the control of *M. tuberculosis* by manipulating the cathepsin expression by pathogenic mycobacteria to favor its intracellular survival.

- The protein encoded by the *CD80* gene (CD80 molecule), the B-lymphocyte activation antigen B7-1 is a membrane receptor that affects the immunological reactivity of T-lymphocytes when its expression decreases. In addition, *CD80* has a role in enhancing the anti-tuberculosis immunity [60].
- The *FCGR1A* gene (Fc fragment of IgG receptor Ia) expression, together with that of the *BLR1* gene has been considered as potential marker for monitoring the extent of TB disease and to predict treatment outcome in children affected by *M. tuberculosis* [61].
- Booty et al. [62] reported that the cytokine IL-21, produced predominantly by activated CD4+ T cells and CD8+ T cells, is an essential signaling marker for host resistance to *M. tuberculosis* infection via the IL-21 receptor (IL-21R).
- Gomes-Pereira et al. [63] reported an increased susceptibility to *M. avium* in Hemochromatosis Protein HFE-Deficient Mice. *HEF* (homeostatic iron regulator) is a fundamental protein involved in the regulation of cellular iron uptake and iron homeostasis. Studies indicate that monocytes with mutated *HFE* have decreased intracellular iron levels [64]. Also, Wang at el. [65] demonstrated that hemochromatosis impacts the regulation of macrophage cytokine translation and, consequently the inflammatory response.
- The *ANO9* gene, also known as *TMEM16J* (anoctamin 9), together with the *SIGIRR* and the *PKP3* genes constitute a polymorphic complex associated with susceptibility to tuberculosis [66]. The *SIGIRR* gene, also known as Toll IL-1 receptor 8, is a regulatory protein acting to inhibit ILRs and TLRs signaling [67]. The *PKP3*, the third part of this complex gene, maps 6.2 Kb from the end of the QTLR_152.

In addition, three QTLRs identified in our study (QTLR_43 on BTA6, QTLR_115, and QTLR_118 on BTA 21) overlap with those found by Richardson et al. [20] in a study on bovine tuberculosis susceptibility performed in a population of Holstein–Friesian bulls (ID: 96694; 96508, 96511, 96525, 96514, 96517, 96411, 96549, and 96497). Also, the QTLR_84 on BTA12 and QTLR_139 on BTA26 are included within the "Bovine respiratory disease susceptibility QTL (ID: 95663)" and the "Heat tolerance QTL (ID: 31198)", respectively.

5. Conclusions

The results presented here reveal novel QTLRs and confirm mapped loci for resistance to tuberculosis in dairy cattle. The novel QTLRs located on BTA 1, 3, 5, 25 and 29 harbor genes related to immune response. Our results confirm QTL regions previously mapped on BTA 2, 6, 13, 21, 22 and 23 related to resistance to bTB in other dairy cattle populations.

Genomic regions and genes identified in the present study with a case-control selective DNA pooling approach were significantly associated with resistance to TB in cattle. The findings of this study could be used to improve the knowledge on the bTB immune response against *Mycobacterium bovis*, and thus provide the basis for genetic control of this disease in cattle.

Author Contributions: Conceptualization, F.M.-S. and S.I.R.-P.; Data curation, M.D.-A., G.J.C.-A., S.E.H.-R. and L.F.G.; Formal analysis, S.G.-R., M.G.S. and A.B.; Funding acquisition, F.M.-S. and S.I.R.-P.; Investigation, M.G.S.; Methodology, G.J.C.-A. and L.F.G., M.D.-A. and G.J.C.-A.; Supervision, M.G.S., M.D.-A., S.E.H.-R., F.M.-S. and S.I.R.-P.; Writing—original draft, S.G.-R., M.G.S.; Writing—review & editing, A.B., F.M.-S., S.I.R.-P.

Acknowledgments: We knowledge the support from the slaughterhouses of the State of Jalisco for allowing sampling collection, Dulce Anahy Verdugo Escárcega and Susana Sosa Gallegos for their support in sample collection and laboratory analysis, and Erica Gorla for her support in data processing.

References

1. Phillips, C.J.C.; Foster, C.R.W.; Morris, P.A.; Teverson, R. The transmission of *Mycobacterium bovis* infection to cattle. *Res. Vet. Sci.* **2003**, *74*, 1–15. [CrossRef]

2. Abalos, P.; Retamal, P. Tuberculosis: Una zoonosis re-Emergente? *Rev. Sci.* **2004**, *23*, 583–594. [CrossRef]
3. Blischak, J.D.; Tailleux, L.; Mitrano, A.; Barreiro, L.B.; Gilad, Y. Mycobacterial infection induces a specific human innate immune response. *Sci. Rep.* **2015**, *5*, 16882. [CrossRef] [PubMed]
4. Mûller, B.; Hity, M.; Berg, S.; García-Pelayo, M.C.; Dale, J.; Boschiroli, M.L.; Cadmus, S.; Ngandolo, B.N.; Godreuil, S.; Diguimbaye-Djaibé, C.; et al. African 1, an epidemiologically important clonal complex of *Mycobacterium bovis* dominant in Mali, Nigeria, Cameroon and Chad. *J. Bacteriol.* **2009**, *191*, 1951–1960. [CrossRef] [PubMed]
5. Olea-Popelka, F.; Muwonge, A.; Perera, A.; Dean, A.S.; Mumford, E.; Erlacher-Vindel, E.; Forcella, S.; Silk, B.J.; Ditiu, L.; El Idrissi, A. Zoonotic tuberculosis in human beings caused by *Mycobacterium bovis* a call for action. *Lancet Infect. Dis.* **2017**, *17*, 21–25. [CrossRef]
6. Perea-Razo, C.A.; Milián-Suazo, F.; Bárcenas-Reyes, I.; Sosa-Gallegos, S.; Rodríguez-Hernández, E.; Flores-Villalba, S.; Canto-Alarcón, G.J. Whole genome sequencing for detection of zoonotic tuberculosis in Querétaro, Mexico. *J. Infect. Dis. Prev. Med.* **2017**, *5*, 2. [CrossRef]
7. Milián-Suazo, F.; Pérez-Guerrero, L.; Arriaga-Díaz, C.; Romero-Torres, C.; Escartín-Chávez, M. Epidemiología molecular de las tuberculosis bovina y humana en una zona endémica de Querétaro, México. *Salub Publ. Mex.* **2008**, *50*, 1–6.
8. Elias, K.; Hussein, D.; Asseged, B.; Wondwossen, T.; Gebeyehu, M. Status of bovine tuberculosis in Addis Ababa dairy farms. *Rev. Sci. Tech.* **2008**, *27*, 915–923. [CrossRef]
9. Perry, B.D.; Randolph, T.F.; McDermott, J.J.; Sones, K.R.; Thornton, P.K. *Investing in Animal Health Research to Alleviate Poverty*; ILRI (International Livestock Research Institute): Nairobi, Kenya, 2002.
10. De la Rua-Domenech, R.; Goodchild, A.T.; Vordermeier, M.; Hewinson, R.G.; Christiansen, K.H.; Clifton-Hadley, R.S. Ante mortem diagnosis of tuberculosis in cattle: A review of the tuberculin tests. C-interferon assay and other ancillary diagnostic techniques. *Res. Vet. Sci.* **2006**, *81*, 190–210. [CrossRef]
11. Uren, C.; Henn, B.M.; Franke, A.; Wittig, M.; van Helden, P.D.; Hoal, E.G.; Möller, M. A post-GWAS analysis of predicted regulatory s and tuberculosis susceptibility. *PLoS ONE* **2017**, *12*. [CrossRef]
12. Allen, A.R.; Minozzi, G.; Glass, E.J.; Skuce, R.A.; McDowell, S.W.J.; Woolliams, J.A.; Bischop, S.C. Bovine tuberculosis: The genetic basis of host susceptibility. *Proc. Biol. Sci.* **2010**, *277*, 2737–2745. [CrossRef] [PubMed]
13. Hernández-Marín, J.A.; Cortez-Romero, C.; Clemente-Sánchez, F.; Gallegos-Sánchez, J.; Salazar-Ortiz, J.; Tarango-Arámbula, L.A. Risk of transmission of Mycobacterium avium subspecies paratuberculosis (Map) in domestic and wild species. *AGRO Prod.* **2014**, *7*, 65–70.
14. Bermingham, M.L.; More, S.J.; Good, M.; Cromie, A.R.; Higgins, I.M.; Berry, D.P. Genetic correlations between measures of *Mycobacterium bovis* infection and economically important traits in Irish Holstein–Friesian dairy cows. *J. Dairy Sci.* **2010**, *93*, 5413–5422. [CrossRef] [PubMed]
15. Brotherstone, S.; White, I.M.S.; Coffey, M.; Downs, S.H.; Mitchell, A.P.; Clfton-Hadley, R.S.; More, S.J.; Good, M.; Woolliams, J.A. Evidence of genetic resistance of cattle to infection with *Mycobacterium bovis*. *J. Dairy Sci.* **2010**, *93*, 1234–1242. [CrossRef] [PubMed]
16. Carmichael, J. Bovine tuberculosis in the tropics with special reference to Uganda. Part 1. *Vet. J.* **1941**, *97*, 329–339.
17. Ameni, G.; Aseffa, A.; Engers, H.; Young, D.; Gordon, S.; Hewinson, G.; Vordermeier, M. High prevalence and increased severity of pathology of bovine tuberculosis in Holsteins compared to Zebu breeds under field cattle husbandry in central Ethiopia. *Clin. Vaccine Immunol.* **2007**, *14*, 1356–1361. [CrossRef]
18. Kadarmideen, H.N.; Ali, A.A.; Thomson, P.C.; Mûller, B.; Zinsstag, J. Polymorphisms of the *SLC11A1* gene and resistance to bovine tuberculosis in African Zebu cattle. *Anim. Genet.* **2011**, *42*, 656–658. [CrossRef]
19. Sun, L.; Song, Y.; Ria, H.; Yang, H.; Hua, G.; Guo, A.; Yang, L. Polymorphisms in Toll-Like receptor 1 and 9 genes and their association with tuberculosis susceptibility in Chinese Holstein cattle. *Vet. Immunol. Immunopathol.* **2012**, *147*, 195–201. [CrossRef]
20. Richardson, I.A.; Berry, D.P.; Wiencko, H.L.; Higgins, I.M.; More, S.J.; McClure, J.; Lynn, D.J.; Bradley, D.G. A genome wide association study for genetic susceptibility to *Mycobacterium bovis* infection in dairy cattle identifies a susceptibility QTL on chromosome 23. *Genet. Sel. Evol.* **2016**, *48*, 19–23. [CrossRef]

21. Bermingham, M.L.; Bishop, S.C.; Woolliams, J.A.; Pon-Wong, R.; Allen, A.R.; McBride, S.H.; Ryder, J.J.; Wright, D.M.; Skuce, R.A.; McDowell, S.W. Genome wide association study identifies novel loci associated with resistance to bovine tuberculosis. *Heredity* **2014**, *112*, 543–551. [CrossRef]
22. Finlay, E.K.; Berry, D.P.; Wickham, B.; Gormley, E.P.; Bradley, D.G. A genome wide association scan of bovine tuberculosis susceptibility in Holstein-Friesian dairy cattle. *PLoS ONE* **2012**, *7*, 30545. [CrossRef]
23. Minozzi, G.; Buggiotti, L.; Stella, A.; Strozzi, F.; Luini, M.; Williamas, J.L. Genetic loci involved in antibody response to Mycobacterium avium ssp. paratuberculosis in cattle. *PLoS ONE* **2010**, *5*, 11117. [CrossRef]
24. Milián, F.; Harris, B.; Arriaga, C.; Thomsen, B.; Stuber, T.; González, D.; Álvarez, G.; Santillán, M.A.; Morales, A.; Estrada, C. Sensibilidad y especificidad de PCR anidada y spoligotyping como pruebas rápidas de diagnóstico de tuberculosis bovina en tejido fresco. *Rev. Mex. Cienc. Pecu.* **2010**, *1*, 403–415.
25. González-Ruiz, S.; Verdugo-Escárcega, D.A.; Milián-Suazo, F.; Cantó-Alarcón, G.J.; Sosa-Gallegos, L. Prevalencia de *Mycobacterium bovis* en tejidos obtenidos de bovinos Holstein en rastros de los Altos de Jalisco. In Proceedings of the LII Reunión Anual de Investigación Pecuaria, Querétaro, Mexico, 30 November 2016; pp. 372–374.
26. Payeur, B.J.; Jarnagin, L.J.; Marquardt, G.J.; Schaper, A.L.; Martin, M.B. Laboratory methods in veterinary mycobacteriology for the isolation and identification of mycobacteria. In *Natural Veterinary Services Laboratory*; United State Department of Agriculture: Ames, IA, USA, 1993.
27. Darvasi, A.; Soller, M. Selective DNA pooling for determination of linkage between a molecular marker and a quantitative trait locus. *Genetics* **1994**, *138*, 1365–1373.
28. Le Hellard, S.; Ballereau, S.J.; Visscher, P.M.; Torrance, H.S.; Pinson, J.; Morris, S.W.; Thomson, M.L.; Semple, C.A.; Muir, W.J.; Blackwood, D.H.; et al. SNP genotyping on pooled DNAs: Comparison of genotyping technologies and a semi automated method for data storage and analysis. *Nucleic Acids Res.* **2002**, *30*, 74. [CrossRef]
29. Janicki, P.K.; Liu, J. Accuracy of allele frequency estimates in pool DNA analyzed by high-Density Illumina Human 610-Quad microarray. *Intern. J. Genom. Proteom.* **2009**, *5*, 1.
30. Strillacci, M.G.; Frigo, E.; Canavesi, F.; Ungar, Y.; Schiavini, F.; Zaniboni, L.; Reghenzani, L.; Cozzi, M.C.; Samoré, A.B.; Kashi, Y.; et al. Quantitative trait loci mapping for conjugated linoleic acid, vaccenic acid and Δ9-Desaturase in Italian Brown Swiss dairy cattle using selective DNA pooling. *Anim. Genet.* **2014**, *45*, 485–499. [CrossRef]
31. Lipkin, E.; Strillacci, M.G.; Eitam, H.; Yishay, M.; Schiavini, F.; Soller, M.; Bagnato, A.; Shabtay, A. The Use of Kosher Phenotyping for Mapping QTL Affecting Susceptibility to Bovine Respiratory Disease. *PLoS ONE* **2016**, *11*, 0153423. [CrossRef]
32. Peletto, S.; Strillacci, M.G.; Capucchioc, M.T.; Biasibettic, E.; Modesto, P.; Acutis, P.L.; Bagnato, A. Genetic basis of Lipomatous Myopathy in Piedmontese beef cattle. *Livest. Sci.* **2017**, *206*, 9–16. [CrossRef]
33. Macgregor, S. Most pooling variation in array-Based DNA pooling is attributable to array error rather than pool construction error. *Eur. J. Hum. Genet.* **2007**, *15*, 501–504. [CrossRef]
34. Macgregor, S.; Zhao, Z.Z.; Henders, A.; Nicholas, M.G.; Montgomery, G.W.; Visscher, P.M. Highly cost-Efficient genome-Wide association studies using DNA pools and dense SNP arrays. *Nucleic Acids Res.* **2008**, *36*, 35. [CrossRef]
35. Fernando, R.L.; Nettleton, D.; Southey, B.R.; Dekkers, J.C.M.; Rothschild, M.F.; Soller, M. Controlling the proportion of false positives in multiple dependent tests. *Genetics* **2004**, *166*, 611–619. [CrossRef]
36. Nicolazzi, E.L.; Picciolini, M.; Strozzi, F.; Schnabel, R.D.; Lawley, C.; Pirani, A.; Breu, F.; Stella, A. SNPchiMp: A database to disentangle the SNPchip jungle in bovine livestock. *BMC Genom.* **2014**, *15*, 123. [CrossRef]
37. European Variation Archive. 2017. Available online: https://www.ebi.ac.uk/eva/?Home (accessed on 21 September 2017).
38. Ensembl Project. 1999. Available online: http://www.ensembl.org/biomart/martview/502ede1207156b60a738ec6c34389633 (accessed on 18 November 2017).
39. Huang, D.W.; Sherman, B.T.; Lempicki, R.A. Systematic and integrative analysis of large gene lists using DAVID Bioinformatics Resources. *Nat. Protoc.* **2009**, *4*, 44–57. [CrossRef]
40. National Animal Genome Research Program. USDA-NRI. 2003–2018. Available online: https://www.animalgenome.org (accessed on 12 March 2018).

41. Hawn, T.T.; Day, T.A.; Scriba, T.J.; Hatherill, M.; Hanekom, W.A.; Evans, T.G.; Churchyard, G.J.; Kublin, J.G.; Bekker, L.G.; Self, S.G. Tuberculosis Vaccines and Prevention of Infection. *Microbiol. Mol. Biol. Rev.* **2014**, *78*, 650–671. [CrossRef]
42. Tsairidou, S.; Woolliams, J.A.; Allen, A.R.; Skuce, R.A.; McBride, S.H.; Wright, D.M.; Bermingham, M.L.; Pong-Wong, R.; Matika, O.; McDowell, S.W.J. Genomic prediction for Tuberculosis resistance in dairy cattle. *PLoS ONE* **2014**, *9*, 96728. [CrossRef]
43. Richardson, I.W.; Bradley, D.G.; Higgins, I.M.; More, S.J.; McClure, J.; Berry, D.P. Variance components for susceptibility to *Mycobacterium bovis* infection in dairy and beef cattle. *Genet. Sel. Evol.* **2014**, *46*, 77. [CrossRef]
44. Curtis, J.; Luo, Y.; Zenner, H.L.; Cuchet-Lourenc, D.; Wu, C.; Lo, K.; Maes, M.; Alisaaca, A.; Stebbings, E.; Liu, J.C.; et al. Susceptibility to tuberculosis is associated with variants in the ASAP1 gene encoding a regulator of dendritic cell migration. *Nat. Genet.* **2015**, *47*, 523–527. [CrossRef]
45. Sobota, R.S.; Stein, C.M.; Kodaman, N.; Scheinfeldt, L.B.; Maro, I.; Wieland-Alter, W.; Igo, R.P.; Magohe, A.; Malone, L.L.; Chervenak, K. A Locus at 5q33.3 Confers Resistance to Tuberculosis in Highly Susceptible Individuals. *Am. J. Hum. Genet.* **2016**, *98*, 514–524. [CrossRef]
46. Raphaka, K.; Matika, O.; Sánchez-Molano, E.; Mrode, R.; Coffey, M.P.; Riggio, V.; Glas, E.J.; Woolliams, J.A.; Bishop, S.C.; Banos, G. Genomic regions underlying susceptibility to bovine tuberculosis in Holstein-Friesian cattle. *BMC Genet.* **2017**, *18*, 27. [CrossRef]
47. Hasenauer, F.C.; Garbaccio, S.G.; Caffaro, M.E.; Garro, C.; Huertas, P.; Poli, M.A.; Rossetti, C.A. Exploring the association between polymorphisms at 3′UTR SLC11A1 gene microsatellites and resistance to tuberculosis: A case-Control study in *Bos taurus* dairy cattle. *Livest. Sci.* **2018**, *210*, 1–7. [CrossRef]
48. Banos, G.; Winters, M.; Mrode, R.; Mitchell, A.P.; Bishop, S.C.; Woolliams, J.A.; Coffey, M.P. Genetic evaluation for bovine tuberculosis resistance in dairy cattle. *J. Dairy Sci.* **2017**, *100*, 1272–1281. [CrossRef]
49. Kurtulus, S.; Sakuishi, K.; Ngiow, S.F.; Joller, N.; Tan, D.J.; Teng, M.W.; Smyth, M.J.; Kuchroo, V.K.; Anderson, A.C. TIGIT predominantly regulates the immune response via regulatory T cells. *J. Clin. Investig.* **2015**, *125*, 4053–4062. [CrossRef]
50. Joller, N.; Hafler, J.P.; Brynedal, B.; Kassam, N.; Spoerl, S.; Levin, S.D.; Arle, H.; Sharpe, K. TIGIT has T cell-Intrinsic inhibitory functions. *J. Immunol.* **2011**, *186*, 1338–1342. [CrossRef]
51. Whitaker, H.C.; Shiong, L.L.; Kay, J.D.; Grönberg, H.; Warren, A.Y.; Seipel, A.; Wiklund, F.; Thomas, B.; Wiklund, P.; Miller, J.L. N-Acetyl-L-Aspartyl-L-Glutamate peptidase-Like 2 is overexpressed in cancer and promotes a pro-Migratory and pro-Metastatic phenotype. *Oncogene* **2014**, *33*, 5274–5287. [CrossRef]
52. Demy, D.L.; Tauzin, M.; Lancino, M.; Le Cabec, V.; Redd, M.; Murayama, E.; Maridonneau-Parini, I.; Trede, N.; Herbomel, P. Trim33 is essential for macrophage and neutrophil mobilization to developmental or inflammatory cues. *J. Cell. Sci.* **2017**, *130*, 2797–2807. [CrossRef]
53. Weng, L.; Mitoma, H.; Tricot, C.; Boo, M.; Liu, Y.; Zhang, Z.; Liu, Y.J. The E3 Ubiquitin Ligase Tripartite Motif 33 Is Essential for Cytosolic RNA–Induced NLRP3 Inflammasome Activation. *J. Immunol.* **2014**, *193*, 3676–3682. [CrossRef]
54. Fjeldborg, K.; Møller, H.J.; Richelsen, B.; Pedersen, S.B. Regulation of *CD163* mRNA and soluble *CD163* protein in human adipose tissue in vitro. *J. Mol Endocrinol.* **2014**, *53*, 227–235. [CrossRef]
55. National Center for Biotechnology Information. Available online: https://www.ncbi.nlm.nih.gov/gene/100125389 (accessed on 3 April 2018).
56. GeneCards®: The Human Gene Database. Weizmann Institute of Science. Available online: https://www.genecards.org/cgi-bin/carddisp.pl?gene=KIF16B (accessed on 3 April 2018).
57. Newman, J.H.; Holt, T.N.; Hedges, L.K.; Womack, B.; Memon, S.S.; Willers, E.D.; Wheeler, L.; Phillips, J.A.; Hamid, R. High-Altitude pulmonary hypertension in cattle (brisket disease): Candidate genes and gene expression profiling of peripheral blood mononuclear cells. *Pulm. Circ.* **2011**, *1*, 462–469. [CrossRef]
58. Clark, D.L.; Boler, D.D.; Kutzler, L.W.; Jones, K.A.; McKeith, F.K.; Killefer, J.; Carr, T.R.; Dilger, A.C. Muscle gene expression associated with increased marbling in beef cattle. *Anim. Biotechnol.* **2011**, *22*, 51–63. [CrossRef]
59. Pires, D.; Bernard, E.M.; Pombo, J.P.; Carmo, N.; Fialho, C.; Gutierrez, M.G.; Bettencourt, P.; Anes, E. Mycobacterium tuberculosis Modulates miR-106b-5p to Control Cathepsin S Expression Resulting in Higher Pathogen Survival and Poor T-Cell Activation. *Front. Immunol.* **2017**, *8*, 1819. [CrossRef]

60. Bragina, E.Y.; Tiys, E.S.; Rudko, A.A.; Ivanisenko, V.A.; Freidin, M.B. Novel tuberculosis susceptibility candidate genes revealed by the reconstruction and analysis of associative networks. *Infect. Genet. Evol.* **2016**, *46*, 118–123. [CrossRef]
61. Jenum, S.; Bakken, R.; Dhanasekaran, S.; Mukherjee, A.; Lodha, R.; Singh, S.; Haks, M.C.; Ottenhoff, T.H.M.; Kabra, K.; Doherty, T.M. BLR1 and FCGR1A transcripts in peripheral blood associate with the extent of intrathoracic tuberculosis in children and predict treatment outcome. *Sci. Rep.* **2016**, *12*, 6. [CrossRef]
62. Booty, M.G.; Barreira-Silva, P.; Carpenter, S.M.; Nunes-Alves, C.; Jacques, M.K.; Stowell, B.L.; Jayaraman, P.; Beamer, G.; Behar, S.M. IL-21 signaling is essential for optimal host resistance against Mycobacterium tuberculosis infection. *Sci. Rep.* **2016**, *7*, 6. [CrossRef]
63. Gomes-Pereira, S.; Rodrigues, P.N.; Appelberg, R.; Gomes, M.S. Increased susceptibility to Mycobacterium avium in hemochromatosis protein *HFE*-deficient mice. *Infect. Immun.* **2008**, *76*, 4713–4719. [CrossRef]
64. Moalem, S.; Weinberg, E.D.; Percy, M.E. Hemochromatosis and the enigma of misplaced iron: Implications for infectious disease and survival. *Biometals* **2004**, *17*, 135–139. [CrossRef]
65. Wang, L.; Johnson, E.E.; Shi, H.N.; Walker, W.A.; Wessling-Resnick, M.; Cherayil, B.J. Attenuated inflammatory responses in hemochromatosis reveal a role for iron in the regulation of macrophage cytokine translation. *J. Immunol.* **2008**, *15*, 2723–2731. [CrossRef]
66. Horne, D.J.; Randhawa, A.K.; Chau, T.T.; Bang, N.D.; Yen, N.T.; Farrar, J.J.; Dunstan, S.J.; Haen, T.R. Common polymorphisms in the *PKP3-SIGIRR-TMEM16J* gene region are associated with susceptibility to tuberculosis. *J. Infect. Dis.* **2012**, *205*, 586–594. [CrossRef]
67. Riva, F.; Bonavita, E.; Barbati, E.; Muzio, M.; Mantovani, A.; Garlanda, C. *TIR8/SIGIRR* is an Interleukin-1 Receptor/Toll Like Receptor Family Member with Regulatory Functions in Inflammation and Immunity. *Front. Immunol.* **2012**, *3*, 322. [CrossRef]

Effect of Breed on the Level of the Nutritional and Health-Promoting Quality of Semimembranosus Muscle in Purebred and Crossbred Bulls

Paweł Solarczyk, Marcin Gołębiewski, Jan Slósarz, Monika Łukasiewicz, Tomasz Przysucha and Kamila Puppel *

Institute of Animal Science, Warsaw University of Life Sciences, Ciszewskiego 8, 02-786 Warsaw, Poland; pawel_solarczyk@sggw.edu.pl (P.S.); marcin_golebiewski@sggw.edu.pl (M.G.); jan_slosarz@sggw.edu.pl (J.S.); monika_lukasiewicz@sggw.edu.pl (M.Ł.); tomasz_przysucha@sggw.edu.pl (T.P.)

* Correspondence: kamila_puppel@sggw.edu.pl

Simple Summary: Beef is an important natural source of nutrients as well as of bioactive ingredients that improve our health. It is an excellent source of alanine, creatine, carnosine, anserine, and polyunsaturated fatty acid (PUFA), which plays an important preventative role in carcinogenic processes. The strategy for rearing and feeding cattle for slaughter should be directed at reducing saturated fatty acid (SFA) in beef fat and/or increasing PUFA, especially n-3. Therefore, the aim of the study was to determine the influence of breed types on the nutritional and pro-health quality of beef. The experiment was conducted in Poland, on 62 bulls from three breeds: Limousin, Polish Holstein-Friesian, and Polish Holstein-Friesian × Limousin. Bulls were slaughtered at 21–23 months of age, and samples of semimembranosus muscle (300 g) were cut parallel to the muscle axis at 24 h postmortem. It can be concluded that commodity crossbreeding significantly improved the quality of beef, resulting in similar or even better results than purebred cattle.

Abstract: Meat from commercial breed cattle are very often used to crossbreed with dairy breeds. The effect of heterosis is most evident when crossbreeds are genetically different from each other. Therefore, the aim of the study was to determine the influence of breed types on the nutritional and pro-health quality of beef. The experiment was conducted on 62 bulls from three breeds: Limousin, Polish Holstein-Friesian, and Polish Holstein-Friesian (PHF) × Limousin. During the fattening period, the animals were fed ad libitum using the same diet. Bulls were slaughtered at 21–23 months of age. The meat of PHF × Limousin hybrids was characterized by the lowest level of SFA and the highest content of n-3 PUFA fatty acids, carnosine, and α-tocopherol compared to the values obtained for the Polish Holstein-Friesian and Limousin breeds. In the case of PHF × Limousin hybrids, there was a 6% increase in n-3 PUFA, 21% in carnosine, and 66% in α-tocopherol compared to the Polish Holstein-Friesian breed. Commodity crossbreeding significantly improved the quality of beef analyzed in this study, resulting in similar or even better results than purebred cattle. This meant that beef from the hybrids with PHF was of the best nutritional and health-promoting quality.

Keywords: breed; meat; quality; crossbreeding

---

1. Introduction

Breed, gender, and the feeding system are factors that determine, to a large extent, the level of bioactive muscle tissue components, because their contribution is closely correlated with the degree of fat cover, and thus is a consequence of diet and genotype [1,2]. Differences between many breeds of cattle have been reported for Red Angus and Simmental steers [3], Aberdeen Angus, Belgian Blue, and Limousine bulls [4], and for different double muscle genotype bulls [1]. Various feeding strategies are often used to increase the content of polyunsaturated fatty acid (PUFA) n-3 fatty acid and to improve beef intramuscular PUFA n-6/PUFA n-3 ratio [5–9]. Beef is an important natural source of alanine, creatine, carnosine, anserine, and polyunsaturated fatty acid, which plays an important preventative role in carcinogenic processes [3,4]. It should be noted that both carnosine and anserine block the production of advanced end-products of glycation, which lead to diseases such as arteriosclerosis, diabetes, cataracts, and Alzheimer's disease [10,11]. Another important function of these compounds is the formation of complexes with the ions of certain metals, supporting biological activity, which can be exemplified by the inhibition of growth and development of *Helicobacter pylori* [12]. Beef is a source of vitamins soluble in fat. Vitamin A takes part in the processes of growth; it mainly influences the differentiation of the epithelial cells of the oral mucosa, digestive, urinary, and respiratory tracts, and sight organs. Vitamin A catalyzes the oxidation of unsaturated fatty acids, and its presence is essential for the biosynthesis of fat from sugars or from fatty acids and glycerol [13]. The effect of vitamin E is mainly due to its antioxidant properties, thanks to which it protects the body against degenerative diseases [14]. A periodic increase in demand for tocopherols is observed during increased exposure to heavy metals, exposure to free radicals, with a lower supply of other antioxidants, increased physical activity, and in old age [13,15]. Vitamin E prevents the rapid dissipation of ion gradients within muscle reducing rates of tenderization [16,17]. Additionally, Rowe et al. [18] concluded that the use of antioxidants in meat could improve tenderness. Omega-3 and omega-6 fatty acids evoke antibacterial, antiviral, antifungal, antioxidant, and antiparasitic effects [19]. Das [20] reported that the ability of eicosapentaenoic acid (EPA, C20:5 n-3) and docosahexaenoic acid (DHA, C22:6 n-3) to suppress the production of pro-inflammatory cytokines and induce their anti-inflammatory effects results indirectly from their ability to increase mRNA Peroxisome proliferator-activated receptor gamma and protein activity. Additionally, Cheah et al. [21] reported that diets rich in monounsaturated fatty acids (MUFAs) have been shown to have favorable anti-inflammatory and cardiovascular benefits.

Beef is characterized by a moderate and, unlike protein, quite varied fat content, representing 0.7–10% of tissue mass. The composition of intramuscular fat varies from breed to breed, and the proportions between the different types of fiber are different. Late maturing breeds (Belgian Blue, Limousine, and Blonde d'Aquitaine) are characterized by better musculature and lower fat content compared to the parameters achieved by early maturing breeds, e.g., Angus [22]. In addition, Chambaz et al. [23] reported that the Angus breed showed a growth rate similar to Simmental and Charolais while Limousin grew slower, became oldest, and provided the heaviest carcasses and best conformation. The feeding system also influences the fat content of the carcass. The highest content is obtained from intensively fattened animals and the lowest from the extensive fattening method [24,25].

One way to improve low-hereditary functional characteristics is by crossbreeding [26]. This is why there has been a growing interest in this method of animal refinement for several years [27,28]. This method has been recognized as possibly causing heterosis, which is conditioned by the presence of a favorable gene combination. The effect of heterosis is most evident when crossbreeds are genetically different from each other. According to Hansen et al. [28], the effect of heterosis on production traits may amount to as much as 6.5%, while for fertility, health, and survival it may amount to 10%. Meat from commercial breed cattle are very often used to crossbreed with dairy breeds. Carcasses of such hybrids should have a higher proportion of meat and a lower fat content. The beef from these animals is more tender but less marbled than purebred beef cattle. The most commonly used bulls for mating are from breeds such as Limousin, Charolais, Simmental, and Piedmontese, and Hereford, Angus, and Salers are rarely used for this purpose [29]. The offspring of the Limousin and Piedmontese breeds grow rapidly and are well-muscled, and their meat is low in fat and of high quality [30,31].

According to Statistics Poland [32] data, approximately 93% of the cattle population in Poland are dairy cows, and only 1% are cattle of beef breeds. The most popular meat breed in Poland is the Limousin, which is approximately 70% of the population of purebred cows, followed by Charolaise and Hereford. The main criterion for choosing the method of creating a beef herd is economic considerations.

Many farmers who decide to create a breeding herd in a short period of time face the problem of high costs associated with the purchase of breeding material. It is possible to reduce such high expenditures by using other methods which, however, involve many years of work. One solution is to create a herd by means of crossbreeding. It is a long-term process, allowing for the gradual elimination of undesired genes and obtaining animals of as similar phenotype and genotype as possible to the paternal breed. Genetic variability in beef quality has been linked to differences between lines or breeds, variations due to the crossing of breeds, and variations between animals [2]. The research hypothesis assumes that commodity crossbreeding Polish Holstein-Friesian (PHF) × Limousin will significantly improve the quality of beef, resulting in similar or even better results than purebred PHF cattle. What is important is that beef production in Poland is mostly related to this dairy breed. Therefore, the aim of the study was to determine the influence of breed (purebred vs. crossbred cattle) on the nutritional and pro-health quality of beef.

2. Material and Methods

The experiment was conducted on 62 bulls from three breeds: Limousin ($n = 25$), Polish Holstein-Friesian (PHF, $n = 12$), and Polish Holstein-Friesian × Limousin ($n = 25$). The detailed characteristics of the bulls are presented in Table 1.

Table 1. Bull characteristics on the day of slaughter.

Bull Characteristics	Breed					
	Limousin		Polish Holstein-Friesian		PHF × Limousin	
	Mean	SD	Mean	SD	Mean	SD
Number (n)	25		12		25	
Age (d)	608	12.54	602	11.25	602	11.89
Live weight (kg)	695	35.23	534	24.47	668	34.25
Carcass weight (kg)	412	29.25	317	26.15	382	28.65

The bulls were kept on one farm located at Warmia and Masuria. Cattle were harvested at 21–23 months of age, and hot carcass weight was recorded. Then carcasses were chilled at 2–4 °C and samples of semimembranosus muscle (300 g) were cut parallel to the muscle axis at 24 h postmortem.

Slaughter and postslaughter processing were carried out in accordance with Council Regulation (EC) No. 1099/2009 of 24 September 2009 [33].

The animals were kept in alcoves in a free-standing system, in accordance with the minimum standards of cattle maintenance. During the fattening period, the animals were fed the same diet, ad libitum, with a total mixed ration (TMR) (Table 2).

Table 2. Ingredients and chemical composition of feed (as fed).

Ingredients	Content
Corn silage (%)	67.80
Barley (%)	29.20
Supplement * (%)	3.00
Diet composition:	
Dry matter (%)	54.24
Crude protein (g/kg)	128.40
NEm (Mcal/kg)	1.77
NEg (Mcal/kg)	1.15
NDF (g/kg)	343.23
ADF (g/kg)	193.56
Crude fat (g/kg)	19.20

* The supplement was composed of: 56.5% barley, 10% rape meal, 2% urea, 25% limestone, 3% salt, 0.066% vitamin E 500, 1% premix, 0.05% flavor, and 2.5% molasses, which provided 5% of diet in Dry matter (DM), and supplemented 1 kg diet (in DM) with additional 14.67 mg copper, 58.32 mg zinc, 26.73 mg manganese, 0.66 mg iodine, 0.23 mg cobalt, 0.29 mg selenium, 4.825 IU vitamin A, 478 IU vitamin D, and 32 IU vitamin E.

2.1. *Chemical Analysis*

Beef samples were chopped, then placed in a blender and ground until a homogeneous mass was obtained, which was analyzed later using a near infrared spectrophotometer. The basic chemical composition of meat was determined with a Food Scan™ analyzer (Foss Electric, Hillerød, Denmark).

Meat fat extraction was carried out according to the Folch method [34]. Fatty acid methylation was performed according to the trans-esterification method EN ISO 5509 [35]. Individual fatty acids were identified in crude fat using an Agilent 7890A GC (Agilent, Waldbronn, Germany) with HP Chem Station software (Agilent, Waldbronn, Germany), a flame ionization detector (FID), and a Varian Select FAME column (100 m length, 0.25 mm diameter, 0.25 μm film thickness; Varian/Agilent Technologies, Waldbronn, Germany) according to the methodology by Batorska et al. [36]. The analysis involved a programmed run with temperature ramps under the following conditions and temperatures: the injector was held at 240 °C fitted with siltek deactivated split/splitless liner packed with glass wool (Agilent, Waldbronn, Germany). The column had a total flow rate of 25 cm/s. One microliter of sample was injected with a split ratio of 50:1. The oven method was as follows: 130 °C held for one minute, increased to a temperature of 170 °C at the rate of 6.5 °C/min, then increased to a temperature of 215 °C at the rate of 2.5 °C/min held for 12 min. Then, it was increased to a temperature of 230 °C at the rate of 20 °C/min, held for three minutes. Helium was used as the carrier gas. The FID was operated at 300 °C. All samples were analyzed in duplicate. Each peak was identified using pure methyl ester standards (Supelco, Bellefonte, PA, USA).

The determination of α-tocopherol (vitamin E), α-retinol (vitamin A), and β-carotene were established using an Agilent 1100 Series reverse phase high performance liquid chromatograph (Agilent Technologies, Waldbronn, Germany) according to the methodology by Puppel [37]. Separations were performed at ambient temperature using solvent gradient on a ZORBAX Eclipse XDB column (Agilent Technologies, Waldbronn, Germany). The chromatographic conditions were as follows: Solvent A was MeOH (Merck, Darmstadt, Germany) and water (Sigma-Aldrich, St. Louis, MO, USA) in a ratio of 950:50 (v/v). The flow rate was 1.0 mL/min and the detection wavelength was 280 nm. The injection volume of the final solution was 25 μL. All samples were analyzed in duplicate. The identification of peaks was confirmed by a comparison with the standards (Sigma-Aldrich, St. Louis, MO, USA).

The determination of anserine, carnosine, taurine, coenzyme Q10, creatinine, and creatine was established using Agilent 1100 reversed-phase high performance liquid chromatography (RP-HPLC). Separations were performed at ambient temperature using solvent gradient on the Jupiter column C18 300A (Phenomenex, Torrance, CA, USA) according to the methodology by Łukasiewicz et al. [11]. The chromatographic conditions were as follows: Solvent A was acetonitrile (Merck, Darmstadt, Germany), water (Sigma-Aldrich), and trifluoroacetic acid (Sigma-Aldrich, St. Louis, MO, USA) in a ratio of 30:970:1 (v/v/v). Solvent B was acetonitrile, water, and trifluoroacetic acid in a ratio of 970:30:1 (v/v/v). The flow rate was 1.4 mL/min and the detection wavelength was 214 nm. The injection volume of the final solution was 25 μL. All samples were analyzed in duplicate. The identification of peaks was confirmed by a comparison with the standards (Sigma-Aldrich, St. Louis, MO, USA).

2.2. *Statistical Analysis*

The data obtained were subjected to analysis of variance using ANOVA analysis, with breed as fixed factors. Significant means were separated using Duncan (at $p < 0.05$). The distribution of bioactive components was checked using the Shapiro–Wilk test. All tests were processed using the IBM SPSS 23 package [38]. Data were presented as least squares means (LSM) with standard error of the mean.

The following statistical model was used:

$$Yijk = \mu + Ai + eij \tag{1}$$

where: *Yijk* = value of the tested trait; μ = mean; A*i* = effect of the *i* (the breed) (*I* = 1–3); *eij* = standard error.

3. Results and Discussion

Many genetic factors influence the quality of beef; the main one is the cattle breed [22,39,40]. They differ in their content and composition of intramuscular fat, the properties of connective tissue, especially collagen, and the proportion between the types of muscle fibers [22]. Table 3 shows a comparison of the protein, fat, and collagen contents in Limousin, Polish Holstein-Friesian, and PHF × Limousin hybrids.

Table 3. The influence of breed on the formation of the basic chemical composition of muscle tissue.

Component	Breed			SEM	*p*-Value
	Limousin	Polish Holstein-Friesian	PHF × Limousin		
Protein (g/100 g)	21.31 ^{AB}	19.4 ^{AC}	22.41 ^{BC}	0.241	0.000
Fat (g/100 g)	1.85 ^{A}	2.95 ^{AB}	1.89 ^{B}	0.035	0.010
Collagen (mg/100 g)	511.68 ^{AB}	592.24 ^{AC}	492.24 ^{BC}	1.231	0.042

A–C: Means in the same row marked with the same letters differ significantly at: capitals, $p \leq 0.01$. SEM, standard error of least square means (LSM).

The biological and nutritional value of meat protein is determined by the content of intramuscular connective tissue. Greater protein content in muscle tissue was found in the PHF × Limousin hybrids, at 22.41 g/100 g of meat, and the lowest in Polish Holstein-Friesian at 19.4 g/100 g. In the study by Malczyk et al. [41], the protein content was 21.61 g/100 g in the semitendinosus muscle and 21.51 g/100 g in the longest lumbar muscle in Lowland Black and White × Limousin hybrids. It should be noted that Holsteins may require concentrate-rich instead of silage-rich diets to express their full growth potential [42]. Additionally, purebred Holsteins have a low carcass weight compared to beef breeds or crossbreds [43], which was confirmed by the results obtained in the experiment (Table 1). Studies have shown that the concentration of protein (*p*-value 0.000) was significantly influenced by the breed.

Breeders usually choose animals that are high caliber and late maturing, which achieve very good fattening results. Late maturing breeds such as Limousin, Belgian White, and Blue have less fat and better musculature than early maturing breeds, but less marbling. The Italian and French cattle breeds are characterized by a low proportion of fat and bone and high muscle content. They also achieve satisfactory slaughter yields [30]. European beef cattle, Limousin, and Charolais have, among other features, better slaughter performance, less fat with higher musculature, but less marbling than British breeds such as Hereford or Angus [44]. Table 3 shows that muscle tissue in Limousin cattle was characterized by the lowest level of fat (1.85 g/100 g), and the highest level was found in Polish Holstein-Friesian at 2.95 g/100 g of meat. Studies by Zając [45] showed that the highest fat contents, of 5.30% and 5.15%, respectively, were found in the musculus serratus ventralis and the comb muscle. For comparison, the lowest fat content was in the semimembranosus muscle (2.38%) and semiendodermis muscle (2.77%). In the research conducted by Malczyk et al. [41], the level of fat in Black and White cattle was 2.07% in the heel muscle and 5.03% in the lumbar muscle. Additionally, Nogalski et al. [46] found that Sida silage can improve carcass and meat quality characteristics of Polish Holstein-Friesian bulls. The morphology, composition, and amount of intramuscular connective tissue vary depending on the muscle type, breed, and age of the animal [47].

Another important ingredient in meat is collagen. Table 3 shows that the highest content was found in Polish Holstein-Friesians (592.94 mg/100 g) and the lowest in PHF × Limousins (492.24 mg/100 g). The meat from dairy breeds is characterized by relatively high total collagen content compared with meat obtained from beef breeds [48]. In research by Dąbrowska et al. [49], the following collagen levels were found in meat from Black and White × Limousin crossbred bulls, depending on the muscle tissue analyzed: finger rectifier muscle (musculus extensor digitorum) 3032.2 mg, medium gluteus muscle (musculus gluteus medius) 1506.5 mg, large lateral muscle (musculus vastus lateralis) 878.9 mg, semispongiform muscle (musculus semitendinosus) 525.6 mg, and large lumbar muscle (musculus psoas major) 300.4 mg. Studies have shown that the concentration of collagen was significantly influenced by the breed [50].

The health-promoting quality of meat depends on the saturated fatty acid (SFA) content. A high saturated fatty acid diet has long been implicated with an increased risk of cardiovascular disease [21]. Studies have shown that C12:0, C14:0, and C16:0 have atherogenic properties, while C14:0, C16:0, and C18:0 have thrombogenic properties [22]. Table 4 shows the share of SFAs in Polish Holstein-Friesian, Limousin, and PHF × Limousin hybrids in muscle tissue.

Table 4. The influence of breed on the formation of the saturated fatty acid composition of muscle tissue.

Component (g/100 g of Fat)	Breed			SEM	*p*-Value
	Limousin	Polish Holstein-Friesian	PHF × Limousin		
C12:0	0.06	0.09	0.05	0.011	0.991
C14:0	2.26 ^{AB}	1.45 ^{AC}	1.92 ^{BC}	0.132	0.004
C16:0	25.57 ^{Ab}	27.47 ^{AC}	24.22 ^{bC}	0.317	0.025
C18:0	18.40 ^{aB}	19.26 ^{aC}	16.87 ^{BC}	0.153	0.000
SFA	48.30 ^{aB}	49.74 ^{aC}	43.99 ^{BC}	0.752	0.000

aa, AA, etc.: Means in the same row marked with the same letters differ significantly at: small letters, $p \leq 0.05$; capitals, $p \leq 0.01$. SEM, standard error of LSM. SFA, saturated fatty acid.

The highest level of SFA, amounting to 49.74 g/100 g, was found in the muscle tissue of Polish Holstein-Friesian cattle. It should be emphasized that this breed exhibited the highest content of all fatty acids studied: lauric acid (C12:0; 0.09 g/100 g), palmitic acid (C16:0; 27.47 g/100 g), and stearic acid (C18:0; 19.26 g/100 g). The levels of the above-mentioned fatty acids in Limousin meat and their hybrids with Polish Holstein-Friesian were similar, especially for C12:0, C14:0, and C16:0. A significant difference was found in C18:0 acid, where in purebred cattle the level of stearic was 18.40 g/100 g, and in hybrids, 16.87 g/100 g. The lowest total content of SFA (43.99 g/100 g) was observed in the PHF × Limousin hybrids. Studies have shown that the concentration of SFA and C18:0 were significantly influenced by the type of breed (*p*-value 0.000). Almeida et al. [51] showed that the formation of a fatty acid profile is also linked to muscle type. Studies have shown that SFA concentration in the biceps femoris is more than three times higher than in the semimembranosus.

Other fatty acids that influence the nutritional and health-promoting quality of beef are monounsaturated fatty acids (MUFAs) and PUFAs.. The main n-3 PUFA in beef are α-linolenic (18:3 n-3), eicosapentaenoic (20:5 n-3), and docosahexaenoic (22:6 n-3) acids [45]. Table 5 presents the content of selected fatty acids in the muscle tissue of Polish Holstein-Friesian, Limousin, and PHF × Limousin hybrids.

Table 5. The influence of breed on MUFA and PUFA levels in muscle tissue.

Component (g/100 g of Fat)	Breed			SEM	*p*-Value
	Limousin	Polish Holstein-Friesian	PHF × Limousin		
C18:1 trans-11 (TVA)	1.13 ^{ab}	0.83 ^{aC}	1.31 ^{bC}	0.071	0.048
C18:2 n-6 (LA)	8.70 ^{Ab}	6.24 ^{Ac}	7.97 ^{bc}	1.041	0.021
C18:2 cis-9, trans-11 (CLA)	3.26 ^{Ab}	2.59 ^{AC}	3.59 ^{bC}	0.147	0.033
C18:3 n-3 (LNA)	0.59 ^{ab}	0.49 ^{ac}	0.71 ^{bc}	0.087	0.042
C20:5 n-3 (EPA)	0.58 ^{a}	0.42 ^{ab}	0.65 ^{b}	0.064	0.049
C22:6 n-3 (DHA)	0.14 ^{A}	0.07 ^{AB}	0.16 ^{B}	0.045	0.714
n-6 PUFA	11.01 ^{A}	8.54 ^{AB}	10.44 ^{B}	0.121	0.036
n-3 PUFA	2.42 ^{Ab}	2.06 ^{AC}	2.81 ^{bC}	0.175	0.006

aa, AA, etc.: Means in the same row marked with the same letters differ significantly at: small letters, $p \leq 0.05$; capitals, $p \leq 0.01$. SEM, standard error of LSM; PUFA, polyunsaturated fatty acid; MUFA, monounsaturated fatty acid.

Cheah et al. [21] reported that MUFAs may be an ideal substitute for SFA, obviating the adverse effects of SFAs; therefore, the aim should be to increase their share in the diet. The first of the lipid components analyzed was vaccenic acid (C18:1 trans-11; TVA), responsible for the efficiency of tissues and organs. Its highest level was found in PHF × Limousin hybrids (1.31 g/100 g), and its lowest in Polish Holstein-Friesians (0.83 g/100 g).

PUFAs, as essential fatty acids, are only available through dietary consumption [21]. The highest content of LA, 8.70 g/100 g, was found in meat obtained from the Limousins. Slightly lower levels were found in crossbreeds (7.97 g/100 g), and the lowest in Polish Holstein-Friesians (6.24 g/100 g). C18:2 cis-9, trans-11 (CLA) has many functions, which are mainly antioxidant, antiatherosclerotic, and anticancer [52]. The muscle tissue of purebred Limousin and their hybrids with the Polish Holstein-Friesian breed were recorded as 3.26 g/100 g and 3.59 g/100 g, respectively, i.e., more than the 2.59 g/100 g from the Polish Holstein-Friesians. Studies have shown that the concentration of CLA was significantly influenced by the breed.

α-linoleic acid (C18:3 n-3; LNA) plays a key role in hepatic glycolysis, de novo lipogenesis, and fatty acid regulation [53]. The highest level was found in PHF × Limousin hybrids and amounted to 0.71 g/100 g, whereas the lowest was in Polish Holstein-Friesians at 0.49 g/100 g. Other acids analyzed were eicosapentaenoic and docosahexaenoic, which support the functioning of the nervous system. Siscovick et al. [54] reported that the American Heart Association recommends 1 g/day of combined EPA/DHA intake or 2–4 g/day for those with hypertriglyceridemia. Both EPA and DHA were found to be the most abundant in crossbred meat (0.65 g/100 g and 0.16 g/100 g) and the least in Polish Holstein-Friesian meat (0.42 g/100 g and 0.07 g/100 g) (Table 5).

Bioactive dipeptides, including carnosine and anserine, are important components of beef that influence its pro-health value. Table 6 shows the content of bioactive protein fraction components in the muscle tissue of Polish Holstein-Friesians, Limousins, and PHF × Limousin hybrids.

Table 6. The influence of breed on bioactive protein fraction component levels in muscle tissue.

Component (mg/100 g)	Breed			SEM	*p*-Value
	Limousin	Polish Holstein-Friesian	PHF × Limousin		
Anserine	83.64 ^{Ab}	61.22 ^{AC}	81.46 ^{bC}	1.170	0.000
Carnosine	462.48 ^{AB}	387.3 ^{AC}	492.36 ^{BC}	8.226	0.000
Taurine	42.13 ^{AB}	34.28 ^{AC}	48.99 ^{BC}	0.551	0.005
Coenzyme Q10	2.35 ^{Ab}	1.87 ^{AC}	2.67 ^{bC}	0.125	0.044
Creatinine	5.48 ^{AB}	4.12 ^{AC}	6.36 ^{BC}	0.054	0.037
Creatine	448.22 ^{AB}	396.96 ^{AC}	481.25 ^{BC}	7.012	0.000

aa, AA, etc.: Means in the same row marked with the same letters differ significantly at: small letters, $p \leq 0.05$; capitals, $p \leq 0.01$. SEM, standard error of LSM.

Anserine (β-alanyl-L-(N-methyl) histidine) is a methyl carnosine derivative. It is a dipeptide consisting of β-alanine and L-(N-methyl) histidine. It occurs mainly in skeletal muscles and the brain, and in mammalian organisms it acts as an antioxidant. The concentration of carnosine in raw beef is 300–500 mg/100 g of tissue. For comparison, the average carnosine content of pork is 211–419 mg/100 g tissue. Differences in the concentration of carnosine in muscle tissues result primarily from different levels of muscle oxidation. Carnosine concentration is lower in muscles with high proportions of oxidative muscle fibers [11]. Breed, age, gender, and the rearing system also influence this concentration. The highest level of anserine (83.64 mg/100 g) was found in Limousine meat, and the lowest in Polish Holstein-Friesian meat (61.22 mg/100 g). The carnosine content in crossbreeds was the highest at 492.36 mg/100 g and the lowest in Polish Holstein-Friesians at 387.3 mg/100 g. Mateescu et al. [55] conducted research on the content of bioactive dipeptides in the longest back muscle of the Angus (by sex). The highest carnosine level was found in steers at 370 mg/100 g, in heifers at 367 mg/100 g, and in bulls at 366 mg/100 g. The content of anserine was almost the same in all categories of cattle and ranged from 66 to 67 mg/100 g. Carnosine levels were also determined in muscles and selected organs in a study by Purchas and Busboom [56]. Its content in the longest dorsal muscle was 432.6 mg/100 g, in the semitendinous muscle, 452.6 mg/100 g, and in the musculus triceps brachii, 299.1 mg/100 g.

Taurine, full chemical name 2-aminoethylsulfonic acid, belongs to the amino acids and is commonly found in animal tissues. A lack of taurine in the diet results in a decrease in the number of leukocytes, and in the ability of neutrophils to oxygen burst and phagocytosis. The administration of taurine before an inflammatory reaction or after exposure to oxidative stress prevents or reduces the intensity of pro-inflammatory changes [57]. The highest level of taurine, 48.99 mg/100 g, was found in PHF × Limousin hybrids, and the lowest in Polish Holstein-Friesian meat, 34.28 mg/100 g. Purchas et al. [58] reported significant differences between cheek muscle and semitendinosus muscle.

Coenzyme Q10, also called ubiquinone, is a compound found in every cell of the body and plays a key role in it. Lowering the level of coenzyme Q10 favors the development of diseases arising from, among others, as a result of a reactive oxygen species, e.g., cardiovascular disease or cancer [59]. It is known that as a result of a deficiency of coenzyme Q10, the respiratory chain does not function properly and, as a result, there is insufficient production of high energy compounds [60], which in consequence may reduce the efficiency of the cell, tissue, and the whole organism. It was also found that clinical symptoms associated with deficiency of coenzyme Q10 can be eliminated or reduced by replenishing its quantity in the body with pharmaceutical preparations or dietary supplements [61]. The highest level of coenzyme Q10, 2.67 mg/100 g, was found in PHF × Limousin hybrids, and the lowest in Polish Holstein-Friesian meat, 1.87 mg/100 g. Mattila et al. [62] reported 1.6 mg/100 g for an unspecified beef muscle.

Table 7 shows the content of vitamins soluble in fat in the muscle tissue of Polish Holstein-Friesians, Limousins, and PHF × Limousin hybrids. β-carotene is a precursor of retinol, which is necessary for cell division and differentiation and reproduction [63]. Retinol also participates in the regulation of immune function by supporting the production of white blood cells [64]. Studies have shown that the concentrations of β-carotene and α-retinol were significantly influenced by the types of breed. The study showed almost double the level of β-carotene in the PHF × Limousin group than those in the Polish Holstein-Friesian group. Darwish et al. [65] reported that grass-fed steers had significantly higher amounts (five- to seven-fold) of β-carotene, compared to grain-fed animals, due to the high β-carotene content of fresh grasses as compared to cereal grains.

Table 7. The influence of breed on vitamins soluble in fat in muscle tissue.

Component (μg/g)	Breed			SEM	*p*-Value
	Limousin	Polish Holstein-Friesian	PHF × Limousin		
β-carotene	0.29 AB	0.20 AC	0.45 BC	0.003	0.000
α-retinol	0.75 AB	0.66 AC	0.92 BC	0.008	0.018
α-tocopherol	3.14 AB	1.61 AC	4.76 BC	0.098	0.024

aa, AA, etc.: Means in the same row marked with the same letters differ significantly at: capitals, $p \leq 0.01$. SEM, standard error of LSM.

The highest level of α-tocopherol, 4.76 μg/g, was found in PHF × Limousin hybrids, and the lowest in Polish Holstein-Friesian meat, 1.61 μg/g. Liu et al. [66] reported that a minimum of 3 to 3.5 μg/g meat of α-tocopherol is necessary to prevent discoloration. Additionally, Clausen et al. [67] reported that raw meat with approximately 2 μg/g meat of α-tocopherol showed a high degree of lipid oxidation. Therefore, it can be concluded that increased tissue levels of α-tocopherol protected against retail discoloration and lipid oxidation. It should be emphasized that the quality of muscle tissue varies, with this variability being significantly influenced by type of breed.

4. Conclusions

Commodity crossbreeding significantly improved the quality of beef analyzed in this study, resulting in similar or even better results than purebred cattle. The meat of PHF × Limousin hybrids was characterized by the lowest level of SFA and the highest content of omega-3 fatty acids (LNA, EPA, DHA), carnosine, taurine, coenzyme Q10, and vitamins soluble in fat. This meant that beef from the hybrids with PHF was of the best nutritional and health-promoting quality. It should be emphasized that the scheme of crossbreeding Polish Holstein-Friesian or Limousin cattle with other breeds, or in beef herds, should be based on the expectations of the breeder. There are many possibilities from using one or two breeds, or through suppressing crossbreeding. In order for these measures to be profitable, the breeder must consistently follow his breeding strategy. The crossbreeding of beef cattle has two main advantages: hybrid animals show heterosis, and crossbred animals combine the forces of different breeds used to form the cross.

Author Contributions: P.S.—conceptualization, formal analysis, investigation, methodology, writing—original draft, writing—review and editing; K.P.—conceptualization, formal analysis, investigation, methodology, writing—original draft, writing—review and editing; M.G.—data curation; T.P.—methodology; J.S., M.Ł.—formal analysis. All authors have read and agreed to the published version of the manuscript.

Acknowledgments: The paper is a part of the PhD thesis of Paweł Solarczyk.

References

1. Aldai, N.; Dugan, M.E.R.; Najera, A.I.; Osoro, K. N-6 and n-3 fatty acids in different beef adipose tissues depending on the presence or absence of the gene responsible for double-muscling. *Czech. J. Anim. Sci.* **2008**, *53*, 515–522. [CrossRef]
2. Garcia, P.T.; Casal, J.J. Effect of dietary plant lipids on conjugated linoleic acid (CLA) concentrations in beef and lamb meats. In *Soybean: Bio-Active Compounds*; IntechOpen: London, UK, 2003; pp. 135–159.
3. Laborde, F.L.; Mandell, I.B.; Tosh, J.J.; Wilton, J.W.; Buchanan-Smith, J.G. Breed effects on growth performance, carcass characteristics, fatty acid composition, and palatability attributes in finishing steers. *J. Anim. Sci.* **2001**, *79*, 355–365. [CrossRef]
4. Cuvelier, C.; Clinquart, A.; Hocquette, J.F.; Cabaraux, J.F.; Dufrasne, I.; Istasse, L.; Hornick, J.L. Comparison of composition and quality traits of meat from young finishing bulls from Belgian Blue, Limousin and Aberdeen Angus breeds. *Meat Sci.* **2006**, *74*, 522–531. [CrossRef]
5. French, P.; Stanton, C.; Lawless, F.; O'Riordan, E.; Monahan, F.; Caffrey, P.; Moloney, A. Fatty acid composition, including conjugated linoleic acid, of intramuscular fat from steers offered grazed grass, grass silage, or concentrate-based diets. *J. Anim. Sci.* **2000**, *78*, 2849–2855. [CrossRef]
6. Choi, N.; Enser; Wood, J.; Scollan, N. Effect of breed on the deposition in beef muscle and adipose tissue of dietary n-3 polyunsaturated fatty acids. *Anim. Sci.* **2000**, *71*, 509–519. [CrossRef]
7. Vatansever, L.; Kurt, E.; Enser, M.; Nute, G.; Scollan, N.; Wood, J.; Richardson, R. Shelf life and eating quality of beef from cattle of different breeds given diets differing in n-3 polyunsaturated fatty acid composition. *Anim. Sci.* **2000**, *71*, 471–482. [CrossRef]
8. Lourenco, M.; Van Ranst, G.; Vlaeminck, B.; De Smet, S.; Fievez, V. Influence of different dietary forages on the fatty acid composition of rumen digesta as well as ruminant meat and milk. *Anim. Feed Sci. Technol.* **2008**, *145*, 418–437. [CrossRef]
9. French, P.; O'Riordan, E.; Monahan, F.; Caffrey, P.; Mooney, M.; Troy, D.; Moloney, A. The eating quality of meat of steers fed grass and/or concentrates. *Meat Sci.* **2001**, *57*, 379–386. [CrossRef]
10. Warwas, M.; Piwowar, A.; Kopiec, G. Zaawansowane produkty glikacji (AGE) w organizmie—Powstawanie, losy, interakcja z receptorami i jej następstwa. *Farm. Polska* **2010**, *66*, 585–590.
11. Łukasiewicz, M.; Puppel, K.; Balcerak, M.; Slósarz, J.; Gołębiewski, M.; Kuczyńska, B.; Batorska, M.; Więcek, J.; Kunowska-Slósarz, M.; Popczyk, B. Variability of Anserine and Carnosine concentration in the wild boar (*Sus scrofa scrofa*) meat. *Anim. Sci. Pap. Rep.* **2018**, *36*, 185–192.
12. Florek, M.; Barłowska, J.; Litwińczuk, Z. Mleko i mięso zwierząt przeżuwających jako źródło substancji biologicznie czynnych Część II Mięso. *Przeg. Hod.* **2016**, *3*, 4–7. (In Polish)
13. *Witaminy*, 1st ed.; Friedrich, M., Ed.; Wydawnictwo Uczelniane Zachodniopomorskiego Uniwersytetu Technologicznego: Szczecin, Poland, 2016.

14. Lobo, V.; Patil, A.; Phatak, A.; Chandra, N. Free radicals, antioxidants and functional foods: Impact on human health. *Pharmacogn. Rev.* **2010**, *4*, 118–126. [CrossRef]
15. Herrera, E.; Barbas, C. Vitamin E: Action, metabolism and perspectives. *J. Physiol. Biochem.* **2001**, *57*, 43–56. [CrossRef]
16. Robbins, K.; Jensen, J.; Ryan, K.J.; Homco-Ryan, C.; McKeith, F.K.; Brewer, M.S. Dietary vitamin E supplementation effects on the color and sensory characteristics of enhanced beef steaks. *Meat Sci.* **2003**, *64*, 279–285. [CrossRef]
17. Traber, M.G.; Atkinson, J. Vitamin E, antioxidant and nothing more. *Free Radic. Biol. Med.* **2007**, *43*, 4–15. [CrossRef]
18. Rowe, L.; Maddock, K.R.; Lonergan, S.M.; Huff-Lonergan, E. Oxidative environments decrease tenderization of beef steaks through inactivation of m calpain. *J. Anim. Sci.* **2004**, *82*, 3254–3266. [CrossRef]
19. Yoon, B.K.; Jackman, J.A.; Valle-González, E.R.; Cho, N.J. Antibacterial Free Fatty Acids and Monoglycerides: Biological Activities, Experimental Testing, and Therapeutic Applications. *Int. J. Mol. Sci.* **2018**, *19*, 1114. [CrossRef]
20. Das, U.N. Essential Fatty acids—A review. *Curr. Pharm. Biotechnol.* **2006**, *7*, 467–482. [CrossRef]
21. Cheah, M.C.C.; McCullough, A.J.; Goh, G.B.B. Dietary Manipulations for Nonalcoholic Fatty Liver Disease (NAFLD). In *Bioactive Food as Dietary Interventions for Diabetes*, 2nd ed.; Elsevier: Amsterdam, The Netherlands, 2019; Chapter 5, pp. 69–88.
22. Abramowicz, P.; Balcerak, M.; Brzozowski, P.; Gołębiewski, M.; Grodzki, H.; Kuczyńska, B.; Kunowska-Slósarz, M.; Przysucha, T.; Puppel, K.; Slósarz, J.; et al. *Meat Use of Cattle*; Przysucha, T., Gołębiewki, M., Slósarz, J., Eds.; SGGW: Warsaw, Poland, 2018; ISBN 978-83-7583-791-9.
23. Chambaz, A.; Scheeder, M.R.; Kreuzer, M.; Dufey, P.A. Meat quality of Angus, Simmental, Charolais and Limousin steers compared at the same intramuscular fat content. *Meat Sci.* **2003**, *63*, 491–500. [CrossRef]
24. Fredriksson-Eriksson, S.; Pickova, J. Fatty acids and tocopherol levels in M Longissimus dorsi of beef cattle in Sweden—A comparison between seasonal diets. *Meat Sci.* **2007**, *76*, 746–754. [CrossRef]
25. Sadowska, A.; Rakowska, R.; Dybkowska, E.; Świąder, K. Ante-mortem factors that condition nutritional value and sensory quality of beef. *Postęp. Techn. Przetw. Spożyw.* **2016**, *2*, 122–128.
26. Heins, B.J.; Hansen, L.B.; Hazel, A.R.; Seykora, A.J.; Johnson, D.G.; Linn, J.G. Birth traits of pure Holstein calves versus Montbeliarde-sired crossbred calves. *J. Dairy Sci.* **2010**, *93*, 2293–2299. [CrossRef]
27. Sorensen, M.K.; Norberg, E.; Pedersen, J.; Christensen, L.G. Invited review: Crossbreeding in dairy cattle: A Danish perspective. *J. Dairy Sci.* **2008**, *91*, 4116–4128. [CrossRef]
28. Heins, B.J.; Hansen, L.B. Short communication: Fertility, somatic cell score, and production of Normande×Holstein, Montbeliarde×Holstein, and Scandinavian Red × Holstein crossbreds versus pure Holsteins during their first 5 lactations. *J. Dairy Sci.* **2012**, *95*, 918–924. [CrossRef]
29. Hansen, L.B.; Heins, B.J.; Seykora, T. Is crossbreeding the answer for reproductive problems of dairy cattle? In Proceedings of the Southwest Nutrition Conference, Tempe, AZ, USA, 24–25 February 2005; pp. 113–119.
30. MacNeil, M.D.; Short, R.E.; Grings, E.E. Characterization of topcross progenies from Hereford, Limousin, and Piedmontese sires. *J. Anim. Sci.* **2001**, *79*, 1751–1756. [CrossRef]
31. Nogalski, Z. Growth rate and slaughter value of the offspring of Black and White cows and bulls from Kortowo Synthetic Lina. *J. Nat. Sci.* **2002**, *12*, 159–167.
32. *Farm Animals in 2018*; Przypaśniak, J., Tylkowska-Siek, A., Dach-Oleszek, I., Wątroba, E., Eds.; GUS: Warsaw, Poland, 2019.
33. Council of the European Union. Council Regulation (EC) No 1099/2009 of 24 September 2009 on the protection of animals at the time of killing. *Off. J. Eur. Union* **2009**, *303*, 1–30.
34. Association of Official Analytical Chemists. *Official Methods of Analysis of AOAC International*, 15th ed.; AOAC: Washington, DC, USA, 1990; Volume 1.
35. International Organization for Standardization. *EN ISO 5509:2000: Animal and Vegetable Fats and Oils—Preparation of Methyl Esters of Fatty Acids*; ISO: Geneva, Switzerland, 2000.
36. Batorska, M.; Więcek, J.; Kunowska-Slósarz, M.; Puppel, K.; Slósarz, J.; Gołębiewski, M.; Kuczyńska, B.; Popczyk, B.; Rekiel, A.; Balcerak, M. The effect of carcass weight on chemical characteristics and fatty acid composition of *Longissimus dorsi* and *Semimembranosus* muscles of European wild boar (*Sus scrofa scrofa*) meat. *Can. J. Anim. Sci.* **2018**, *98*, 557–564. [CrossRef]

37. Puppel, K. The Influence of Fish Oil and Linseed Supplementation on the Fat and the Protein Fraction Content of Cow's Milk. Ph.D. Thesis, Warsaw University of Life Sciences, Warsaw, Poland, 2011.
38. IBM Corp. *IBM SPSS Statistics for Windows*; Version 23.0; IBM Corp.: Armonk, NY, USA, 2020.
39. De Smet, S.; Raes, K.; Demeyer, D. Meat fatty acid composition as affected by fatness and genetic factors: A review. *Anim. Res.* **2004**, *53*, 81–98. [CrossRef]
40. Pesonen, M.; Honkavaara, M.; Huuskonen, A. Effect of breed on production, carcass traits and meat quality of Aberdeen Angus, Limousin and Aberdeen AngusxLimousin bulls offered a grass silage-grain-based diet. *Agric. Food Sci.* **2012**, *21*, 361–369. [CrossRef]
41. Malczyk, E.; Marchel, J.; Dudek, M.; Cierach, M. Basic composition and tenderness of beef hybrids between the meat breed and the dairy utility breed. *Inżynier. Przetw. Spożyw.* **2012**, *3*, 29–32.
42. Murphy, B.; Kelly, A.; Prendiville, R. Alternative finishing strategies for Holstein-Friesian bulls slaughtered at 15 months of age. *Agric. Food Sci.* **2018**, *27*, 28–37. [CrossRef]
43. Keane, M.G.; Moloney, A.P. Comparison of pasture and concentrate finishing of Holstein Friesian, Aberdeen Angus × Holstein Friesian and Belgian Blue × Holstein Friesian steers. *Irish J. Agric. Food Res.* **2010**, *49*, 11–26.
44. Domaradzki, P.; Florek, M.; Litwińczuk, A. Factors influencing the quality of beef. *Wiad. Zootechn.* **2016**, *54*, 160–170.
45. Zając, M. Comparison of the Quality of Selected Bovine Muscles. Ph.D. Thesis, University of Agriculture in Krakow, Krakow, Poland, 2007.
46. Nogalski, Z.; Starczewski, M.; Purwin, C.; Pogorzelska-Przybyłek, P.; Sobczuk-Szul, M.; Modzelewska-Kapituła, M. CarCass and meat quality traits in young bulls fed Virginia fanpetals silage. *Ann. Anim. Sci.* **2020**, *20*, 1127–1140. [CrossRef]
47. Purslow, P.P. Intramuscular connective tissue and its role in meat quality. *Meat Sci.* **2005**, *70*, 435–447. [CrossRef] [PubMed]
48. Domaradzki, P.; Florek, M.; Litwińczuk, A. Total and soluble collagen contents in skeletal muscles of different cattle categories of Polish Holstein-Friesian breed. *Episteme* **2013**, *21*, 177–185.
49. Dąbrowska, E.; Jankowska, B.; Kwiatkowska, A.; Cierach, M. Zawartość kolagenu w mięśniach tylnej ćwierćtuszy wołowej. *Inżyn. Aparat. Chem.* **2011**, *50*, 18–19.
50. Gagaoua, M.; Terlouw, E.M.C.; Micol, D.; Hocquette, J.-F.; Moloney, A.P.; Nuernberg, K.; Bauchart, D.; Boudjellal, A.; Scollan, N.D.; Richardson, I.; et al. Sensory quality of meat from eight different types of cattle in relation with their biochemical characteristics. *J. Integr. Agric.* **2016**, *15*, 1550–1563. [CrossRef]
51. Almeida, J.C.; Perassolo, M.S.; Camargo, J.L.; Bragagnolo, N.; Gross, J.L. Fatty acid composition and cholesterol content of beef and chicken meat in Southern Brazil. *Braz. J. Pharm. Sci.* **2006**, *42*, 109–117. [CrossRef]
52. Bocca, C.; Bozzo, F.; Francica, S.; Colombatto, S.; Miglietta, A. Involvement of PPARγ and E-cadherin/β-catenin pathway in the antiproliferative effect of conjugated linoleic acid in MCF-7 cells. *Int. J. Cancer* **2007**, *121*, 248–256. [CrossRef] [PubMed]
53. Chitturi, S.; Abeygunasekera, S.; Farrell, G.C.; Holmes-Walker, J.; Hui, J.M.; Fung, C.; Karim, R.; Lin, R.; Samarasinghe, D.; Liddle, C.; et al. NASH and insulin resistance: Insulin hypersecretion and specific association with the insulin resistance syndrome. *Hepatology* **2002**, *35*, 373–379. [CrossRef] [PubMed]
54. Siscovick, D.S.; Barringer, T.A.; Fretts, A.M.; Wu, J.H.Y.; Lichtenstein, A.H.; Costello, R.B.; Kris-Etherton, P.M.; Jacobson, T.A.; Engler, M.B.; Alger, H.M.; et al. Omega-3 polyunsaturated fatty acid (fish oil) supplementation and the prevention of clinical cardiovascular disease: A science advisory from the AHA. *Circulation* **2017**, *135*, 867–884. [CrossRef]
55. Mateescu, R.G.; Garmyn, A.J.; Neil, M.A.O.; Tait, R.G., Jr.; Abuzaid, A.; Mayes, M.S.; Garrick, D.J.; Van Eenennaam, A.L.; Van Overbeke, D.L.; Hilton, G.G.; et al. Genetic parameters for carnitine, creatine, creatinine, carnosine, and anserine concentration in longissimus muscle and their association with palatability traits in Angus cattle. *J. Anim. Sci.* **2013**, *90*, 4248–4255. [CrossRef] [PubMed]
56. Purchas, R.W.; Busboom, J.R. The effect of production system and age on levels of iron, taurine, carnosine, coenzyme Q10 and creatine in beef muscles and liver. *Meat Sci.* **2005**, *70*, 589–596. [CrossRef]
57. Schuller-Levis, G.B.; Gordon, R.E.; Wang, C.; Park, E. Taurine reduces lung inflammation and fibrosis caused by bleomycin. In *Taurine Advances in Experimental Medicine and Biology*, 5th ed.; Springer: Boston, MA, USA, 2003; Volume 526, pp. 395–402.

58. Purchas, R.W.; Rutherfurd, S.M.; Pearce, P.D.; Vather, R.; Wilkinson, B.H.P. Concentrations in beef and lamb of taurine, carnosine, coenzyme Q 10, and creatine. *Meat Sci.* **2004**, *66*, 629–637. [CrossRef]
59. Overvad, K.; Diamant, B.; Holm, L.; Holmer, G.; Mortensen, S.A.; Stender, S. Coenzyme Q10 in health and disease. *Eur. J. Clin. Nutr.* **1999**, *53*, 764–770. [CrossRef]
60. Rötig, A.; Appelkvist, E.L.; Geromel, V.; Chretien, D.; Kadhom, N.; Edery, P.; Rustin, P. Quinone-responsive multiple respiratory-chain dysfunction due to widespread coenzyme Q10 deficiency. *Lancet* **2000**, *356*, 391–395. [CrossRef]
61. James, A.M.; Smith, R.A.; Murphy, M.P. Antioxidant and prooxidant properties of mitochondrial Coenzyme Q. *Arch. Biochem. Biophys.* **2004**, *423*, 47–56. [CrossRef]
62. Mattila, P.; Lehtonen, M.; Kumpulainen, J. Comparison of in-line connected diode array and electrochemical detectors in the high-performance liquid chromatographic analysis of coenzymes Q9 and Q10 in food materials. *J. Agric. Food Chem.* **2000**, *48*, 1229–1233. [CrossRef]
63. Scott, L.W.; Dunn, J.K.; Pownall, H.J.; Brauchi, D.J.; McMann, M.C.; Herd, J.A.; Harris, K.B.; Savell, J.W.; Cross, H.R.; Gotto, A.M. Effects of beef and chicken consumption on plasma lipid levels in hypercholesterolemic men. *Arch. Intern. Med.* **1994**, *154*, 1261–1267. [CrossRef] [PubMed]
64. Beauchesne-Rondeau, E.; Gascon, A.; Bergeron, J.; Jacques, H. Plasma lipids and lipoproteins in hypercholesterolemic men fed a lipid-lowering diet containing lean beef, lean fish, or poultry. *Am. J. Clin. Nutr.* **2003**, *77*, 587–593. [CrossRef] [PubMed]
65. Darwish, W.S.; Ikenaka, Y.; Morshdy, A.E.; Eldesoky, K.I.; Nakayama, S.; Mizukawa, H.; Ishizuka, M. β-carotene and retinol contents in the meat of herbivorous ungulates with a special reference to their public health importance. *J. Vet. Med. Sci.* **2016**, *78*, 351–354. [CrossRef] [PubMed]
66. Liu, Q.; Scheller, K.K.; Arp, S.C.; Schaefer, D.M.; Frigg, M. Color coordinates for assessment of dietary vitamin E effects on beef color stability. *J. Anim. Sci.* **1996**, *74*, 106–116. [CrossRef] [PubMed]
67. Clausen, I.; Jakobsen, M.; Ertbjerg, P.; Madsen, N.T. Modified atmosphere packaging affects lipid oxidation, myofibrillar fragmentation index and eating quality of beef. *Packag. Technol. Sci.* **2009**, *22*, 85–96. [CrossRef]

5

Improvement of Disease Resistance in Livestock: Application of Immunogenomics and CRISPR/Cas9 Technology

Md. Aminul Islam [1,2,3], Sharmin Aqter Rony [4], Mohammad Bozlur Rahman [5], Mehmet Ulas Cinar [6,7], Julio Villena [2,8], Muhammad Jasim Uddin [1,9,*] and Haruki Kitazawa [2,3,*]

1 Department of Medicine, Faculty of Veterinary Science, Bangladesh Agricultural University, Mymensingh 2202, Bangladesh; aminul.vmed@bau.edu.bd
2 Food and Feed Immunology Group, Graduate School of Agricultural University Science, Tohoku University, Sendai 980-8572, Japan; jcvillena@cerela.org.ar
3 Livestock Immunology Unit, International Research and Education Centre for Food and Agricultural Immunology (CFAI), Graduate School of Agricultural Science, Tohoku University, Sendai 980-8572, Japan
4 Department of Parasitology, Faculty of Veterinary Science, Bangladesh Agricultural University, Mymensingh 2202, Bangladesh; s.a.rony@bau.edu.bd
5 Department of Livestock Services, Krishi Khamar Sarak, Farmgate, Dhaka 1215, Bangladesh; mbozlur@gmail.com
6 Department of Animal Science, Faculty of Agriculture, Erciyes University, 38039 Kayseri, Turkey; mucinar@erciyes.edu.tr
7 Department of Veterinary Microbiology & Pathology, College of Veterinary Medicine, Washington State University, Pullman, WA 99164, USA
8 Laboratory of Immunobiotechnology, Reference Centre for Lactobacilli, (CERELA), Tucuman 4000, Argentina
9 School of Veterinary Science, Gatton Campus, The University of Queensland, Brisbane 4072, Australia
* Correspondence: m.uddin2@uq.edu.au (M.J.U.); haruki.kitazawa.c7@tohoku.ac.jp (H.K.);

Simple Summary: Disease resistance is the ability of animals to inhibit the growth of invading pathogens within the body, which is influenced by the interaction of the host immune system, host genetics, and the pathogens. Resistant animals can be produced by molecular breeding by introducing the genomic marker responsible for disease resistance or immunocompetence. Immunogenomics is an information science that enables the genome-scale investigation of host immune response to pathogenic infection thereby identification of the genomic marker for disease resistance. Once the genomic marker is determined, it could be implemented in producing disease resistance animals by applying the advanced reproductive biotechnology like genome editing. The technical ease and decreasing cost over time might enhance the application of genome editing techniques for producing disease resistance livestock.

Abstract: Disease occurrence adversely affects livestock production and animal welfare, and have an impact on both human health and public perception of food–animals production. Combined efforts from farmers, animal scientists, and veterinarians have been continuing to explore the effective disease control approaches for the production of safe animal-originated food. Implementing the immunogenomics, along with genome editing technology, has been considering as the key approach for safe food–animal production through the improvement of the host genetic resistance. Next-generation sequencing, as a cutting-edge technique, enables the production of high throughput transcriptomic and genomic profiles resulted from host-pathogen interactions. Immunogenomics combine the transcriptomic and genomic data that links to host resistance to disease, and predict the potential candidate genes and their genomic locations. Genome editing, which involves insertion, deletion, or modification of one or more genes in the DNA sequence, is advancing rapidly and may be poised to become a commercial reality faster than it has thought. The clustered regulatory interspaced short palindromic repeats (CRISPR)/CRISPR-associated protein 9 (Cas9) [CRISPR/Cas9] system has recently emerged as a powerful tool for genome editing in agricultural food production including livestock disease management. CRISPR/Cas9 mediated insertion of *NRAMP1* gene for producing tuberculosis resistant cattle, and deletion of *CD163* gene for producing porcine reproductive and respiratory syndrome (PRRS) resistant pigs are two groundbreaking applications of genome editing in livestock. In this review, we have highlighted the technological advances of livestock immunogenomics and the principles and scopes of application of CRISPR/Cas9-mediated targeted genome editing in animal breeding for disease resistance.

Keywords: next generation sequencing; transcriptomics; bioinformatics; genome editing; disease resistance; livestock

1. Introduction

Foods from the livestock are a vital source of high-quality protein. Efficient production of animal-originated food is one of the major issues for global food safety, a long desire for a healthy population. The occurrence of infectious diseases in livestock affects not only the farm production, economics, and animal health-welfare; but it also increases the risk of zoonoses. Therefore, the outbreak of infectious diseases in food animals is a major threat to food safety and public health. The emergence of antimicrobial drug resistance along with the unavailability of effective vaccines and spontaneous genetic mutation of infectious pathogens are the major perils for breaking down the disease control strategies [1]. On the other hand, there is a growing consumer demand to produce organic animal food by securing animal welfare standards. Raising disease-free healthy livestock is the key to produce safe meat and milk. Good husbandry practices including optimum housing, ration, use of probiotics, biosecurity, and vaccination should be taken into account for the maintenance of health and production of farmed animals [2]. However, the improvement of host genetic resistance to disease may potentially contribute to the profitability through improved animal welfare and reduced antibiotic usage in livestock production [3].

Disease resistance is the host's ability to restrict or inhibit the establishment of infections and/or pathological processes of infectious pathogens [4]. Interactions among the host immune system and invading pathogens, and host genome determine the fate of infection and disease pathogenesis (Figure 1). Innate immunity is the frontline host defense against invading pathogens, and genes associated with the induction of innate immune responses are considered as the potential candidates for disease resistance [5]. Innate immune responses provide immediate and non-specific defense against a wider range of pathogens; therefore, innate immune response traits are the first choice to be incorporated in the disease-resistant breeding plans. Notably, the heritability of the innate immune response is medium to moderate [6]. The contribution of host genetic factors to disease occurrence is one of the fundamental issues in understanding disease pathogenesis and host resistance. The variation in the genetic resistance to disease is due largely to the variability in the host's immune response to infection. Thus, information on immunology and genomics together would better characterize the disease phenotype [4]. The application of genomic technologies to understand the immunology is termed as immunogenomics. Immunogenomics include integrated analysis of immunologic and genomic data on host response to infectious pathogens, and thereby contribute to identifying potential candidate genes for disease resistance in livestock [7]. The single nucleotide polymorphisms (SNPs) within the candidate gene associated with host immunocompetence to infection can subsequently be considered as a DNA marker for disease resistance.

Genome editing is a bio-engineering technology that involves insertion, deletion, or modification of a specific section of DNA sequence in the genome. The genome-editing technology encompasses nuclease enzyme for cutting DNA sequence, in addition to a targeting mechanism that guides the enzyme to a particular site on the genome [8]. The clustered regulatory interspaced short palindromic repeats (CRISPR)/CRISPR-associated protein 9 (Cas9) [CRISPR/Cas9] system is one of the latest genome-editing tools that has been widely used over the last couple of years (reviewed by Pellagatti et al. [9]). Genome editing in livestock has become a commercial reality due to the emergence of CRISPR/Cas9 technology. Advance use of CRISPR/Cas9 could facilitate the improvement of disease resistance in livestock through (a) enhancing the frequency of favorable trait-associated alleles, (b) introgression of favorable alleles from other breeds/species, and (c) by generating de novo favorable alleles [10]. However, the main challenge is the identification of genome-editing targets for a disease-resistant trait, which will require a combination of high-quality annotated livestock genomes, well-powered genome-wide association studies, and robust knowledge of molecular genetics of pathogen-host immune system interactions. In this review, we have systematically explained how the gift of immunogenomics could be applied to grasp the disease resistance candidate genes and use of the biological scissor, CRISPR/Cas9 technology, for insertion or deletion of desired genes in the host genome (Figure 1). The prospects, regulations, and social acceptance of genome editing technology concerning improving the livestock health and production are also discussed.

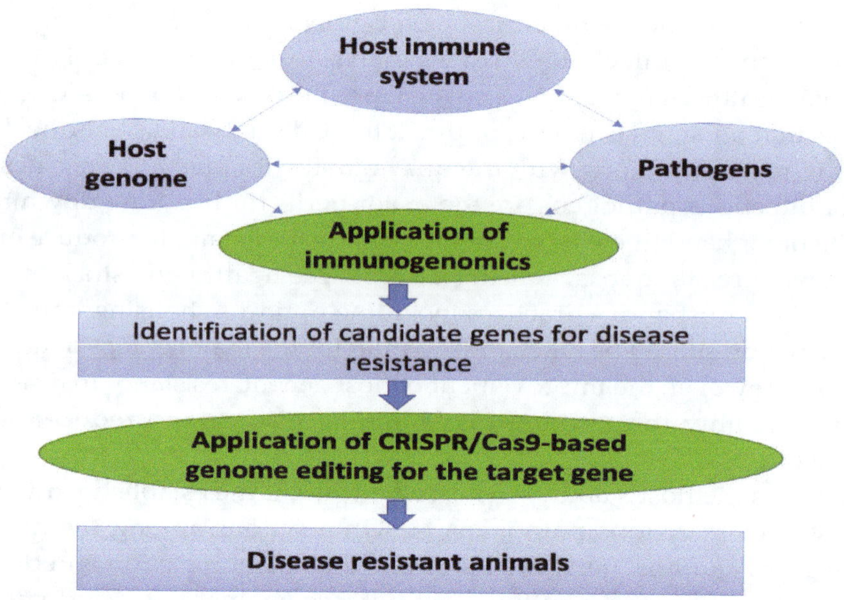

Figure 1. Schematic diagram showing the applications of immunogenomics and genome editing to produce disease-resistant animals. Severity and pathogenesis of disease depend on the interaction of the host immune system and the invading pathogens, where host genetic has potential influence. Immunogenomics employ the integrated bioinformatics tools to explore the influence of host genetic on the interaction between the host immune system and invading pathogens and subsequently identify the candidate gene (s) for disease resistance. The CRISPR/Cas9 mediated genome editing technology could subsequently be employed for targeted modification of the host genome to produce disease-resistant animals.

2. Disease Resistance: The Phenotype

Host-pathogen interactions result in either death or survival of the affected animal. Survivors either remain healthy and unaffected by the pathogens or experience a course of a disease that recover afterward. The immune system plays a crucial role in maintaining a balance between health and disease pathogenesis. In general, disease resistance demonstrates the host's ability to limit or prevent the replication of invading pathogens [11,12], and the relationship between the host and pathogens is better understood from an ecological point of view [13]. This concept includes several ways through which a host becomes comparatively more robust. For example, to display less possibility of infection, to have a reduced proliferation rate once infected, to possess a reduced rate of shedding or transmission [4]. It is not easy to measure the disease resistance trait, which is a major challenge for the investigator. It is possible that phenotype of disease resistance is relative rather than absolute and altered resistance impacts on the population as a whole because few attributes favor the individual host in certain cases, but other attributes (such as lower rate of transmission and infection) favor other population members. There is another associated phenotype called disease resilience, the capacity of the host to suppress the establishment or development of infection. Disease resilience is a physiological state in which an infected animal is capable of sustaining an acceptable degree of efficiency despite the burden of the pathogen [14]. The prospects and possibilities of using disease resilience in animal breeding programs are reviewed by Berghof et al. [15]. In addition, tolerance is another closely related phenotype that indicates the ability of the host to maintain the body homeostasis in the presence of replicating pathogens, with limited pathological consequences [12]. In a mixed population, the presence of asymptomatic and disease tolerant individuals may increase the genetic resistance of individual hosts, but there is a risk of increasing the prevalence of disease on the farm. Therefore, the disease resistance phenotype could consider to be incorporated into the host genetic improvement strategy.

Absolute quantification of the disease resistance phenotype under field condition is very difficult due to logistic and economic constraints, which is one of the major rate-limiting steps in animal breeding for disease resistance. Therefore, targeting immunocompetence trait is the indirect approach for improving disease resistance in livestock, and thereby producing safe milk and meat in the age of antibiotic resistance. Immunocompetent animals possess higher metabolic function and resilience to a wider range of infectious diseases, thereby improving the production performance in terms of quality and quantity. The host resistance to infectious diseases in livestock could be enhanced by incorporating resistance genes in the host genetics. The most economically important diseases in different livestock species could be considered first in the breeding goals for more sustainable production of disease-resistant animals [3]. Some infectious diseases of economic importance are mastitis, foot and mouth disease (FMD), tuberculosis, John's disease, and tick-borne diseases in cattle, Peste des petits ruminant (PPR) in goats, porcine reproductive and respiratory syndrome (PRRS), African swine fever in pigs, and gastrointestinal (GI) parasite infection in cattle and sheep [16].

Breeds of different animal species have a great influence on the innate resistance to infectious disease. Native breeds usually exert a higher degree of resistance to pathogens than the high-yielding exotic breed of the same species, which is believed to be due to the baseline immune competence, mainly innate immunity which could be transmitted down the progeny via genetic information and colostrum. Indigenous breeds of cattle (*Bos indicus*) were found to have a higher resistance to tick infestation and tick-borne diseases compared to high-yielding crossbred cattle as evidenced by higher hemolytic complement activity [17]. Native breed's resilience to local pathogens could be gained through evolution and adaptability when raised in the extensive farming system [18]. On contrary, intensive farming may weaken hosts' innate immunity. The relative difference in immunocompetence to infectious disease was reported among porcine breeds [19,20]. The genetic components associated with disease resistance should incorporate into the breeding program. Advances in tools and techniques for studying immunology and genetics of livestock and data analyses by immunogenomics enabled animal scientists to implement the molecular breeding technique including marker-assisted selection, genomic selection, and targeted genome editing for sustainable livestock production.

3. Advances of Immunogenomics

Immunogenomics is an information science that deals with big data from immunology and genomics. Immunogenomics integrates the molecular interactions among the host genome, immune system, and the invading pathogens. Understanding the function of the mammalian immune system has been broadening since the intersection of immunology and high-throughput sequencing technologies. Immunogenomics combines the transcriptome, DNA variants, polymorphisms/SNPs, and quantitative trait loci (QTL) mapping data resulted from host-pathogen interactions through a series of integrated bioinformatics [7]. Thus, immunogenomics have been considered as an efficient omics tool for identifying disease resistance genes or DNA markers [7]. Transcriptome profile provides an overview of expressed genes associated with particular phenotypes and is used as guidelines for subsequent analyses by proteomics, metabolomics, epigenomics, and other omics approaches. Since transcriptome can explore the relationship between genotype and phenotype of an organism, it has been considered as the most informative assay to start with for the functional genomics. Microarray and next-generation sequencing (NGS) are the cutting-edge technologies for transcriptomics or immunogenomics in many areas of the life sciences [21]. In parallel to the revolutionary progress of NGS technology, some advanced tools for cell biology studies are equally impactful. For example, flow cytometry and mass spectrometry/cytometry can provide a better picture of the phenotypic diversity among immune cell subsets [22]. Besides, the development of the induced pluripotent stem cell (iPSC) model from peripheral T cells has opened up another exciting avenue of immunology research [23].

3.1. Sequencing Technology

As a cutting-edge tool for immunogenomics, the NGS platform has rapidly evolved over the past 15 years, and exponentially increased amounts of sequence data generated per instrument run at ever-decreasing costs [24]. NGS-based RNA sequencing (RNA-Seq) can quantify all sorts of RNA species including messenger RNA (mRNA), microRNA, small interfering RNA, and long non-coding RNA, which enables the researcher to discover novel RNA forms and variants. The NGS methodology has been extended through the development of single-cell RNA sequencing (scRNA-seq) and in-situ RNA sequencing [24–26]. A single cell is the smallest structural and functional unit of a living organism, as such a particular cell represents a specific unit of molecular coding across the DNA, RNA, and protein expression [27]. Therefore, the omics-based investigations are highly expected to be carried out at the single-cell level for more precise results. The scRNA-seq has tremendous progress in the last couple of years owing to overcoming the difficulties of isolation of a single cell population [28]. The technological progress and application of the single-cell sequencing platform about cancer research have been well-summarized in Huang et al. [28]. The scRNA-seq has recently advanced along with the development of whole-genome sequencing such as scRNA methylation sequencing and single-cell assay for transpose-accessible chromatin sequencing (Single-cell ATAC-seq) [28]. Recently, the direct RNA sequencing using high throughput nanopore sequencing technology has emerged as the latest state-of-the-art RNA-Seq technique [29]. However, the single-molecule, long-read sequencing-based NGS technology is coming soon which may replace the ongoing platforms [30].

Currently, Illumina and Thermo Fisher's (Ion Torrent) standard and commonly used NGS platforms are based on short-read sequencing technologies [31]. To build sequencing ready libraries with an average length of 300 bp (ranging from 200–700 bp), short-read RNA-seq requires either fragmentation followed by reverse transcription or full-length cDNA synthesis followed by fragmentation. Since most mammalian RNA transcripts are 1–2 kb in length [32], getting complete RNA sequencing information relies on agreement with the annotated whole transcriptomic sequence or de novo transcriptome assembly approaches. In addition, genes have more than a transcriptional isoform that confronts the performance of the NGS in accurate gene expression quantification. The mRNA molecules transcribed from the same locus are referred to as transcriptional isoforms because mRNA can be produced from different transcriptional start sites, terminated at different polyadenylation sites, or as a result of alternative splicing [33]. Due to the limitations of short-read sequencing, it is difficult to assemble all expressed isoform for each gene and quantify the expression of all the isoforms with currently available bioinformatics tools [34,35]. To address these limitations, two commercial companies have recently launched the single-molecule, long-read sequencing technology-based NGS platform: Pacific Bioinformatics (PacBio), and Oxford Nanopore Technologies (ONT). With these technologies, the read length achieved (~15 kb for PacBio and >30 kb for ONT) exceeds the length of most mammalian transcripts. Combined with the benefit of full-length cDNA synthesis [36]. Especially SMARer (Switching Mechanism at RNA Termini) technology, long-read technologies are commercially available from Clontech (Mountain view, CA, USA), makes full-length mRNA sequencing possible with more precise transcriptomic studies. While a very powerful approach to unraveling the full spectrum of gene expression profiles is represented by long-read technologies, the relatively high costs of these technologies have prevented the broader spectrum of use. Oikinomopoulos et al. [30] reviewed the recent scientific and methodological developments in transcriptome profiling using the newly introduced single-molecule, long-read sequencing technology.

3.2. *Bioinformatics Tools*

While in the NGS platform, sequencing has become relatively straightforward with overcoming the technological limitations, the processing of upstream samples and downstream data analyses are still labor-intensive. To make a meaningful biological analysis, big data obtained from microarray and RNA-seq experiments requires high-power statistics and rigorous bioinformatics. Although most of the RNA-Seq data analysis algorithms can be run either in a Unix environment or inside the R/Bioconductor environment [37] from a command-line interface, some web-based menu-driven interfaces (e.g., Galaxy (www.usegalaxy.org), Geneious (www.geneious.com)) also support NGS data analysis. For the identification of DNA variants/SNPs associated with features like disease resistance, NGS sequence reading has been an area of rapid development [38]. Data from DNA variants (SNPs) or genome-wide association studies can be incorporated to explore the association between genomic architecture and the traits of interest once the potential candidate genes have become available from transcriptome analysis. The Animal QTL database (QTLdb) has been developed to bridge genotypes and phenotypes by repositing all publicly accessible QTLs and SNP/gene association data on animal species [39]. Approximately 191,422 QTLs have been curated to date, including 142,261 for cattle, 30,580 for pigs, 12,246 for chicken, 3305 for sheep and 2446 for horses (https://www.animalgenome.org/cgi-bin/QTLdb/index, Release 41, 26 April 2020). In order to analyze, annotate and visualize such genomic data for complex phenotype, such as immune repertoires, including disease resistance, bioinformatics software tools are essential components [40].

The keystone of immunogenomics is data integration. Accordingly, the scientific community can benefit from data sharing strategies that facilitate the integration of datasets among research groups. However, reliable methods for data integration are needed and require a broad range of expertise such as in mathematical and statistical models, computational methods, visualization strategies, and deep understanding of complex phenotypes. The commonly used tools and databases for immunogenomics of animals are summarized in Table 1.

Table 1. Bioinformatic tools or database commonly used for transcriptomics or immunogenomics studies aiming to identify the key regulatory genes in animals.

Bioinformatics Tools/Databases	Potential Implications	References
'Bowtie', 'msa'	Sequence-read alignment,	https://cran.r-project.org/
R/Bioconductor, limma, DESeq2	Differential gene expression analyses	https://cran.r-project.org/
GSEA-Gene Set Enrichment Analysis	Gene set enrichment analysis	[41] https://www.gsea-msigdb.org/gsea/index.jsp
DAVID	Gene ontology and pathway analysis	[42] https://david.ncifcrf.gov/
KEEG-Kyoto Encyclopedia of Genes and Genomes	Gene ontology and pathway analysis	https://www.genome.jp/kegg/

Table 1. *Cont.*

Bioinformatics Tools/Databases	Potential Implications	References
InnateDB	Database for gene ontology, pathway analysis and prediction interactome	[43] https://www.innatedb.com/
REACTOME	Database for gene ontology and pathway analysis	[44] https://reactome.org/
QTLdb	Database of quantitative trait loci of animals	[39] https://www.animalgenome.org/cgi-bin/QTLdb/index
BovineMine	Annotation and functions of gene	[45] http://128.206.116.13:8080/bovinemine/begin.do
bioDBnet-Biological database network	Interconnected access to many types of biological databases, conversion of gene or protein identifies	[46] https://biodbnet-abcc.ncifcrf.gov/
STRING	Functional protein association network analysis and visualization	[47] https://string-db.org/
NetworkAnalyst	Co-regulatory gene or protein network analysis and visualization	[48] https://www.networkanalyst.ca/
WGCNA	Weighted gene co-expression network analysis	[49] https://cran.r-project.org/
Cytoscape	Creation and visualization gene network	[50] https://cytoscape.org/

While in silico genomics tools and databases for the human genome have been developed well, those for the genomes of livestock are still growing. Thus, an ID conversion tool, such as bioDBnet [46], is required to convert gene ID to human orthologous identifiers to perform the downstream functional analysis using human database. BovineMine, for instance, is a useful database and web portal for data mining for the annotation of bovine genes and genomes [45]. Standardize laboratory workflows, raw data formats, experimental designs, and methods of biostatistical analyses are, however, required. The technological shortcomings of immunogenomics are being resolved and are likely to be put in the life sciences among the largest 'big data' enterprises [51]. The Functional Annotation of ANimal Genomes (FAANG www.faang.org) was developed in this regard to support the standard protocol for core research, data research and meta-data analysis of standards for swine immunogenomics studies [52]. In addition, the 1000 Bull Genome Project has provided the bovine research community with a huge volume of data on bovine variants that will be useful for GWAS and the identification of causal mutations (http://1000bullgenomes.com). These initiatives pave the way for a systemic incorporation of the findings of bovine immunogenomics studies and for making them available online.

4. Applications of Immunogenomics in Livestock Disease Management

Sustainable management of livestock diseases requires breeding techniques that protect the environment, animal welfare, and public health, as well as providing adequate financial rewards for farmers. Several efforts are in progress to develop a disease-resistant stock through molecular breeding. By dissecting the genetic makeup, a typical first stage of molecular breeding by marker-assisted selection, genomic selection, or genome editing is to determine the extent in genetic variation on the individual trait. Simple understanding of host immunology and genetics better characterize the disease-resistant phenotype. The advent of immunogenomics provides more accurate identification of candidate biomarkers for disease resistance, which makes it easier to enhance disease resistance by genome editing techniques.

In a real-life situation, the direct estimation of disease resistance phenotype is very difficult because a precise animal identification and disease regression method and infection challenge routines are required [53]. The disease resistance phenotype is typically quantified in the direct disease model by calculating the magnitude of the infection, such as burden of the inside-host pathogen (e.g., viral load), and these are technically difficult to incorporate in the intensive commercial production system. In addition, the direct measurement techniques target the host's resistance to a particular infection. However, when introduced by molecular breeding, it can result in increased susceptibility to other infections [54]. Appropriate indirect methods are therefore highly desirable for estimating disease resistance. One method may be to estimate the phenotype of disease resistance by defining the genomic marker associated with the immunocompetence of the host produced from vaccination that is inheritable and linked to improved health and production performance [55,56]. Vaccination does not cause disease, but it allows memory T-lymphocytes, B-lymphocytes, and antibodies to be formed by the host immune system, enabling hosts to defend the subsequent infection [57]. The most suitable candidates for disease resistance traits are possibly genes regulating the first few hours of the host's response during innate immunity to infection or vaccination [5,58]. Due to the rapid onset and wider range of defense, innate immune traits have the potentials to be used in the selection of livestock for disease resistance [53], and the innate immune traits display significant genetic variation among the breeds of livestock species [6,59]. Thus, as a possible indirect indicator of disease resistance, enhancing innate immunocompetence is of great importance.

To identify the potential biomarkers for immunocompetence as indirect measures of disease resistance in livestock, the study population could be divided into two contrast phenotypes correlated to disease resistance (Figure 2). The contrast phenotypes may be achieved by either taking animals with the extreme immune response phenotype following vaccination (extremely high antibody titre vs. extremely low antibody titre) or vaccinated vs. control animals. In order to obtain adequate statistical power from the experiment, the use of an optimum number of animals as biological replicates for each group should be considered. Schurch et al. [60] proposed that for the detection of substantially differentially expressed gene between two contrast phenotypes using RNA sequencing technology, at least six biological replicates should be used. The single population of target primary cells should be separated once the experimental group is fixed in order to prevent cell-type-specific gene expression. Then, a pure single-cell population should be subjected to the extraction of total RNA and genomic DNA separately. To scan the full spectrum of gene expression between the contrast phenotypes, the quality-assured total RNA samples can be subjected to holistic transcriptome profiling by RNA-seq. The RNA samples could be used for profiling for proteomics and metabolomics. On the other hand, SNP sequencing and genotyping, quantitative trait loci (QTL) mapping, and genome-wide association study (GWAS) may also be subjected to DNA samples, and epigenomics analysis targeting the phenotype of disease resistance. Rigorous integrated bioinformatics framework on all sets of omics data together helps us to identify the molecular biomarkers for intended immunocompetence trait. Those could be suggested as the targets for CRISPR/Cas9 mediated genome editing technology after functional validation of the identified biomarkers in the independent population.

Applications of immunogenomics in human disease particularly in cancer have much progress such as the in-silico prediction of human leukocyte antigen (HLA) gene has been accelerated through a combination of high-throughput sequencing technology and specialized computational approaches [61]. Immunogenomics have been employed to explore the porcine resistance to Gram-negative bacterial infection in porcine [7] and gastrointestinal nematode infection in ruminant [62]. Knowledge of immunogenomics has been applied in the identification of several immune response genes in livestock based on their association with resistance or susceptibility in several diseases and their proven function in disease pathogenesis [16]. Several GWAS have been performed aiming to identify the QTLs or SNP profiles associated with resistance or susceptibility to bovine mastitis [63], and milk somatic cell count as an indicator of mastitis [64,65]. Many immune response genes are associated with mastitis resistance including cytokines IL-4, IL-8, IL-13, and IL-17 [66,67]. Nevertheless, further fine-tuning of the genomics tools and in silico omics software recourses in near future would enable the identification of disease resistance candidate biomarkers in a more precise way.

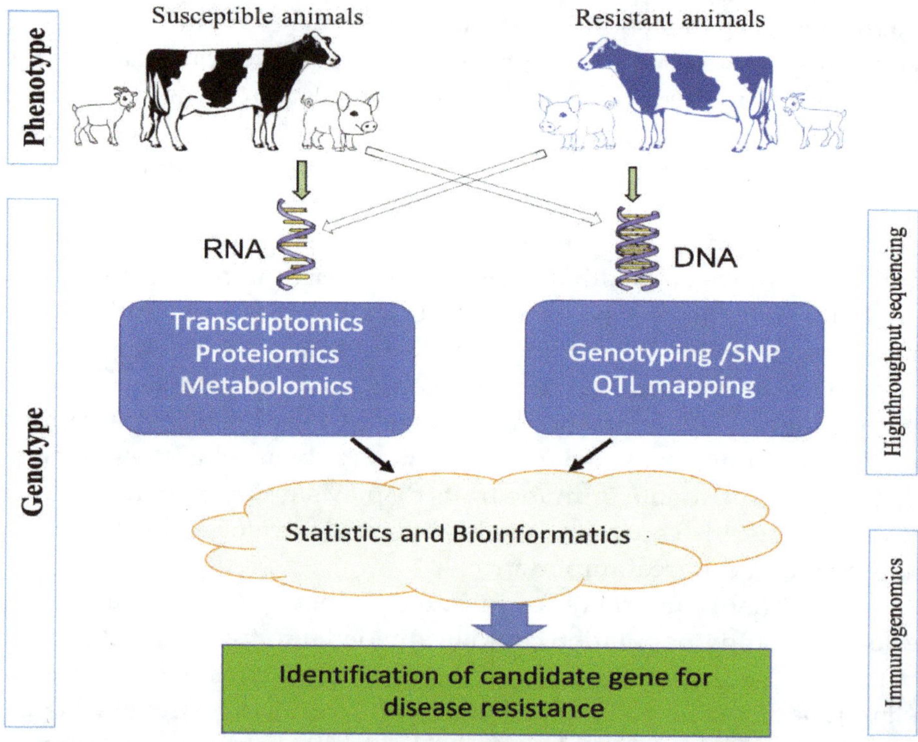

Figure 2. A working pipeline of (in vivo, in vitro, and in silico) immunogenomics for identification of disease resistance candidate gene/marker as prospective targets for genome editing. Isolation of single-cell population of a target from both phenotypic groups followed by RNA and DNA extraction separately. The RNA samples could be employed for proteomics and metabolomics profiling. On the other hand, DNA samples could also be subjected to single nucleotide polymorphisms (NSP) sequencing and genotyping, quantitative trait loci (QTL) mapping, and genome-wide association study, and epigenomics study targeting the disease resistance phenotype. Rigorous integrated bioinformatics application on all sets of omics data together enables us to identify the molecular biomarker for the target immunocompetence trait. After functional validation of the identified biomarkers in the independent population, those could be recommended as the targets for CRISPR/Cas9 mediated genome editing technology.

5. Advances of Genome Editing Technology

The premier seed for the possibility of a desired improvement of the mammalian genome has sown by Palmiter and Brinster in 1988 [68]. The active insertion into the mouse embryos by pronuclear microinjection of a foreign DNA fragment, a growth hormone gene called metallothionein-I, resulted in the rapid growth of the animals as targeted [68]. This technique of genome engineering based on cells was restricted to injecting plasmids or gene fragments into the embryos pronucleus. Subsequent advances in genome engineering have been achieved by the introduction of transposons or retroviral vectors [69], followed by the development of homing endonuclease (HEs), natural meganuclease capable of introducing double-strand breaks (DSBs) at 14–40 bp target sites [70]. Nevertheless, in vivo application of HE-based genome modification has been limited due to their off-target cutting propensity. In general, modern genome editing relies on DNA insertion, deletion, or substitution in the genome of a living organism using programmable nuclease-based editors (Figure 3). Zinc finger nuclease (ZFNs) [71,72] and transcription activator-like effector nuclease (TALENs) [73] were the most widely used genome editors until recently. Zinc fingers (ZFs) are among the most well-characterized DNA-binding protein domains found in the nature that have enhanced the programmed modification repertoire of enable any target genome to be accurately cut and repair [72]. A second group of naturally occurring proteins containing a DNA-binding domain and formed by proteobacteria of the genus Xanthomonas is transcription activator-like effector (TALE) [73]. A pair of ZFNs must bind regions flanking the target locus for genome editing to form a FokI dimer, which is required to induce DSBs (Figure 3A) [74]. Similarly, TALENs are also modular proteins that contain two domains: a customizable DNA-binding domain (TALE) and the FokI nuclease domain. The TALE-binding DNA sequence is cut by dimerization and thus produces DSBs in a similar manner to ZFNs (Figure 3B) [75]. However, both ZFNs and TALENs are limited by targeting multiple sites in the same genome. The comprehensive interaction of ZFNs with protein-DNA and the highly repetitive nature of TALENs warrant the advent of new instruments.

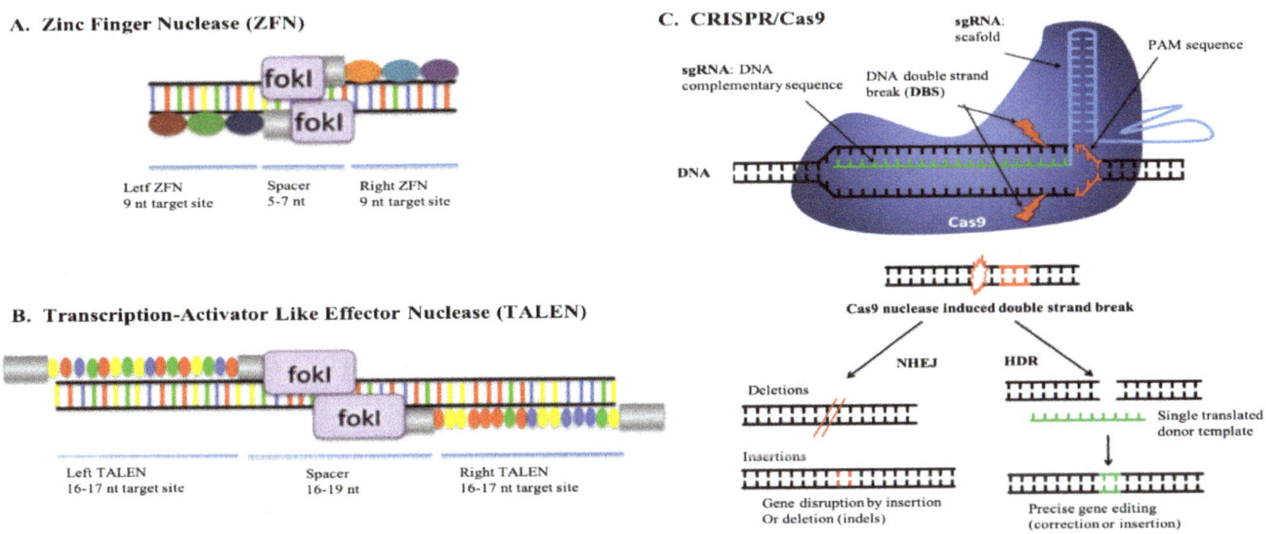

Figure 3. Nuclease-based genome editors. (**A**). Zinc Finger Nuclease (**B**). Transcription-Activator Like Effector Nuclease (TALEN). (**C**). Schematic diagram showing genome editing using CRISPR/Cas9 system. The Cas9 induces DNA double-strand break (DSB) which are repaired either by imperfect nonhomologous end-joining (NHEJ) to generate insertion or deletion (indels) or if a repair is provided, by homology-directed repair (HDR) (Adapted from Moore et al. [71], and Pellagatti et al. [9].

The clustered regulatory interspaced short palindromic repeats (CRISPR)/Cas9 system, which was built from an inherent antiviral mechanism found in bacteria [76], is the latest addition to the genome toolbox. In comparison to a classical genetic modification that involves moving genes from species to another, the CRISPR/Cas9 system relies on the use of molecular 'scissors' to introduce changes in existing DNA sequences [75,77]. The CRISPR/Cas9 system uses a single guided RNA (sgRNA) to help the Cas9 nuclease to classify the particular genomic sequence, unlike the ZFNs and TALENs, which use proteins to recognize specific sequences in the genome (Figure 3C). In the presence of sgRNA complementary sequence and the Porto-spacer adjacent motif (PAM) sequence [9], the Cas9 protein binds to the sgRNA scaffold and generates a DSB. The DSB activates the machinery for the repair of endogenous cellular DNA that catalyzes non-homologous end joining (NHEJ) and homology direct repair (HDR) (Figure 3C). The NEHJ pathway is preferably used by most cell types, which is possibly an error-prone mechanism that generally results in minor insertions or deletions at the site of repair. NEHJ also produces a mutation and induces encoded protein fragmentation or functional gene knockout by producing DNA break in the coding sequence of a gene. On the other hand, the HDR pathway can be activated through flooding the target cell with a DNA repair template, which allows the implementation of specific sequence changes proximal to the cut site ranging from single base changes to the insertion of transgenes. In order to make minor change, a synthetic single-stranded oligodeoxynucleotide is used, whereas larger modification requires the plasmid/dsDNA template. Finally, two simultaneous breaks are produced and transcriptional profiles are altered either by removing regulatory elements or by deleting exons. Protein domains are subsequently deleted, leaving the remaining reading frame intact [78]. One of the CRISPR/Cas9 system's key advantage is that the Cas9 nuclease is not covalently fused to a DSB, so it is possible to use same protein to attack multiple target sites by combining it with a different sgRNA package. Besides, most of the necessary reagents can be made in the molecular biology laboratory, while Cas9 nuclease and sgRNA molecules can be purchased commercially. The CRISPR/Cas9 system has made the genome-editing technique a practical reality in recent years due to its methodological simplicity, performance, precision, flexibility, and a greater degree of accuracy.

A variety of techniques are available to produce the genetically modified animals depending on the species and cell type used to deliver the Cas9 genome-editor (reviewed by Harwood et al. [79]). The technique of sperm mediated gene transfer (SMGT) is used to deliver the genome-edited reagents into a zygote. Manipulation of spermatogonial stem cells (SSCs) or primordial germ cells (PGCs) is often used for the development of genome-edited organisms. For the development of genome-manipulated animals, the pronuclear and intracytoplasmic injection of genome editors into zygotes accompanied by either direct transfer to surrogates or in vitro maturation and embryo transfer could be applied. In addition, somatic cell nuclear transfer (SCNT) is another approach that enables precise edits to be selected in somatic cells before nuclear transfer to surrogates or in vitro maturation. The injection of edited embryonic or iPSC into blastocyst may also be used for the development of chimeric animals examined by Harwood et al. [79]. Like the genome-editor tool use, the techniques follow is also important to achieve the intended efficiency and precision in generating genome-edited animal species. The introduction of genome editing in the research animal model for the treatment of human disease has also made tremendous progress, in addition to the development of CRISPR/Cas9 techniques in animal disease management. Recent reviews have summarized the methodological advances of CRISPR/Cas-9 mediated genome editing in large animals (pigs, monkeys, dogs, rabbits, mice, rats) with a focus on the creation of model animals for studying human diseases [80,81].

6. Applications of Genome Editing in Livestock Disease Management

The CRISPR/Cas9-based genome editing has been applied in livestock for several specific (but not limited to) purposes: (a) for inactivation or alteration of expression of targeted genes in the model animals to confirm their functions (b) for producing research animals for studying human disease pathogenesis in controlled setup and evaluate potential therapies, (c) and producing genetically modified animals for industrial, pharmaceutical, and biotechnological implications [82]. Nevertheless, the success of the gene-editing system in controlling animal diseases would be affected by several factors. For instance, the proportion of gene-edited animals and how they are distributed within and across the population. According to epidemiological theory, a certain proportion of gene-edited animals required to achieve herd immunity, and to prevent disease transmission within the population [83]. Disease-specific epidemiological modeling could provide information on the required number of genome-edited animals for preventing certain disease/infectious agents. Such modeling should consider the influence of population structure, demographic characteristics, diverse environmental factors, and management strategies that affect the disease transmission dynamics to estimate the size of the population for genome editing. The latest advance in genome editing with programmable nucleases, such as CRISPR/Cas9, has opened up new avenues for animal breeding targeted with disease resistance. However, the efficiency of genome editing varies due to the variation in reproductive physiology among different livestock species. Genome editing in cattle accompanied by major challenges due to high market value, a small number of offspring, and longer gestation period (9 months gestation, 12–18 months to reach puberty). While pigs, sheep, and goats have several advantages as they are smaller, cheaper, and produce more offspring at a time, shorter gestation lengths, and shorter ages of puberty. Over time, genome editing has been successfully applied in livestock species to improve different traits like growth, production performance, and resistance to certain diseases.

Myostatin (*MSTN)* gene is known to be associated with growth and skeletal muscle development. *MSTN* was targeted in the earlier attempts of genetic manipulation in farm animals because the disruption of this single gene has significant effects on meat production, an economically important trait. To date, genome editing has been successfully applied to knockout the *MSTN* from the genomes of cattle, pigs, sheep, and goats (reviewed by Petersen [8]). In cattle, the introduction of antibiotic lysostaphin by SCNT resulted in secretion of milk protein that has bactericidal activity against mastitis-causing bacteria *Staphylococcus aureus* [84]. The gene encoded with bovine whey protein ß-lactoglobulin (BLG), which is a major milk protein and a dominant allergen, was successfully knocked out in the bovine genome using ZFNs technique [85]. Another genome editing study has described the production of swine with mutation RELA (p56) gene using ZFNs, which confer the tolerance of African swine fever [86]. Production of a hornless strain of dairy cattle (Holstein Frisian) by inserting the pooled gene (P) of beef cattle (Angus) through the HDR pathway of gene editing has also been reported [87]. With the evolution of CRISPR/Cas9-based genome editing and a deeper understating of how to gear up its potential, it is now possible to introduce extremely precise changes to the genome with better accuracy and efficiency than any previous attempts. The CRISPR/Cas9 mediated insertion of *NRAMP1* gene for producing tuberculosis resistant cattle and deletion of *CD163* gene for producing porcine reproductive and respiratory syndrome (PRRS) resistant pigs are two groundbreaking application of genome editing technique in livestock. Hereinbelow, we summarized some prominent examples of implication of CRISPR/Cas9-based genome editing to produce disease-resistant livestock (Table 2).

Table 2. Reported application of genome editing techniques for disease resistance livestock breeding.

Species	Disease	Targets of Genome Modification	Reference
Goat	Mastitis	Lysozyme (human)	[88]
Cattle	Mastitis	Lysostaphin (*Staphylococcus simulans*)	[84]
	Enzootic pneumonia	Cluster of differentiation 18 (CD18)	[89]
	Tuberculosis	The natural resistance to infection with intracellular pathogens 1 (NRAMP1) gene	[90]
Pigs	African swine fever	RELA	[86]
	PRRS	Histone deacetylase HDAC6	[91]
		Cluster of differentiation 163 (CD163)	[92,93]

6.1. *Porcine Reproductive and Respiratory Syndrome (PRRS) in Pigs*

PRRS is considered the most economically important infectious disease of the swine industry worldwide affecting the production, reproduction, health, and welfare of pigs. The global transcriptome profiling of peripheral blood mononuclear cells revealed that pigs can induce innate and subsequent adaptive immune response to PRRS virus infection or vaccination [92,93]. The host transcriptomic response to PRRSV has been found to have substantial genetic variation [19,20]. The cluster of differentiation 163 (CD163) is a cell surface receptor gene, which is a member of scavenger receptor cysteine-rich superfamily (SRCR) having one intracellular domain and nine extracellular SRCR domains [94]. The CD163 facilitates the PRRS virus to enter into the pulmonary alveolar macrophage through endocytosis, where the virus replicates and induces disease pathogenesis [94,95]. Whitworth et al. [96] reported for the first time that CRISPR/Cas9 mediated CD163-knockout pigs were fully protected against the clinical outcome of PRRS virus infection with a single isolate [96]. A subsequent experiment demonstrated that the SRCR5 domain is crucial for establishing viral infection [97]. The implication of reproductive biotechnology for the production of genome-modified pigs might therefore significantly reduce the PRRS-associated economic losses in the pork industry.

6.2. *African Swine Fever Resistance in Pig*

Another economically relevant infectious disease caused by the African swine fever virus (ASFV) in pigs is African swine fever (ASF). Many areas of sub-Saharan Africa are endemic to the ASF. It has been detected recently in Eastern Europe, from where it is rapidly spreading to both Western Europe and China. Native wild swine breeds including the Warthog, have been reported to be resilient to ASFV infection, whereas domestic pigs experience cytokine storm-related lethal hemorrhagic fever. Significant variation in the expression of the RELA gene between resilient and susceptible pigs is associated with host response to ASFV infection [98]. The RELA is a part of the Nuclear Factor kappa Beta (NFkB) transcription factor, considered to play an important role in stress management and immune defense. By using the ZFN-based genome editing technique [99], the sequence of RELA gene in domestic pigs could be translated to that of Warthog pigs. However, the phenotypic data supporting the genetic resistance to ASFV infection yet to be reported.

6.3. *Tuberculosis Resistance in Cattle*

Bovine tuberculosis (bTB) is a chronic bacterial disease that is crippling and caused by *Mycobacterium bovis* in cattle. With a wide host range, *M. bovis* infection create considerable hardship for livestock producers with estimates of more than 50 million cattle infected worldwide [100]. This zoonotic infection can be transmitted to humans mainly through the ingestion of milk products that are not pasteurized, resulting in a 10–15% prevalence of human TB [99]. Compulsory testing accompanied by the slaughter of test-positive animals, which accounts for as huge economic loss, is an important means of bTB regulation. The bTB is as a crucial target for genome editing for producing tuberculosis resistant cattle, due to its economic and zoonotic importance, endemic existence, and failure of conventional control strategies. As a strong candidate gene for tuberculosis resistance, natural resistance to infection with intracellular pathogens 1 (*NRAMP1*) gene has been reported by several studies. In a recent study, Cas9 nickase (nCas9) was used by scientist to insert the *NRAMP1* into the genome of the bovine fetal fibroblast [90]. These engineered fibroblast cells were then used as donor cells in somatic cell nuclear transfer, where the *NRAMP1*-containing donor cell nucleus was inserted into the cow's ovum. Before being transferred to recipient cows following a physiologically natural estrous cycle, ova were then nurtured in the laboratory up to embryos. The inserted *NRAMP1* gene was correctly expressed and provided cattle by showing a higher degree of resistance to *M. bovis* infection [90]. It has also been reported that resistance against *M. bovis* infection could be achieved in cattle through TALEN-mediated insertion of mouse SP110 gene into an intergenic region of the bovine genome [101].

6.4. *Enzootic Pneumonia Resistance in Cattle*

Pasteurellosis in cattle also called shipping fever or enzootic pneumonia is a respiratory disease complex mostly found in recently weaned, single-sucked beef calves after housing or transport to a new house. Following infection, *P. hameolytica* secretes a leukotoxin that is cytotoxic and it binds to the uncleaved signal peptide of the CD18 protein on the surface of leukocytes. However, the mature CD18 lacks the signal peptide in the leukocytes of other species (e.g., mouse and human) that do not suffer from this disease. ZFNs have been used to introduce a single amino acid change in the bovine CD18 protein and leukocytes from the resultant cattle were able to inhibit the *P. hameolytica* leukotoxin-induced cytotoxicity [102].

7. Ethics, Regulations, and Social Acceptance of Genome-Edited Livestock Products

Manipulation of genomes in farm animals is becoming a lucrative and materialistic alternative. However, problems such as regulatory legislation, market pay off, and performance acceptability of users are still unresolved. The societal attitude towards genome-edited animal products worldwide will depend on whether the handling was carried out with due regard to the ethical value of target customer community and the issue of animal welfare [103]. The resulting foods after genome-edited livestock should appear on the commercial market ready to be distributed to consumers immediately, with the required legislative approval of a country. However, the contested factors linked to genetically modified (GM) as well as cloned animals suggest that food derived from genome-edited animals is socially rejected or unable to accept it. Psychological studies have shown that several factors such as the consumer's perceived risks of the consumer, the recognized benefits and/or the confidence in regulatory legislation, can cause the acceptability of GM animals by researchers [104]. The public's skeptical view of GMOs (GM organisms) is partly related to the degree of skepticism of both researchers and state policymakers [105]. Off-target mutagenesis seems to be a big problem due to the widespread use of the CRISPR/Cas9 tool. In relation to the breeding of disease resistant animals, the problem is of more serious concern. The debate on closed animals, stimulated by so many tests, prompted the study of off-target mutation. Exploration of off-target mutations tends to be crucial from the point of view of animal health and ethics to the broader implications of genome-editing techniques in animal breeding [103]. Therefore, in addition to scientific ethics, ethical concerns of animal health and welfare to minimize the imminence of off-target mutations are required to enhance public understanding. This could advocate the social acceptance of genome-edited livestock products gradually.

8. Potentials and Prospects of CRISPR/Cas9 Technology in Livestock Production

The CRISPR/Cas9 exhibits the potentials for substantial improvement over the gene-editing technologies in the ease of application, speed, efficiency, and cost involved. The genome-editing technique has been extensively used for elucidating the gene function in disease pathogenesis and host immune responses. Indeed, the CRISPR/Cas9-based correction of gene mutation in a mouse model of human disease and the primary adult stem cells derived from patients suffering monogenic hereditary defects are being considered the cornerstones for future gene therapy technique [9]. The CRISPR/Cas9-mediated knockout libraries could also potentially be applied to target regions of interest in the noncoding regulatory segment of the genome, such as promoter and enhancer. Moreover, the application of CRISPR/Cas9 in genome-wide studies will facilitate the holistic screening of disease resistance markers. The CRISPR/Cas9 technique would also enable a much wider range of modifications, for instance, gene knockout, base-pair substitution, targeted insertion/deletion of larger genomic regions, and modulation of gene expression [8]. Despite many challenges, remarkable advancements in the field of gene therapy and CRISPR/Cas9-based genome editing technique have been observed in recent years, which paves the way for the development of sustainable disease control strategies for humans, crops, fish, and livestock. Though unlikely in crops, where the whole population can rapidly be replaced, the application of genome editing in the livestock population is a more complex and time-consuming process. Moreover, increasing the efficiency of the CRISPR/Cas9-based repairing process, particularly to increase the rate of gene correction and reduce resultant off-target effects and the development of more effective delivery methods would require for its wider application.

9. Conclusions

Raising immunocompetent healthy livestock is crucial for the sustainable production of safe food. Understanding the genetics behind the host immunocompetence to infectious pathogens is the key to improve the level of disease resistance through molecular breeding approaches. Exploring the variation of host innate immunocompetence to economically important infectious diseases among indigenous, exotic, and cross-bred animals of the same species can be of important starting point toward estimating the genetic components of disease resistance phenotype. The cutting-edge techniques for immunological and molecular genetics study may create a direct linkage between disease-resistant phenotype and the host genotype. Continuous advancement of open-source in silico omics tools will identify the potential genomic marker, the target for genome editing for disease resistance in livestock. The application of modern reproductive biotechnology, such as CRISPR/Cas9 mediated genome editing, is a breakthrough tool for improving disease resistance in livestock due to its high precision. Minimizing the risk of off-target mutations would restore the animal welfare standard and increase consumer acceptance of food products derived from genome-edited livestock.

Author Contributions: M.A.I., M.J.U., and H.K. designed the study. M.A.I., S.A.R., M.B.R. collected the literature. M.A.I. wrote the original draft. S.A.R., M.B.R., M.U.C., J.V., M.J.U., and H.K. critically reviewed the manuscript. All authors have read and agreed to the published version of the manuscript.

Acknowledgments: Authors are thankful to the Karl Schellander of the Institute of Animal Science, University of Bonn, Bonn, Germany for his insightful advice in planning this work.

References

1. Aslam, B.; Wang, W.; Arshad, M.I.; Khurshid, M.; Muzammil, S.; Rasool, M.H.; Nisar, M.A.; Alvi, R.F.; Aslam, M.A.; Qamar, M.U.; et al. Antibiotic resistance: A rundown of a global crisis. *Infect. Drug Resist.* **2018**, *11*, 1645–1658. [CrossRef] [PubMed]
2. Villena, J.; Aso, H.; Rutten, V.P.M.G.; Takahashi, H.; van Eden, W.; Kitazawa, H. Immunobiotics for the Bovine Host: Their Interaction with Intestinal Epithelial Cells and Their Effect on Antiviral Immunity. *Front. Immunol.* **2018**, *9*, 326. [CrossRef]
3. Davies, G.; Genini, S.; Bishop, S.C.; Giuffra, E. An assessment of opportunities to dissect host genetic variation in resistance to infectious diseases in livestock. *Animal* **2009**, *3*, 415–436. [CrossRef] [PubMed]
4. Bishop, S.C.; Woolliams, J.A. Genomics and disease resistance studies in livestock. *Livest. Sci.* **2014**, *166*, 190–198. [CrossRef] [PubMed]
5. Loving, C.L.; Osorio, F.A.; Murtaugh, M.P.; Zuckermann, F.A. Innate and adaptive immunity against Porcine Reproductive and Respiratory Syndrome Virus. *Vet. Immunol. Immunopathol.* **2015**, *167*, 1–14. [CrossRef] [PubMed]
6. Flori, L.; Gao, Y.; Laloe, D.; Lemonnier, G.; Leplat, J.-J.; Teillaud, A.; Cossalter, A.-M.; Laffitte, J.; Pinton, P.; de Vaureix, C.; et al. Immunity traits in pigs: Substantial genetic variation and limited covariation. *PLoS ONE* **2011**, *6*, e22717. [CrossRef]
7. Zhao, S.; Zhu, M.; Chen, H. Immunogenomics for identification of disease resistance genes in pigs: A review focusing on Gram-negative bacilli. *J. Anim. Sci. Biotechnol.* **2012**, *3*, 34. [CrossRef]
8. Petersen, B. Basics of genome editing technology and its application in livestock species. *Reprod. Domest. Anim.* **2017**, *52* (Suppl. 3), 4–13. [CrossRef]
9. Pellagatti, A.; Dolatshad, H.; Valletta, S.; Boultwood, J. Application of CRISPR/Cas9 genome editing to the study and treatment of disease. *Arch. Toxicol.* **2015**, *89*, 1023–1034. [CrossRef]
10. Tait-Burkard, C.; Doeschl-Wilson, A.; McGrew, M.J.; Archibald, A.L.; Sang, H.M.; Houston, R.D.; Whitelaw, C.B.; Watson, M. Livestock 2.0—Genome editing for fitter, healthier, and more productive farmed animals. *Genome Biol.* **2018**, *19*, 204. [CrossRef] [PubMed]
11. Bishop, S.C.; Stear, M.J. Modeling of host genetics and resistance to infectious diseases: Understanding and controlling nematode infections. *Vet. Parasitol.* **2003**, *115*, 147–166. [CrossRef]
12. Bishop, S.C. A consideration of resistance and tolerance for ruminant nematode infections. *Front. Genet.* **2012**, *3*, 168. [CrossRef] [PubMed]
13. Grenfell, B.T.; Dobson, A.P. *Ecology of Infectious Diseases in Natural Populations*; Cambridge University Press: Cambridge, UK, 1995.
14. Albers, G.A.; Gray, G.D.; Piper, L.R.; Barker, J.S.; Le Jambre, L.F.; Barger, I.A. The genetics of resistance and resilience to Haemonchus contortus infection in young merino sheep. *Int. J. Parasitol.* **1987**, *17*, 1355–1363. [CrossRef]
15. Berghof, T.V.L.; Poppe, M.; Mulder, H.A. Opportunities to Improve Resilience in Animal Breeding Programs. *Front. Genet.* **2019**, *9*, 692. [CrossRef] [PubMed]
16. Pal, A.; Chakravarty, A.K. *Genetics and Breeding for Disease Resistance in Livestock*; Imprint Academic Press: Cambridge, MA, USA, 2019; p. 384. [CrossRef]
17. Robbertse, L.; Richards, S.A.; Maritz-Olivier, C. Bovine Immune Factors Underlying Tick Resistance: Integration and Future Directions. *Front. Cell. Infect. Microbiol.* **2017**, *7*, 522. [CrossRef] [PubMed]

18. Bronzo, V.; Lopreiato, V.; Riva, F.; Amadori, M.; Curone, G.; Addis, M.F.; Cremonesi, P.; Moroni, P.; Trevisi, E.; Castiglioni, B. The Role of Innate Immune Response and Microbiome in Resilience of Dairy Cattle to Disease: The Mastitis Model. *Animals* **2020**, *10*, 1397. [CrossRef] [PubMed]
19. Pröll, M.J.; Neuhoff, C.; Schellander, K.; Uddin, M.J.; Cinar, M.U.; Sahadevan, S.; Qu, X.; Islam, M.A.; Müller, N.A.; Drosten, C.; et al. Transcriptome profile of lung dendritic cells after in vitro porcine reproductive and respiratory syndrome virus (PRRSV) infection. *PLoS ONE* **2017**, *12*, e0187735. [CrossRef]
20. Islam, M.A.; Neuhoff, C.; Rony, S.A.; Grosse-Brinkhaus, C.; Uddin, M.J.; Hoelker, M.; Tesfaye, D.; Tholen, E.; Schellander, K.; Proll-Cornilissen, M.J. PBMCs transcriptome profiles identified breed-specific transcriptome signatures for PRRSV vaccination in German Landrace and Pietrain pigs. *PLoS ONE* **2019**, *14*, e0222513. [CrossRef]
21. Chris, T. Transcriptomics today: Microarrays, RNA-seq, and more. *Science* **2015**, *349*, 544–546.
22. Spitzer, M.H.; Nolan, G.P. Mass Cytometry: Single Cells, Many Features. *Cell* **2016**, *165*, 780–791. [CrossRef]
23. Nishimura, T.; Kaneko, S.; Kawana-Tachikawa, A.; Tajima, Y.; Goto, H.; Zhu, D.; Nakayama-Hosoya, K.; Iriguchi, S.; Uemura, Y.; Shimizu, T.; et al. Generation of rejuvenated antigen-specific T cells by reprogramming to pluripotency and redifferentiation. *Cell Stem Cell* **2013**, *12*, 114–126. [CrossRef] [PubMed]
24. Mardis, E.R. DNA sequencing technologies: 2006–2016. *Nat. Protoc.* **2017**, *12*, 213–218. [CrossRef] [PubMed]
25. Lee, J.H.; Daugharthy, E.R.; Scheiman, J.; Kalhor, R.; Yang, J.L.; Ferrante, T.C.; Terry, R.; Jeanty, S.S.F.; Li, C.; Amamoto, R.; et al. Highly multiplexed subcellular RNA sequencing in situ. *Science* **2014**, *343*, 1360–1363. [CrossRef] [PubMed]
26. Lowe, R.; Shirley, N.; Bleackley, M.; Dolan, S.; Shafee, T. Transcriptomics technologies. *PLoS Comput. Biol.* **2017**, *13*, e1005457. [CrossRef] [PubMed]
27. Coskun, A.F.; Eser, U.; Islam, S. Cellular identity at the single-cell level. *Mol. BioSyst.* **2016**, *12*, 2965–2979. [CrossRef]
28. Huang, X.; Li, X.; Qin, P.; Zhu, Y.; Xu, S.; Chen, J. Technical Advances in Single-Cell RNA Sequencing and Applications in Normal and Malignant Hematopoiesis. *Front. Oncol.* **2018**, *8*, 582. [CrossRef]
29. Garalde, D.R.; Snell, E.A.; Jachimowicz, D.; Sipos, B.; Lloyd, J.H.; Bruce, M.; Pantic, N.; Admassu, T.; James, P.; Warland, A.; et al. Highly parallel direct RNA sequencing on an array of nanopores. *bioRXiv* **2016**. [CrossRef]
30. Oikonomopoulos, S.; Bayega, A.; Fahiminiya, S.; Djambazian, H.; Berube, P.; Ragoussis, J. Methodologies for Transcript Profiling Using Long-Read Technologies. *Front. Genet.* **2020**, *11*, 606. [CrossRef]
31. Goodwin, S.; Mcpherson, J.D.; Mccombie, W.R. Coming of age: Ten years of next-generation sequencing technologies. *Nat. Rev. Genet.* **2016**, *17*, 333–351. [CrossRef]
32. Harrow, J.; Frankish, A.; Gonzalez, J.M.; Tapanari, E.; Diekhans, M.; Kokocinski, F.; Aken, B.L.; Barrell, D.; Zadissa, A.; Searle, S.; et al. GENCODE: The reference human genome annotation for the ENCODE Project. *Genome Res.* **2012**, *22*, 1760–1774. [CrossRef]
33. Matlin, A.J.; Clark, F.; Smith, C.W. Understanding alternative splicing: Towards a cellular code. *Nat. Rev. Mol. Cell Biol.* **2005**, *6*, 386–398. [CrossRef] [PubMed]
34. Engstrom, P.G.; Steijger, T.; Sipos, B.; Grant, G.R.; Kahles, A.; Ratsch, G.; Goldman, N.; Hubbard, T.J.; Harrow, J.; Guigó, R.; et al. Systematic evaluation of spliced alignment programs for RNA-seq data. *Nat. Methods* **2013**, *10*, 1185–1191. [CrossRef] [PubMed]
35. Steijger, T.; Abril, J.F.; Engstrom, P.G.; Kokocinski, F.; Hubbard, T.J.; Guigo, R.; Harrow, J.; Bertone, P.; The RGASP Consortium. Assessment of transcript reconstruction methods for RNA-seq. *Nat. Methods* **2013**, *10*, 1177–1184. [CrossRef] [PubMed]
36. Cartolano, M.; Huettel, B.; Hartwig, B.; Reinhardt, R.; Schneeberger, K. cDNA library enrichment of full-length transcripts for smrt long read sequencing. *PLoS ONE* **2016**, *11*, e0157779. [CrossRef]
37. Huber, W.; Carey, V.J.; Gentleman, R.; Anders, S.; Carlson, M.; Carvalho, B.S.; Bravo, H.C.; Davis, S.; Gatto, L.; Girke, T.; et al. Orchestrating high-throughput genomic analysis with Bioconductor. *Nat. Methods* **2015**, *5*, 115–121. [CrossRef]
38. Krøigard, A.B.; Thomassen, M.; Lænkholm, A.-V.; Kruse TALarsen, M.J. Evaluation of Nine Somatic Variant Callers for Detection of Somatic Mutations in Exome and Targeted Deep Sequencing Data. *PLoS ONE* **2016**, *11*, e0151664. [CrossRef]
39. Hu, Z.-L.; Carissa, A.P.; James, M.R. Building a livestock genetic and genomic information knowledgebase through integrative developments of Animal QTLdb and CorrDB. *Nucleic Acids Res.* **2019**, *47*, D701–D710. [CrossRef]

40. Greiff, V.; Bhat, P.; Cook, S.C.; Menzel, U.; Kang, W.; Reddy, S.T. A bioinformatic framework for immune repertoire diversity profiling enables detection of immunological status. *Genome Med.* **2015**, *7*, 49. [CrossRef]
41. Subramanian, A.; Tamayo, P.; Mootha, V.K.; Mukherjee, S.; Ebert, B.L.; Gillette, M.A.; Paulovich, A.; Pomeroy, S.L.; Golub, T.R.; Lander, E.S.; et al. Gene set enrichment analysis: A knowledge-based approach for interpreting genome-wide expression profiles. *Proc. Natl. Acad. Sci. USA* **2005**, *102*, 15545–15550. [CrossRef]
42. Huang, D.W.; Sherman, B.T.; Lempicki, R.A. Systematic and integrative analysis of large gene lists using DAVID bioinformatics resources. *Nat. Protoc.* **2009**, *4*, 44–57. [CrossRef]
43. Breuer, K.; Amir, K.F.; Matthew, R.L.; Carol, C.; Anastasia, S.; Raymond, L.; Geoffrey, L.; Robert, E.W.H.; Fiona, S.L.B.; David, J.L. InnateDB: Systems biology of innate immunity and beyond—Recent updates and continuing curation. *Nucleic Acids Res.* **2013**, *41*, D1228–D1233. [CrossRef] [PubMed]
44. Fabregat, A.; Jupe, S.; Matthews, L.; Sidiropoulos, K.; Gillespie, M.; Garapati, P.; Haw, R.; Jassal, B.; Korninger, F.; May, B.; et al. The Reactome Pathway Knowledgebase. *Nucleic Acids Res.* **2018**, *46*, D649–D655. [CrossRef] [PubMed]
45. Elsik, C.G.; Unni, D.R.; Diesh, C.M.; Tayal, A.; Emery, M.L.; Nguyen, H.N.; Hagen, D.E. Bovine Genome Database: New tools for gleaning function from the Bos taurus genome. *Nucleic Acids Res.* **2016**, *44*, D834–D839. [CrossRef] [PubMed]
46. Mudunuri, U.; Che, A.; Yi, M.; Stephens, R.M. bioDBnet: The biological database network. *Bioinformatics* **2009**, *25*, 555–556. [CrossRef]
47. Szklarczyk, D.; Gable, A.L.; Lyon, D.; Junge, A.; Wyder, S.; Huerta-Cepas, J.; Simonovic, M.; Doncheva, N.T.; Morris, J.H.; Bork, P.; et al. STRING v11: Protein-protein association networks with increased coverage, supporting functional discovery in genome-wide experimental datasets. *Nucleic Acids Res.* **2019**, *47*, D607–D613. [CrossRef]
48. Zhou, G.; Soufan, O.; Ewald, J.; Hancock, R.E.W.; Basu, N.; Xia, J. NetworkAnalyst 3.0: A visual analytics platform for comprehensive gene expression profiling and meta-analysis. *Nucleic Acids Res.* **2019**, *47*, W234–W241. [CrossRef]
49. Langfelder, P.; Horvath, S. WGCNA: An R package for weighted correlation network analysis. *BMC Bioinform.* **2008**, *9*, 559. [CrossRef]
50. Shannon, P.; Markiel, A.; Ozier, O.; Baliga, N.S.; Wang, J.T.; Ramage, D.; Amin, N.; Schwikowski, B.; Ideker, T. Cytoscape: A software environment for integrated models of biomolecular interaction networks. *Genome Res.* **2003**, *13*, 2498–2504. [CrossRef]
51. Holt, R.A. Immunogenomics: A foundation for intelligent immune design. *Genome Med.* **2015**, *7*, 116. [CrossRef]
52. Tuggle, C.K.; Giuffra, E.; White, S.N.; Clarke, L.; Zhou, H.; Ross, P.J.; Acloque, H.; Reecy, J.M.; Archibald, A.; Bellone, R.R.; et al. GO-FAANG meeting: A Gathering on Functional Annotation of Animal Genomes. *Anim. Genet.* **2016**, *47*, 528–533. [CrossRef]
53. Doeschl-Wilson, A.B.; Bishop, S.C.; Kyriazakis, I.; Villanueva, B. Novel methods for quantifying individual host response to infectious pathogens for genetic analyses. *Front. Genet.* **2012**, *3*, 266. [CrossRef] [PubMed]
54. Wilkie, B.; Mallard, B. Selection for high immune response: An alternative approach to animal health maintenance? *Vet. Immunol. Immunopathol.* **1999**, *72*, 231–235. [CrossRef]
55. Rowland, R.R.; Lunney, J.; Dekkers, J. Control of porcine reproductive and respiratory syndrome (PRRS) through genetic improvements in disease resistance and tolerance. *Front. Genet.* **2012**, *3*, 260. [CrossRef]
56. Clapperton, M.; Diack, A.B.; Matika, O.; Glass, E.J.; Gladney, C.D.; Mellencamp, M.A.; Hoste, A.; Bishop, S.C. Traits associated with innate and adaptive immunity in pigs: Heritability and associations with performance under different health status conditions. *Genet. Sel. Evol.* **2009**, *41*, 54. [CrossRef] [PubMed]
57. Siegrist, C.-A. *Vaccine: General Aspects of Vaccinations*; Elsevier Health Sciences Saunders: Amsterdam, The Netherlands, 2012; pp. 17–36.
58. Glass, E.J. The molecular pathways underlying host resistance and tolerance to pathogens. *Front. Genet.* **2012**, *3*, 263. [CrossRef]
59. Edfors-Lilja, I.; Wattrang, E.; Magnusson, U.; Fossum, C. Genetic variation in parameters reflecting immune competence of swine. *Vet. Immunol. Immunopathol.* **1994**, *40*, 1–16. [CrossRef]
60. Schurch, N.J.; Schofield, P.; Gierliński, M.; Cole, C.; Sherstnev, A.; Singh, V.; Wrobel, N.; Gharbi, K.; Simpson, G.G.; Owen-Hughes, T.; et al. How many biological replicates are needed in an RNA-seq

experiment and which differential expression tool should you use? *RNA* **2016**, *22*, 839–851, [published correction appears in RNA. 2016, 22(10):1641]. [CrossRef]
61. Liu, X.S.; Mardis, E.R. Applications of Immunogenomics to Cancer. *Cell* **2017**, *168*, 600–612. [CrossRef]
62. Sweeney, T.; Hanrahan, J.P.; Ryan, M.T.; Good, B. Immunogenomics of gastrointestinal nematode infection in ruminants—Breeding for resistance to produce food sustainably and safely. *Parasite Immunol.* **2016**, *38*, 569–586. [CrossRef]
63. Sodeland, M.; Kent, M.P.; Olsen, H.G.; Opsal, M.A.; Svendsen, M.; Sehested, E.; Hayes, B.J.; Lien, S. Quantitative trait loci for clinical mastitis on chromosomes 2, 6, 14 and 20 in Norwegian Red cattle. *Anim. Genet.* **2011**, *42*, 457–465. [CrossRef]
64. Meredith, B.K.; Berry, D.P.; Kearney, F.; Finlay, E.K.; Fahey, A.G.; Bradley, D.G.; Lynn, D.J. A genome-wide association study for somatic cell score using the Illumina high-density bovine beadchip identifies several novel QTL potentially related to mastitis susceptibility. *Front. Genet.* **2013**, *4*, 229. [CrossRef] [PubMed]
65. Wijga, S.; Bastiaansen, J.W.; Wall, E.; Strandberg, E.; de Haas, Y.; Giblin, L.; Bovenhuis, H. Genomic associations with somatic cell score in first-lactation Holstein cows. *J. Dairy Sci.* **2012**, *95*, 899–908. [CrossRef] [PubMed]
66. Lewandowska-Sabat, A.M.; Gunther, J.; Seyfert, H.M.; Olsaker, I. Combining quantitative trait loci and heterogeneous microarray data analyses reveals putative candidate pathways affecting mastitis in cattle. *Anim. Genet.* **2012**, *43*, 793–799. [CrossRef] [PubMed]
67. Islam, M.A.; Takagi, M.; Fukuyama, K.; Komatsu, R.; Albarracin, L.; Nochi, T.; Suda, Y.; Ikeda-Ohtsubo, W.; Rutten, V.; Eden, V.W.; et al. Transcriptome analysis of inflammatory responses of bovine mammary epithelial cells: Exploring immunomodulatory target genes for bovine mastitis. *Pathogens* **2020**, *9*, 200. [CrossRef] [PubMed]
68. Palmiter, R.D.; Brinster, R.L.; Hammer, R.E.; Trumbauer, M.E.; Rosenfeld, M.G.; Birnberg, N.C.; Evans, R.M. Dramatic growth of mice that develop from eggs microinjected with metallothionein-growth hormone fusion genes. *Nature* **1982**, *300*, 611–615. [CrossRef]
69. Ivics, Z.; Hackett, P.B.; Plasterk, R.H.; Izsvák, Z. Molecular reconstruction of Sleeping Beauty, a Tc1-like transposon from fish, and its transposition in human cells. *Cell* **1997**, *91*, 501–510. [CrossRef]
70. Chevalier, B.S.; Stoddard, B.L. Homing endonucleases: Structural and functional insight into the catalysts of intron/intein mobility. *Nucleic Acids Res.* **2001**, *29*, 3757–3774. [CrossRef]
71. Moore, F.E.; Reyon, D.; Sander, J.D.; Martinez, S.A.; Blackburn, J.S.; Khayter, C.; Ramirez, C.L.; Joung, J.K.; Langenau, D.M. Improved Somatic Mutagenesis in Zebrafish Using Transcription Activator-Like Effector Nucleases (TALENs). *PLoS ONE* **2012**, *7*, e37877. [CrossRef]
72. Belfort, M.; Bonocora, R.P. Homing endonucleases: From genetic anomalies to programmable genomic clippers. *Methods Mol. Biol.* **2014**, *1123*, 1–26. [CrossRef]
73. Joung, J.K.; Sander, J.D. TALENs: A widely applicable technology for targeted genome editing. *Nat. Rev. Mol. Cell Biol.* **2013**, *14*, 49–55. [CrossRef]
74. Kim, Y.G.; Cha, J.; Chandrasegaran, S. Hybrid restriction enzymes: Zinc finger fusions to Fok I cleavage domain. *Proc. Natl. Acad. Sci. USA* **1996**, *93*, 1156–1160. [CrossRef] [PubMed]
75. Christian, M.; Cermak, T.; Doyle, E.L.; Schmidt, C.; Zhang, F.; Hummel, A.; Bogdanove, A.J.; Voytas, D.F. Targeting DNA double-strand breaks with TAL effector nucleases. *Genetics* **2010**, *186*, 757–761. [CrossRef] [PubMed]
76. Ran, F.A.; Hsu, P.D.; Wright, J.; Agarwala, V.; Scott, D.A.; Zhang, F. Genome engineering using the CRISPR-Cas9 system. *Nat. Protoc.* **2013**, *8*, 2281–2308. [CrossRef] [PubMed]
77. Doudna, J.A.; Charpentier, E. Genome editing. The new frontier of genome engineering with CRISPR-Cas9. *Science* **2014**, *346*, 1258096. [CrossRef]
78. Shao, Y.; Guan, Y.; Wang, L.; Qiu, Z.; Liu, M.; Chen, Y.; Wu, L.; Li, Y.; Ma, X.; Liu, M.; et al. CRISPR/Cas-mediated genome editing in the rat via direct injection of one-cell embryos. *Nat. Protoc.* **2014**, *9*, 2493–2512. [CrossRef]
79. Harwood, W.; Proudfoot, C.; Burkard, C. Genome editing for disease resistance in livestock. *Emerg. Top. Life Sci.* **2017**, *1*, 209–219. [CrossRef]
80. Lee, H.; Yoon, D.E.; Kim, K. Genome editing methods in animal models. *Anim. Cells Syst.* **2020**, *24*, 8–16. [CrossRef]

81. Zhao, J.; Lai, L.; Ji, W.; Zhou, Q. Genome editing in large animals: Current status and future prospects. *Nat. Sci. Rev.* **2019**, *6*, 402–420. [CrossRef]
82. Shrock, E.; Güell, M. *CRISPR in Animals and Animal Models*; Academic Press: Cambridge, MA, USA, 2017; pp. 95–114. [CrossRef]
83. Anderson, R.M.; May, R.M. *Infectious Diseases of Humans: Dynamics and Control*; Oxford University Press: New York, NY, USA, 1991; Available online: https://global.oup.com/academic/product/infectious-diseases-of-humans-9780198540403?cc=gb&lang=en& (accessed on 26 July 2020).
84. Wall, R.J.; Powell, A.M.; Paape, M.J.; Kerr, D.E.; Bannerman, D.D.; Pursel, V.G.; Wells, K.D.; Talbot, N.; Hawk, H.W. Genetically enhanced cows resist intramammary Staphylococcus aureus infection. *Nat. Biotechnol.* **2005**, *23*, 445–451. [CrossRef]
85. Yu, S.; Luo, J.; Song, Z.; Ding, F.; Dai, Y.; Li, N. Highly efficient modification of beta-lactoglobulin (BLG) gene via zinc-finger nucleases in cattle. *Cell Res.* **2011**, *21*, 1638–1640. [CrossRef]
86. Carlson, D.F.; Tan, W.; Lillico, S.G.; Stverakova, D.; Proudfoot, C.; Christian, M.; Fahrenkrug, S.C. Efficient TALEN-mediated gene knockout in livestock. *Proc. Natl. Acad. Sci. USA* **2012**, *109*, 17382–17387. [CrossRef] [PubMed]
87. Carlson, D.F.; Lancto, C.A.; Zang, B.; Kim, E.S.; Walton, M.; Oldeschulte, D.; Fahrenkrug, S.C. Production of hornless dairy cattle from genome-edited cell lines. *Nat. Biotechnol.* **2016**, *34*, 479–481. [CrossRef] [PubMed]
88. Maga, E.A.; Cullor, J.S.; Smith, W.; Anderson, G.B.; Murray, J.D. Human lysozyme expressed in the mammary gland of transgenic dairy goats can inhibit the growth of bacteria that cause mastitis and the cold-spoilage of milk. *Foodborne Pathog. Dis.* **2006**, *3*, 384–392. [CrossRef] [PubMed]
89. Gao, Y.; Wu, H.; Wang, Y.; Liu, X.; Chen, L.; Li, Q.; Cui, C.; Liu, X.; Zhang, J.; Zhang, Y. Single Cas9 nickase induced generation of NRAMP1 knockin cattle with reduced off-target effects. *Genome Biol.* **2017**, *18*, 13. [CrossRef] [PubMed]
90. Tuggle, C.K.; Waters, W.R. Tuberculosis-resistant transgenic cattle. *Proc. Natl. Acad. Sci. USA* **2015**, *112*, 3854–3855. [CrossRef]
91. Lu, T.; Song, Z.; Li, Q.; Li, Z.; Wang, M.; Liu, L.; Tian, K.; Li, N. Overexpression of histone deacetylase 6 enhances resistance to porcine reproductive and respiratory syndrome virus in pigs. *PLoS ONE* **2017**, *12*, e0169317. [CrossRef]
92. Islam, M.A.; Große-Brinkhaus, C.; Pröll, M.J.; Uddin, M.J.; Rony, S.A.; Tesfaye, D.; Tholen, E.; Hölker, M.; Schellander, K.; Neuhoff, C. Deciphering transcriptome profiles of peripheral blood mononuclear cells in response to PRRSV vaccination in pigs. *BMC Genom.* **2016**, *17*, 641. [CrossRef]
93. Islam, M.A.; Große-Brinkhaus, C.; Pröll, M.J.; Uddin, M.J.; Rony, S.A.; Tesfaye, D.; Tholen, E.; Hoelker, M.; Schellander, K.; Neuhoff, C. PBMC transcriptome profiles identifies potential candidate genes and functional networks controlling the innate and the adaptive immune response to PRRSV vaccine in Pietrain pig. *PLoS ONE* **2017**, *12*, e0171828. [CrossRef]
94. Van Gorp, H.; Van Breedam, W.; Delputte, P.L.; Nauwynck, H.J. The porcine reproductive and respiratory syndrome virus requires trafficking through CD163-positive early endosomes, but not late endosomes, for productive infection. *Arch. Virol.* **2009**, *154*, 1939–1943. [CrossRef]
95. Duan, X.; Nauwynck, H.J.; Favoreel, H.W.; Pensaert, M.B. Identification of a putative receptor for porcine reproductive and respiratory syndrome virus on porcine alveolar macrophages. *J. Virol.* **1998**, *72*, 4520–4523. [CrossRef]
96. Whitworth, K.M.; Rowland, R.R.; Ewen, C.L.; Trible, B.R.; Kerrigan, M.A.; Cino-Ozuna, A.G.; Samuel, M.S.; Lightner, J.E.; McLaren, D.G.; Mileham, A.J.; et al. Gene-edited pigs are protected from porcine reproductive and respiratory syndrome virus. *Nat. Biotechnol.* **2016**, *34*, 20–22. [CrossRef]
97. Burkard, C.; Lillico, S.G.; Reid, E.; Jackson, B.; Mileham, A.J.; Ait-Ali, T.; Whitelaw, C.B.; Archibald, A.L. Precision engineering for PRRSV resistance in pigs: Macrophages from genome edited pigs lacking CD163 SRCR5 domain are fully resistant to both PRRSV genotypes while maintaining biological function. *PLoS Pathog.* **2017**, *13*, e1006206. [CrossRef] [PubMed]
98. Palgrave, C.J.; Gilmour, L.; Lowden, C.S.; Lillico, S.G.; Mellencamp, M.A.; Whitelaw, C.B.A. Species-specific variation in RELA underlies differences in NF-κB activity: A potential role in african swine fever pathogenesis. *J. Virol.* **2011**, *85*, 6008–6014. [CrossRef] [PubMed]

99. Lillico, S.G.; Proudfoot, C.; King, T.J.; Tan, W.; Zhang, L.; Mardjuki, R.; Paschon, D.E.; Rebar, E.J.; Urnov, F.D.; Mileham, A.J.; et al. Mammalian interspecies substitution of immune modulatory alleles by genome editing. *Sci. Rep.* **2016**, *6*, 21645. [CrossRef] [PubMed]
100. Michel, A.L.; Müller, B.; van Helden, P.D. Mycobacterium bovis at the animal–human interface: A problem, or not? *Vet. Microbiol.* **2010**, *140*, 371–381. [CrossRef] [PubMed]
101. Wu, H.; Wang, Y.; Zhang, Y.; Yang, M.; Lv, J.; Liu, J.; Zhang, Y. TALE nickase-mediated SP110 knockin endows cattle with increased resistance to tuberculosis. *Proc. Natl. Acad. Sci. USA* **2015**, *112*, E1530–E1539. [CrossRef] [PubMed]
102. Shanthalingam, S.; Tibary, A.; Beever, J.E.; Kasinathan, P.; Brown, W.C.; Srikumaran, S. Precise gene editing paves the way for derivation of Mannheimia haemolytica leukotoxin-resistant cattle. *Proc. Natl. Acad. Sci. USA* **2016**, *113*, 13186–13190. [CrossRef]
103. Ishii, T. Genome-edited livestock: Ethics and social acceptance. *Anim. Front.* **2017**, *7*. [CrossRef]
104. Bruce, A. Genome edited animals: Learning from GO crops? *Transgenic Res.* **2017**, *26*, 385–398. [CrossRef]
105. Araki, M.; Ishii, T. Towards social acceptance of plant breeding by genome editing. *Trends Plant Sci.* **2015**, *20*, 145–149. [CrossRef]

6

Genetics of Arthrogryposis and Macroglossia in Piemontese Cattle Breed

Liliana Di Stasio [1,*], Andrea Albera [2], Alfredo Pauciullo [1], Alberto Cesarani [3], Nicolò P. P. Macciotta [3] and Giustino Gaspa [1]

[1] Department of Agricultural, Forest and Food Sciences, University of Torino, Largo Baccini 2, 10095 Grugliasco (TO), Italy; alfredo.pauciullo@unito.it (A.P.); giustino.gaspa@unito.it (G.G.)
[2] Associazione Nazionale Allevatori Bovini di Razza Piemontese, strada provinciale Trinita' 31/A, 12061 Carrù (CN), Italy; andrea.albera@anaborapi.it
[3] Department of Agriculture, University of Sassari, Via De Nicola 9, 07100 Sassari, Italy; acesarani@uniss.it (A.C.); macciott@uniss.it (N.P.P.M.)
* Correspondence: liliana.distasio@unito.it

Simple Summary: The study was carried out in order to investigate the genetic background of arthrogryposis and macroglossia in the Piemontese cattle breed, for which limited information is available so far. The genotyping of affected and healthy animals with a high-density chip and the subsequent genome-wide association study did not evidence a single strong association with the two pathologies. Therefore, for arthrogryposis, the results do not support the existence of a single-gene model, as reported for other breeds. Rather, 23 significant markers on different chromosomes were found, associated to arthrogryposis, to macroglossia, or to both pathologies, suggesting a more complex genetic mechanism underlying both diseases in the Piemontese breed. The significant single nucleotide polymorphisms (SNPs) allowed the identification of some genes (*NTN3*, *KCNH1*, *KCNH2*, and *KANK3*) for which a possible role in the pathologies can be hypothesized. The real involvement of these genes needs to be further investigated and validated.

Abstract: Arthrogryposis and macroglossia are congenital pathologies known in several cattle breeds, including Piemontese. As variations in single genes were identified as responsible for arthrogryposis in some breeds, we decided: (i) to test the hypothesis of a similar genetic determinism for arthrogryposis in the Piemontese breed by genotyping affected and healthy animals with a high-density chip and applying genome-wide association study (GWAS), F_{ST} and canonical discriminant analysis (CDA) procedures, and (ii) to investigate with the same approach the genetic background of macroglossia, for which no genetic studies exist so far. The study included 125 animals (63 healthy, 30 with arthrogryposis, and 32 with macroglossia). Differently from what reported for other breeds, the analysis did not evidence a single strong association with the two pathologies. Rather, 23 significant markers on different chromosomes were found (7 associated to arthrogryposis, 11 to macroglossia, and 5 to both pathologies), suggesting a multifactorial genetic mechanism underlying both diseases in the Piemontese breed. In the 100-kb interval surrounding the significant SNPs, 20 and 26 genes were identified for arthrogryposis and macroglossia, respectively, with 12 genes in common to both diseases. For some genes (*NTN3*, *KCNH1*, *KCNH2*, and *KANK3*), a possible role in the pathologies can be hypothesized, being involved in processes related to muscular or nervous tissue development. The real involvement of these genes needs to be further investigated and validated.

Keywords: Piemontese breed; arthrogryposis; macroglossia; genetic model

---

1. Introduction

Arthrogryposis and macroglossia have long been known as congenital abnormalities observed in several cattle breeds [1,2]. Arthrogryposis is characterized by joints contractures with different degrees of severity, which can affect one to four legs, with various associated clinical signs, the most frequent being cleft palate [3]. More than one etiologic event, such as plant toxicosis [4], prenatal viral infections, and a possible hereditary component, have been reported as responsible for the disease occurrence [5]. Less information is available for macroglossia, which consists in the swelling of the tongue that may interfere with the calf's ability to nurse. The defect is thought to have a genetic basis, but no scientific evidence is available so far.

For both defects, double muscling is considered as a predisposing factor. Already back in the 1963, Lauvergne et al. [6] listed rickets-like troubles and macroglossia among the clinical signs displayed by the hypertrophied animals. The observation that the manipulation of the myostatin gene and, more specifically, the downregulation of its expression resulted in a series of adverse effects, including leg problems and macroglossia, which seems to confirm the negative influence of double muscling [7]. Moreover, macroglossia is one of the primary features of the human Wiedemann-Beckwith syndrome (OMIM 130650), which is clinically similar to muscular hypertrophy in cattle [8].

Both arthrogryposis and macroglossia have been reported for decades in the hypertrophied Piemontese cattle breed. Since the end of 1980s, the National Association of the Piemontese cattle Breeders (ANABORAPI) started to select against these two pathologies by culling Artificial Insemination (AI) bulls with a high percentage of affected progeny. A decrease from 2.74% to 0.34% and from 2.36% to 0.28% in the occurrence of arthrogryposis and macroglossia, respectively, were obtained in the period 1990–2017 (Supplemental Figure S1) as a consequence of this selection strategy (ANABORAPI).

These data seem to support the hypothesis of a genetic background for the defects, but the few investigations in the Piemontese breed did not give conclusive results. Huston et al. [3] suggested that, in the Piemontese, arthrogryposis could be determined by an incompletely penetrant recessive allele, with higher penetrance in males, which seems to be consistent with the ANABORAPI data (Supplemental Figure S1). However, a genome-wide association study carried out on Piemontese calves affected by arthrogryposis and macroglossia genotyped with a medium density (50 K) single nucleotide polymorphism (SNP) BeadChip did not detect clear signals of association for both pathologies [9]. On the contrary, recent studies detected variations in single genes as responsible for arthrogryposis in Angus [10], Swiss Holstein [11], Belgian Blue [12], and Red Danish [13] cattle breeds.

Therefore, the aims of this study were: (i) to test the hypothesis of a similar monogenic determinism for arthrogryposis in the Piemontese cattle breed by genotyping affected and healthy animals with a high-density chip never used in previous studies and applying genome-wide association study (GWAS), F_{ST} and canonical discriminant analysis (CDA) procedures, and (ii) to investigate with the same approach the genetic background of macroglossia, for which no information is available so far.

2. Materials and Methods

2.1. Ethics Statement

No animals were used in the present study. The biological samples belonged to collections available from the ANABORAPI institutional activity. For this reason, the Animal Care and Use Committee approval was not necessary.

2.2. Animals, Genotyping, and Data Editing

Animals affected by arthrogryposis or macroglossia were found and sampled by the veterinarians of the ANABORAPI during the routine inspections in the farms registered in the Herd Book of the Piemontese breed. The phenotypic expression of arthrogryposis in the Piemontese breed is very variable, ranging from moderate contracture of the legs to more severe expressions that can be only surgically corrected. As this variability could represent a confounding factor, only animals with extreme expressions of the defect (Supplemental Figure S2a) were considered. Moreover, as in about 3% of the affected animals the two pathologies coexist, only animals affected by a single pathology, arthrogryposis or macroglossia (Supplemental Figure S2), were included in the study, in order to avoid a further confounding effect.

Blood samples were collected from a total of 98 Piemontese male veals: 17 affected by arthrogryposis (Ar), 18 affected by macroglossia (Ma), and 63 healthy (He). The Ar, Ma, and He subjects were distributed in 17, 15, and 59 herds, respectively. All these animals were genotyped with the customized GeneSeek® Genomic Profiler™ Bovine 150 K (Lincoln, NE, USA). As it was difficult to collect a larger number of affected animals for their low incidence due the selection policy, we decided to include 31 additional subjects (16 affected by arthrogryposis and 15 by macroglossia) previously genotyped with the Illumina® BovineSNP50v2 (San Diego, CA, USA). Both 150 K and 50 K markers were mapped on the ARS-UCD1.2 and subjected to quality checks (QC). The QC was performed using PLINK v.1.923 [14] independently for each dataset using the following filters: SNPs with missing rate > 0.02, minor allele frequency (MAF) < 0.05 or deviating from Hardy-Weinberg equilibrium (p-values < 10^{-6}) were discarded; moreover, only autosomal SNPs with known genomic positions were considered for further analysis. On the subjects' side, both SNP missingness per individual (>0.02) and individual heterozygosity deviations caused an animal to be removed from the datasets. After data editing, 94 and 31 veals were left in 150 K and 50 K, respectively. Then, the default settings of Beagle software [15] were applied for imputing the 50-K genotypes at 150 K on the whole dataset, obtaining a group of 125 animals (63 He, 30 Ar, and 32 Ma). This dataset was then split into two subsets of 93 (He + Ar) and 95 (He + Ma) individuals each that underwent a new round of QC with the aforementioned settings. A total of 100,791 and 100,907 SNPs were analyzed for the Ar and Ma subsets, respectively.

2.3. Statistical Analysis

A genome-wide association study (GWAS) was conducted using two separate case-control designs for the two syndromes following the approaches of [16,17]. The individuals involved in this study were weakly or not related. The genomic relationship matrix off-diagonal elements were, on average, −0.03, −0.03, and −0.02 for Ar, Ma, and He animals, respectively. The negative relatedness values signify that the individuals have genotypes less similar in expectation than the average. The affected and healthy animals were respectively assigned to cases or controls prior to test the allelic associations (–assoc flag in PLINK) performed by a X^2 test. Genomic-control adjusted p-values were plotted against the genomic position for the two analyzed diseases. To tackle the multiple testing issue that arises when thousands of hypotheses are simultaneously tested, we decided to consider as significant the associations with false discovery rate (FDR) [18] below 0.05 using the –adjust flag in PLINK [14]. On the same two datasets, F_{ST} analysis was conducted using the Weir and Cockerham [19] estimator implemented in PLINK, and those SNPs exceeding the 99.9th percentile threshold were retained. Then, the F_{ST} outliers were merged with SNPs resulting from the GWAS, obtaining two sets of SNPs associated to Ar and Ma, respectively. In order to corroborate the GWAS results, the canonical discriminant analysis (CDA) was run on the top significant SNPs associated to both diseases, jointly considering all the animals and using the CANDISC procedures of SAS software (Sas Institute, Cary, NC, USA). The correlation structure between the top ranked SNPs was used to derive new variables, namely canonical discriminant variables (CAN), able to maximize the separation between predefined groups [20]. If S is the $n \times p$ matrix of the p SNP genotypes (coded as 0, 1, or 2 for the "aa", "Aa", or "AA" genotypes, respectively) measured in n animals belonging to k groups (three in our cases: Ar, Ma, and He), the ith CAN may be calculated as

$$\mathrm{CAN_i} = \mathrm{w_{i1}s_1} + \mathrm{w_{i2}s_2} + \cdots + \mathrm{w_{ip}s_p} \tag{1}$$

where s_i are the centered SNP genotypes and $\mathrm{w_{ip}}$ are the raw canonical coefficients for the p analyzed SNP (i.e., the weights of each SNP in the discriminant function). The vectors of coefficients w were obtained with a procedure that involves the eigen-decomposition of a linear transformation of between- and within-group SNP (co)variance matrices [20].

2.4. Candidate Gene Detection

Annotated genes were retrieved in the region of 100-kilo base pairs (kb) (50-kb down- and upstream, respectively) surrounding each SNP highlighted by the combined use of GWAS and F_{ST}. The National Center for Biotechnology Information (NCBI) (http://www.ncbi.nlm.nih.gov) and UCSC Genome Browser Gateway (http://genome.ucsc.edu/) databases were used.

3. Results

3.1. Genome-wide Association Study and F_{ST}

The results of the genome-wide case-control study are shown in Figure 1, which reports the −log10 of genomic-control adjusted p-values for the two diseases; in green are highlighted the SNPs that exceeded the chosen threshold. The factor λ was 1.11 and 1.17 for Ar and Ma, respectively, indicating a slight inflation of the statistical test. Quantile-quantile (QQ) plots of the ordered p-values for the Ar and Ma case-control GWAS (Supplemental Figure S3) showed that few SNPs strongly deviate from the diagonal identity lines for both diseases.

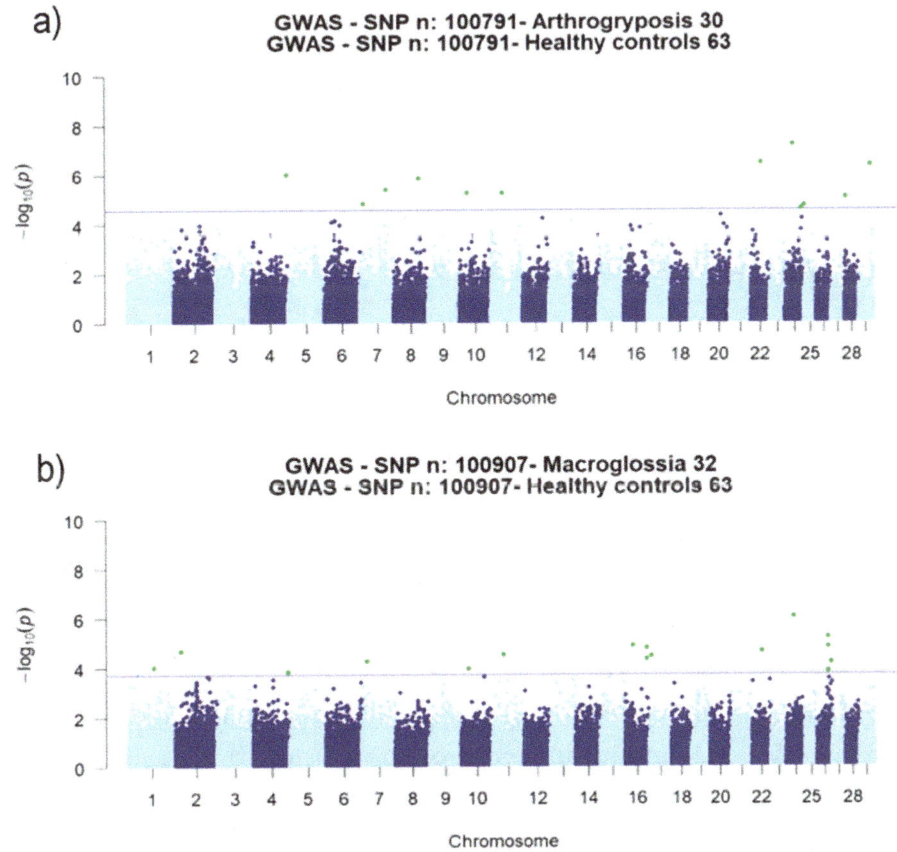

Figure 1. Manhattan plots. (**a**) Healthy vs. arthrogryposis and (**b**) healthy vs. macroglossia. GWAS: genome-wide association study and SNP: single nucleotide polymorphism.

The F_{ST} analysis enabled to highlight 102 and 101 outlier SNPs for Ar and Ma, respectively, (Supplemental Tables S1 and S2) that overcame the 99.9th percentile threshold (Ar vs. He: 0.1401 and Ma vs. He: 0.1425) (Supplemental Figure S4). The combined GWAS and F_{ST} approaches were able to identify 23 SNPs that were considered in a further analysis. In particular, seven SNPs were exclusively associated with arthrogryposis (on *Bos taurus* chromosomes, BTAs, 7, 8, 24, 25, 28, and 29) and 11 exclusively with macroglossia (on BTAs 1, 2, 7, 16, 17, and 26), whereas five markers (on BTAs 4, 11, 22, and 24) were in common to both pathologies (Table 1). Consistently, those SNPs presented MAF values markedly deviating in the two groups of animals, as also highlighted by the F_{ST} values (from 0.217 to 0.336 and from 0.200 to 0.319 for Ar and Ma, respectively) compared with healthy samples (Supplemental Table S3).

Table 1. Relevant markers found by the genome-wide association study (GWAS) and F_{ST} analysis and raw canonical coefficients (CC) associated to significant single nucleotide polymorphisms (SNPs). Within-class average scores for the two discriminant functions (Can1 and Can2). CC: canonical coefficients.

SNP	GWAS		Raw CC	
	BTA [1]	Disease [2]	Can1	Can2
ARS-BFGL-NGS-13673	1	Ma	0.63	0.52
ARS-USDA-AGIL-chr2-17084934-000418	2	Ma	0.27	0.59
ARS-USDA-AGIL-chr4-114395607-000108	4	Ar, Ma	−0.19	0.05
ARS-USDA-AGIL-chr7-12174899-000752	7	Ar	−0.18	−0.14
Hapmap44668-BTA-119022	7	Ar	0.62	−0.26
ARS-USDA-AGIL-chr7-18201332-000761	7	Ma	0.66	0.88
ARS-USDA-AGIL-chr8-84099468-000783	8	Ar	−0.15	−0.72
ARS-USDA-AGIL-chr10-25594159-000176	10	Ar, Ma	−0.37	0.15
ARS-USDA-AGIL-chr11-36809347-000009	11	Ar, Ma	−0.16	0.22
ARS-BFGL-NGS-15423	16	Ma	0.02	0.02
BovineHD1600007856	16	Ma	0.37	0.25
BovineHD4100012725	16	Ma	0.72	−0.11
ARS-USDA-AGIL-chr17-6999864-000318	17	Ma	−0.09	−0.17
ARS-USDA-AGIL-chr22-32285822-000477	22	Ar, Ma	0.19	−0.08
BovineHD2400015279	24	Ar	−0.57	0.56
ARS-USDA-AGIL-chr24-25995108-000530	24	Ar, Ma	−0.17	−0.47
ARS-USDA-AGIL-chr25-1930875-000536	25	Ar	−0.12	0.45
BovineHD4100017966	26	Ma	−0.02	−0.78
BovineHD2600011259	26	Ma	0.31	0.42
BovineHD2600011282	26	Ma	0.42	0.5
BovineHD2600014129	26	Ma	0.59	0.85
BovineHD2800000629	28	Ar	0.56	−1.17
ARS-USDA-AGIL-chr29-39842168-000583	29	Ar	−0.40	−0.65
Within-class average				
Arthrogryposis		Ar	1.23	−1.55
Macroglossia		Ma	2.03	1.13
Healthy control		He	−1.62	0.16

[1] *Bos taurus* chromosome; [2] Ar: arthrogryposis and Ma: macroglossia.

3.2. Canonical Discriminant Analysis

The analysis of the squared Mahalanobis distances computed using the top significant SNPs indicated that affected (Ar or Ma) and healthy controls statistically differ ($p < 0.001$) as well as Ar and Ma did within affected animals (Supplemental Table S4).

The results of the CDA carried out using the significant markers identified by the GWAS and F_{ST} are presented in Figure 2 and Table 1. The two canonical functions explained 75% and 25% of the variance, respectively. When the individual samples were plotted in the new coordinate system defined by the first two discriminant functions, a clear, albeit imperfect, separation between the affected (regardless of the pathology) and the healthy subjects was highlighted (Figure 2). The animals with positive CAN1 scores are mostly the affected animals. In addition, CAN2 allowed to separate the subjects affected by arthrogryposis (with negative scores on CAN2) from those affected by macroglossia (with positive scores), as confirmed by the within-class (Ar, Ma, or He) average scores for CAN1 and CAN2 (Table 1).

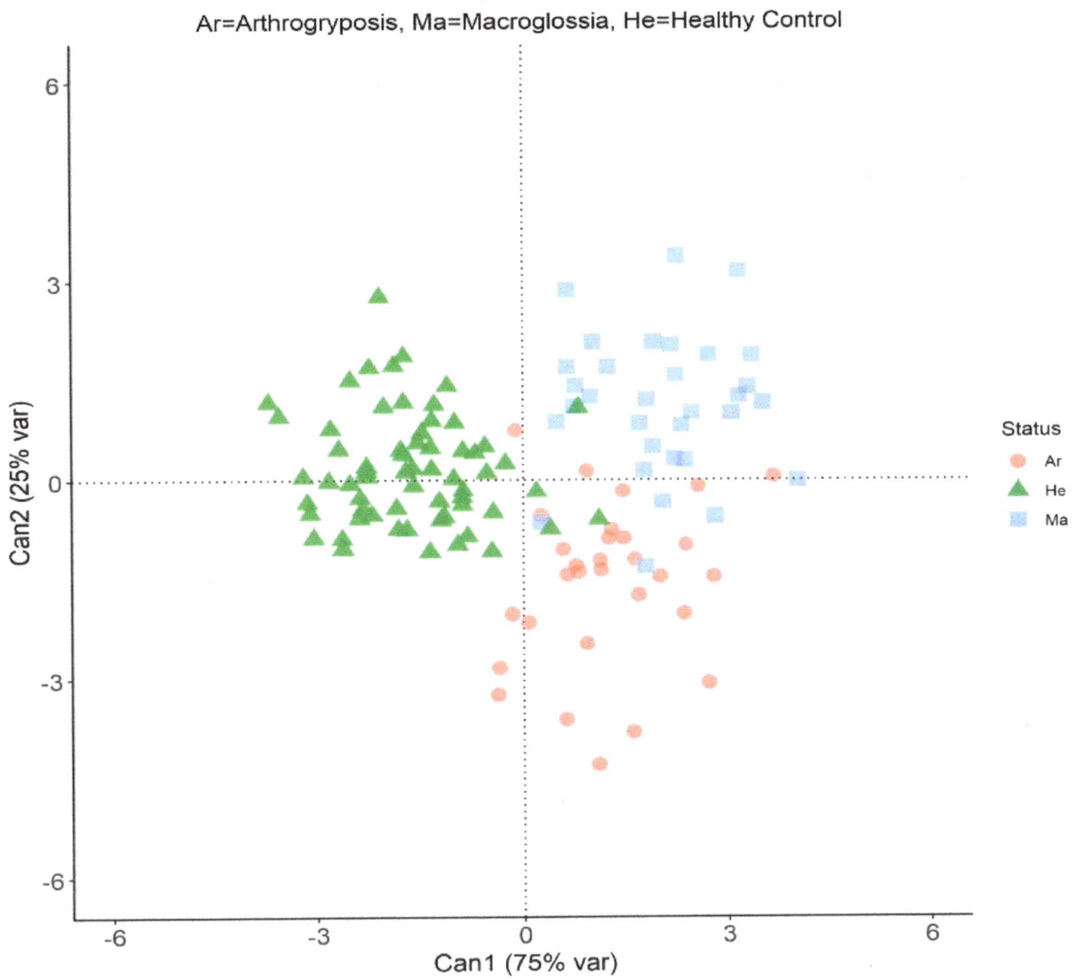

Figure 2. Plot of the individual scores on the two canonical variables (Can1 and Can2) depicted in different colors and symbols according to their health status.

The raw canonical coefficients for the identified SNPs had mainly large positive weights for Ma (ranging from −0.09 to 0.72) and negative weights for Ar, even with some exceptions (from −0.57 to 0.62). A rather elusive pattern was ascertained looking at the most deviating canonical weight; conversely, the selected SNPs jointly were able to discriminate between groups of animals. This seems also confirmed looking at the canonical correlation between the SNP genotype and CAN variables (Supplemental Figure S5).

3.3. Candidate Gene Detection

The lists of genes that mapped in the interval of 100 kb surrounding the significant SNPs and that may be putatively associated with the diseases are reported in Tables 2 and 3. As for arthrogryposis, a total of 20 genes were identified in the considered interval, and eight of them included a significant marker, while, for macroglossia, 26 genes were mapped in the highlighted regions, with 10 of them including a marker. Of the identified genes, 12 were in common to both investigated diseases (Tables 2 and 3).

Table 2. Genes near the SNPs associated to arthrogryposis. The genes including a marker are in bold.

BTA	SNP		Gene		
	Name	Position	Symbol	Name	Location
4	ARS-USDA-AGIL-chr4-114395607-000108	113,596,650	*KCNH2*	Potassium voltage-gated channel, sub-family H, member 2	113,526,185..113,562,025
			NOS3	Nitric oxide synthase 3	113,577,075..113,595,527
			ATG9B	**Autophagy-related 9B**	113,594,821..113,605,878
			ABCB8	ATP binding cassette subfamily B member 8	113,605,775..113,623,178
			ASIC3	acid sensing ion channel subunit 3	113,624,088..113,629,085
7	ARS-USDA-AGIL-chr7-12174899-000752	11,085,449	***ZNF333***	**zinc finger protein 333**	11,071,151..11,102,144
			ADGRE3	adhesion G protein-coupled receptor E3	11,116,555..11,181,632
	Hapmap44668-BTA-119022	85,227,970	//	no genes in the considered interval	
8	ARS-USDA-AGIL-chr8-84099468-000783	82,677,581	***ERCC6L2***	**ERCC excision repair 6 like 2**	82,557,942..82,712,671
10	ARS-USDA-AGIL-chr10-25594159-000176	25,539,231	***OR4E2***	**olfactory receptor, family 4, subfamily E, member 2**	25,539,229..25,540,170
			OR10G2	olfactory receptor, family 10, subfamily G, member 2	25,587,007..25,587,963
11	ARS-USDA-AGIL-chr11-36809347-000009	36,957,396	***ACYP2***	**acylphosphatase 2**	36,831,155..37,010,456
			TSPYL6	**TSPY like 6**	36,954,224..36,957,858
22	ARS-USDA-AGIL-chr22-32285822-000477	32,169,050	***FRMD4B***	**FERM domain containing 4B**	32,022,767..32,382,939
24	ARS-USDA-AGIL-chr24-25995108-000530	25,684,356	*DSG2*	desmoglein 2	25,602,973..25,653,973
			DSG3	**desmoglein 3**	25,666,298..25,699,081
			DSG4	desmoglein 4	25,725,711..25,755,364
	BovineHD2400015279	53,288,962	//	no genes in the considered interval	
25	ARS-USDA-AGIL-chr25-1930875-000536	1,929,340	*CCNF*	cyclin F	1,947,654..1,965,422
			TEDC2	tubulin epsilon and delta complex 2	1,966,625..1,970,947
			NTN3	netrin 3	1,975,804..1,978,415
28	BovineHD2800000629	2,661,658	//	no genes in the considered interval	
29	ARS-USDA-AGIL-chr29-39842168-000583	39,215,494	*PAG9*	pregnancy-associated glycoprotein 9	39,237,412..39,246,707
1	ARS-BFGL-NGS-13673	86,784,250	//	no genes in the considered interval	
2	ARS-USDA-AGIL-chr2-17084934-000418	17,077,000	***ZNF385B***	**zinc finger protein 385B**	16,957,646..17,442,243
			TRNAC-ACA	transfer RNA cysteine	17,082,352..17,082,423

Table 3. Genes near the SNPs associated to macroglossia. The genes including a marker are in bold.

BTA	SNP		Gene		
	Name	Position	Symbol	Name	Location
4	ARS-USDA-AGIL-chr4-114395607-000108	113,596,650	*KCNH2*	potassium voltage-gated channel, sub-family H, member 2	113,526,185..113,562,025
			NOS3	nitric oxide synthase 3	113,577,075..113,595,527
			ATG9B	**autophagy related 9B**	113,594,821..113,605,878
			ABCB8	ATP binding cassette subfamily B member 8	113,605,775..113,623,178
			ASIC3	acid-sensing ion channel subunit 3	113,624,088..113,629,085
7	ARS-USDA-AGIL-chr7-18201332-000761	16,970,401	*CERS4*	ceramide synthase 4	16,897,965..16,933,292
			CD320	CD320 molecule	16,952,355..16,957,071
			NDUFA7	NADH:ubiquinone oxidoreductase subunit A7	16,960,703..16,967,936
			RPS28	ribosomal protein S28	16,968,061..16,969,193
			KANK3	**KN motif and ankyrin repeat domains 3**	16,969,360..16,980,814
			ANGPTL4	angiopoietin like 4	17,005,585..17,012,655
10	ARS-USDA-AGIL-chr10-25594159-000176	25,539,231	***OR4E2***	**olfactory receptor, family 4, subfamily E, member 2**	25,539,229..25,540,170
			OR10G2	olfactory receptor, family 10, subfamily G, member 2	25,587,007..25,587,963
11	ARS-USDA-AGIL-chr11-36809347-000009	36,957,396	***ACYP2***	**acylphosphatase 2**	36,831,155..37,010,456
			TSPYL6	**TSPY like 6**	36,954,224..36,957,858
16	BovineHD1600007856	27,494,192	***NVL***	**nuclear valosin-containing protein-like**	27,322,130..27,502,627
			CNIH4	cornichon family AMPA receptor auxiliary protein 4	27,529,034..27,543,276
	ARS-BFGL-NGS-15423 BovineHD4100012725	72,258,249 72,266,300	***KCNH1***	**potassium voltage-gated channel subfamily H member 1**	72,205,829..72,642,416
17	ARS-USDA-AGIL-chr17-6999864-000318	7,013,884	***LRBA***	**lipopolysaccharide responsive beige-like anchor protein**	6,799,299..7,556,716
22	ARS-USDA-AGIL-chr22-32285822-000477	32,169,050	***FRMD4B***	**FERM domain containing 4B**	32,022,767..32,382,939
24	ARS-USDA-AGIL-chr24-25995108-000530	25,684,356	*DSG2*	desmoglein 2	25,602,973..25,653,973
			DSG3	**desmoglein 3**	25,666,298..25,699,081
			DSG4	desmoglein 4	25,725,711..25,755,364
26	BovineHD4100017966 BovineHD2600011259 BovineHD2600011282	40,441,709 40,460,199 40,517,972	***PLPP4***	**phospholipid phosphatase 4**	40,509,729..40,656,785
	BovineHD2600014129	48,680,201	//	no genes in the considered interval	

4. Discussion

The present study provides new data on the genetics of arthrogryposis and the first insight into the analysis of macroglossia in the Piemontese breed. An important systematic bias in GWAS often reported in the literature is caused by population stratification due to ethnic/breed admixture and/or close relationships among individuals of case-control studies [21,22]. In our case, a limited inflation of the statistical tests was observed; thus, a genomic-control approach was adopted, since the individuals included in the design belonged to the same breed and were weakly or not related [21].

Interestingly, the combined use of case-control GWAS, F_{ST}, and CDA highlighted several markers potentially associated with the investigated syndromes. The use of multiple approaches is generally advised in genome-wide analysis [17,23,24]. The use of CDA was recently proposed as an effective tool for improving the discovery rate either alone or in a combination with GWAS, especially when the sample size is reduced [25].

As for arthrogryposis, the results depict a situation different from what was observed in the other investigated breeds [10–13], where variations in single genes were identified as responsible for the disease. In fact, our data did not evidence a single strong association with the pathology, while they highlighted a number of significant markers located on different chromosomes, suggesting a polygenic mechanism underlying the disease. The joint role of these markers is supported by their ability to separate the three groups of animals according to their health status.

None of the markers for arthrogryposis identified in the Piemontese breed are located within or near the genes reported as causing the disease in the other breeds. In this respect, it is important to underline that also the causal variations found in those breeds were of different types and in different genes: a large deletion encompassing three genes (BTA 16) in Angus [10], a missense mutation in the *MYBPC1* gene (BTA 5) in Swiss Holstein [11], a splicing variant in the *PIGH* gene (BTA 10) in Belgian Blue [12], and a small deletion in the *CHRNB1* gene (BTA 19) in Red Danish [13]. This implies that the genetic determinism of arthrogryposis is not the same in the affected breeds. On the other hand, it must be considered that a large variability in the phenotypic expression of what is called "arthrogryposis" was observed in the breeds studied so far, from lethal consequences, as in Belgian Blue or Angus breeds, to less severe problems, as in the Piemontese. Additionally, at least six types of arthrogryposis with different clinical signs and grades of severity were reviewed by Huston et al. [3] in cattle. Such heterogeneity makes it difficult to clearly define the trait that could explain the differences observed at the genetic level. In all cases, however, the findings of the different studies are compatible with the autosomal recessive mode of inheritance suggested since the earliest studies. The incidences of the two pathologies in the Piemontese breed in the last decades also showed a trend compatible with the case of selection against the recessive phenotype, and this led us to hypothesize the existence of a monogenic determinism similar to what was observed in the other cattle breeds. However, the present data do not support this hypothesis, suggesting that a more complex mechanism is responsible for the disease in the Piemontese breed.

For macroglossia, no previous genetic data exist. The results of the current study highlight a situation comparable to that obtained for arthrogryposis, so that a multifactorial mechanism can be hypothesized also for macroglossia.

The identified SNPs were located within or close to 33 genes, of which 9 and 13 were exclusive for arthrogryposis and macroglossia, respectively, and 11 common to the two pathologies. This is worthy of note, considering that, in the Piemontese breed, both pathologies are sometimes observed in the same animal. Thus, the findings of this study might suggest that the putative candidate genes common to both diseases could be involved in basic physiological processes common to both defects.

In the case of arthrogryposis, seven of the relevant SNPs mapped in coding genes, whereas, for macroglossia, 11 SNPs were located within coding genes. In some cases, it is unclear from the gene annotations their possible involvement in the pathologies. Instead, for other genes, a possible role can be hypothesized, as their products are part of processes related to muscular or nervous tissue developments whose defects are included among the common causes of the pathologies here considered [26].

Among these genes, Netrin3 (*NTN3*) encodes a member (NTN3) of a family of extracellular proteins that act as chemotropic guidance cues for migrating cells and axons during neural development [27]. In mice, it was demonstrated that NTN3 is expressed in muscle cells, and therefore, it may play a role in guiding peripheral axons to their corrected muscle targets [28].

Additionally, *KCNH1* (potassium voltage-gated channel subfamily H member 1) and *KCNH2* (potassium voltage-gated channel subfamily H member 2) genes code for proteins that belong to a complex protein superfamily widely distributed during embryonic development and involved in a wide variety of cell functions. In mice, the two genes are co-expressed in the skeletal muscle during embryogenesis, including the cranial, thoracic, and limb regions [29]. In man, KCNH1 was shown to be involved in myoblast fusion, a complex process that includes withdrawal from the cell cycle, cell-cell interactions, adhesion, alignment, and a final membrane fusion to form the multinucleated skeletal muscle fiber [30].

A possible role can be also suggested for the *KANK3* (KN motif and ankyrin repeat domains 3) gene strongly expressed in different body compartments, including the skeletal muscle, and involved in the control of cytoskeleton formation by negatively regulating actin polymerization [31].

5. Conclusions

The overall findings indicate that the genetic determinism of arthrogryposis and macroglossia in the Piemontese breed is more complex than previously believed. In fact, the results do not support the existence of a single-gene model, while suggesting a multifactorial genetic mechanism underlying the investigated pathologies. Several markers significantly associated with both diseases were found, and genes possibly affecting the traits were identified. The real involvement of these genes needs to be further investigated and validated.

Supplementary Materials:
Figure S1: Trend of arthrogryposis and macroglossia in the Piemontese breed: Incidence from 1990 to 2017. Figure S2: Affected Piemontese veals: (**a**) arthrogryposis and (**b**) macroglossia. Figure S3: Quantile-quantile plot for the case-control genome-wide analysis (in red, the identity line). Figure S4: Distribution of F_{ST} values and threshold line of the 99.9th percentile of the ranked F_{ST} values for arthrogryposis and macroglossia vs. the healthy control. Figure S5: Canonical correlation between Can1, Can2, and the original SNP results significantly associated with the disease status, represented by different colors. SNPs associated with arthrogryposis (Ar), macroglossia (Ma), or both (Ar_Ma). Table S1: F_{ST} outliers (99.9% of ranked F_{ST}, threshold value: 0.140158) from the arthrogryposis vs. healthy control comparison (n = 102). Table S2: F_{ST} outliers (99.9% of ranked F_{ST}, threshold value: 0.1425518) from the macroglossia vs. healthy control comparison (n = 101). Table S3: Statistics of the significant markers in common between the GWAS and F_{ST} analysis. Table S4: Quadratic distance between the animals affected and healthy controls for each comparison.

Author Contributions: Conceptualization, L.D.S. and A.A.; formal analysis, G.G., A.C., and N.P.P.M.; investigation, L.D.S., A.A., and A.P.; resources, L.D.S.; data curation, G.G.; writing—original draft preparation, L.D.S. and G.G.; writing—review and editing, L.D.S., A.A., A.P., A.C., N.P.P.M., and G.G.; supervision, L.D.S.; and funding acquisition, L.D.S. All authors have read and agreed to the published version of the manuscript.

References

1. Hutt, F.B. A hereditary lethal muscle contracture in cattle. *J. Hered.* **1934**, *25*, 41–46. [CrossRef]
2. Leipold, H.W.; Cates, W.F.; Radostis, O.M.; Howell, W.E. Arthrogryposis and associated defects in newborn calves. *Am. J. Vet. Res.* **1970**, *31*, 1367–1374. [PubMed]
3. Huston, K.; Saperstein, G.; Steffen, D.; Millar, P.; Lauvergne, J.J. Clinical, pathological and other visible traits loci except coat colour (category 2). In *Mendelian Inheritance in Cattle 2000*; Millar, P., Lauvergne, J.J., Dolling, C., Eds.; EAAP Publication: Wageningen, The Netherlands, 2000; Volume 101, pp. 164–175.
4. Shupe, J.L.; Binns, W.; James, L.F.; Keeler, R.F. Lupine, a cause of crooked calf disease. *J. Am. Vet. Med. Assoc.* **1967**, *151*, 198–203.

5. Anderson, D.E.; Desrochers, A.; St. Jean, G. Management of Tendon Disorders in Cattle. *Vet. Clin. N. Am. Food Anim. Pract.* **2008**, *24*, 551–566. [CrossRef]
6. Lauvergne, J.J.; Vissac, B.; Perramon, A. Étude du caractère culard. I. Mise au point bibliographique. Annales de zootechnie, INRA/EDP. *Sciences* **1963**, *12*, 133–156.
7. Webb, E.C.; Casey, N.H. Physiological limits to growth and the related effects on meat quality. *Livest. Sci.* **2010**, *130*, 33–40. [CrossRef]
8. Best, L.G.; Gilbert-Barness, E.; Gerrard, D.E.; Gendron-Fitzpatrick, A.; Opitz, J.M. "Double-Muscle" trait in cattle: A possible model for Wiedemann-Beckwith Syndrome. *Fetal Pediatr. Pathol.* **2006**, *25*, 9–20. [CrossRef]
9. Biscarini, F.; Del Corvo, M.; Stella, A.; Alber, A.; Ferencakovic, M.; Pollo, G. Busqueda de las mutaciones causales para artrogriposis y macroglosia en vacuno de raza piemontesa: Resultados preliminares. In Proceedings of the XV Jornadas sobre Producción Animal, Zaragoza, Spain, 14–15 May 2013; Volume II, pp. 538–540.
10. Beever, J.E.; Marron, B.M. Screening for Arthrogryposis Multiplex in Bovines. U.S. Patent 20,110,151,440 A1, 23 June 2011.
11. Wiedemar, N.; Riedi, A.K.; Jagannathan, V.; Drögemüller, C.; Meylan, M. Genetic abnormalities in a calf with congenital increased muscular tonus. *J. Vet. Intern. Med.* **2015**, *29*, 1418–1421. [CrossRef]
12. Sartelet, A.; Li, W.; Pailhoux, E.; Richard, C.; Tamma, N.; Karim, L.; Fasquelle, C.; Druet, T.; Coppieters, W.; Georges, M.; et al. Genome-wide next-generation DNA and RNA sequencing reveals a mutation that perturbs splicing of the phosphatidylinositol glycan anchor biosynthesis class H gene (PIGH) and causes arthrogryposis in Belgian Blue cattle. *BMC Genom.* **2015**, *16*, 316–323. [CrossRef]
13. Agerholm, J.S.; McEvoy, F.J.; Menzi, F.; Jagannathan, V.; Drögemüller, C.A. CHRNB1 frameshift mutation is associated with familial arthrogryposis multiplex congenita in Red dairy cattle. *BMC Genom.* **2016**, *17*, 479. [CrossRef]
14. Chang, C.C.; Chow, C.C.; Tellier, L.C.A.M.; Vattikuti, S.; Purcell, S.M.; Lee, J.J. Second-generation PLINK: Rising to the challenge of larger and richer datasets. *GigaScience* **2015**, 4. [CrossRef] [PubMed]
15. Browning, B.L.; Browning, S.R. Genotype imputation with millions of reference samples. *Am. J. Hum. Genet.* **2016**, *98*, 116–126. [CrossRef] [PubMed]
16. Kijas, J.W.; Hadfield, T.; Naval Sanchez, M.; Cockett, N. Genome-wide association reveals the locus responsible for four-horned ruminant. *Anim. Genet.* **2016**, *47*, 258–262. [CrossRef] [PubMed]
17. Mastrangelo, S.; Sottile, G.; Sardina, M.T.; Sutera, A.M.; Tolone, M.; Di Gerlando, R.; Portolano, B. A combined genome-wide approach identifies a new potential candidate marker associated with the coat color sidedness in cattle. *Livest. Sci.* **2019**, *225*, 91–95. [CrossRef]
18. Benjamini, Y.; Hochberg, Y. Controlling the false discovery rate: A practical and powerful approach to multiple testing. *J. R. Stat. Soc. B Methodol.* **1995**, *57*, 289–300. [CrossRef]
19. Weir, B.S.; Cockerham, C.C. Estimating F-statistics for the analysis of population structure. *Evolution* **1984**, *38*, 1358–1370.
20. Sorbolini, S.; Gaspa, G.; Steri, R.; Dimauro, C.; Cellesi, M.; Stella, A.; Marras, G.; Ajmone Marsan, P.; Valentini, A.; Macciotta, N.P.P. Use of canonical discriminant analysis to study signatures of selection in cattle. *Genet. Sel. Evol.* **2016**, *48*, 58. [CrossRef]
21. Aulchencko, Y.S. Effects of Population Structure in Genome-wide Association Studies in Analysis of complex Disease Association Study. In *Analysis of Complex Disease Association Studies*, 1st ed.; Zeggini, E., Morris, A., Eds.; Accademic Press: London, UK, 2011; Chapter 9; pp. 123–156. ISBN 9780123751430.
22. Price, A.L.; Patterson, N.J.; Plenge, R.M.; Weinblatt, M.E.; Shadick, N.A.; Reich, D. Principal components analysis corrects for stratification in genome-wide association studies. *Nat. Genet.* **2006**, *38*, 904–909. [CrossRef]
23. Cornetti, L.; Tschirren, B. Combining genome-wide association study and FST-based approaches to identify targets of Borrelia-mediated selection in natural rodent hosts. *Mol. Ecol.* **2020**, *29*, 386–1397. [CrossRef]
24. Cesarani, A.; Sechi, T.; Gaspa, G.; Usai, M.G.; Sorbolini, S.; Macciotta, N.P.P.; Carta, A. Investigation of genetic diversity and selection signatures between Sarda and Sardinian Ancestral black, two related sheep breeds with evident morphological differences. *Small Rumin. Res.* **2019**, *177*, 68–75. [CrossRef]
25. Manca, E.; Cesarani, A.; Gaspa, G.; Sorbolini, S.; Macciotta, N.P.; Dimauro, C. Use of the Multivariate Discriminant Analysis for Genome-Wide Association Studies in Cattle. *Animals* **2020**, *10*, 1300. [CrossRef] [PubMed]

26. Windsor, P.A.; Kessell, A.E.; Finnie, J.W. Neurological diseases of ruminant livestock in Australia. V: Congenital neurogenetic disorders of cattle. *Aust. Vet. J.* **2011**, *89*, 394–401. [CrossRef] [PubMed]
27. Sathyanath, R.; Kennedy, T.E. The Netrin Protein Family. *Genome Biol.* **2009**, *10*, 239. [CrossRef]
28. Wang, H.; Copeland, N.G.; Gilbert, D.J.; Jenkins, N.A.; Tessier-Lavigne, M. Netrin-3, a Mouse Homolog of Human NTN2L, Is Highly Expressed in Sensory Ganglia and Shows Differential Binding to Netrin Receptors. *J. Neurosci.* **1999**, *19*, 4938–4947. [CrossRef]
29. De Castro, M.P.; Aránega, A.; Franco, D. Protein Distribution of Kcnq1, Kcnq2, and Kcnq3 Potassium Channel Subunits during Mouse embryonic Development. *Anat. Rec.* **2006**, *288*, 304–315. [CrossRef]
30. Occhiodoro, T.; Bernheim, L.; Liu, J.H.; Bijlenga, P.; Sinnreich, M.; Bader, C.R.; Fischer-Lougheed, J. Cloning of a Human Ether-a-Go-Go Potassium Channel Expressed in Myoblasts at the Onset of Fusion. *FEBS Lett.* **1998**, *434*, 177–182. [CrossRef]
31. Zhu, Y.; Kakinuma, N.; Wang, Y.; Kiyama, R. Kank Proteins: A New Family of Ankyrin-Repeat Domain-Containing Proteins. *BBA-Gen. Subj.* **2008**, *1780*, 128–133. [CrossRef]

7

Embryonic Thermal Manipulation Affects the Antioxidant Response to Post-Hatch Thermal Exposure in Broiler Chickens

Khaled M. M. Saleh [1], Amneh H. Tarkhan [1] and Mohammad Borhan Al-Zghoul [2,*]

1 Department of Applied Biological Sciences, Faculty of Science and Arts, Jordan University of Science and Technology, P.O. Box 3030, Irbid 22110, Jordan; khaledmousa93@gmail.com (K.M.M.S.); amneht92@gmail.com (A.H.T.)

2 Department of Basic Medical Veterinary Sciences, Faculty of Veterinary Medicine, Jordan University of Science and Technology, P.O. Box 3030, Irbid 22110, Jordan

* Correspondence: alzghoul@just.edu.jo;

Simple Summary: The broiler chicken is one of the most important livestock species in the world, as it occupies a major role in the modern human diet. Due to uneven artificial selection pressures, the broiler has increased in size over the past few decades at the expense of its ability to withstand oxidative damage, the latter of which is often a byproduct of thermal stress. In order to attenuate the effects of heat stress, thermal manipulation (TM), which involves changes in incubation temperature at certain points of embryonic development, is increasingly being presented as a way in which to improve broiler thermotolerance. Therefore, the objective of this study was to investigate how TM might affect broiler response to post-hatch thermal stress in the context of the genes that help combat oxidative damage, namely the catalase, NADPH oxidase 4 (*NOX4*), and superoxide dismutase 2 (*SOD2*) genes. Expression of all three aforementioned genes differed significantly between TM and control chickens after exposure to cold and heat stress. Conclusively, TM may act as a viable mode of preventative treatment for broilers at risk of thermally induced oxidative stress.

Abstract: Thermal stress is a major source of oxidative damage in the broiler chicken (*Gallus gallus domesticus*) due to the latter's impaired metabolic function. While heat stress has been extensively studied in broilers, the effects of cold stress on broiler physiologic and oxidative function are still relatively unknown. The present study aimed to understand how thermal manipulation (TM) might affect a broiler's oxidative response to post-hatch thermal stress in terms of the mRNA expression of the catalase, NADPH oxidase 4 (*NOX4*), and superoxide dismutase 2 (*SOD2*) genes. During embryonic days 10 to 18, TM was carried out by raising the temperature to 39 °C at 65% relative humidity for 18 h/day. To induce heat stress, room temperature was raised from 21 to 35 °C during post-hatch days (PD) 28 to 35, while cold stress was induced during PD 32 to 37 by lowering the room temperature from 21 to 16 °C. At the end of the thermal stress periods, a number of chickens were euthanized to extract hepatic and splenic tissue from the heat-stressed group and cardiac, hepatic, muscular, and splenic tissue from the cold-stressed group. Catalase, *NOX4*, and *SOD2* expression in the heart, liver, and spleen were decreased in TM chickens compared to controls after both cold and heat stress. In contrast, the expression levels of these genes in the breast muscles of the TM group were increased or not affected. Moreover, TM chicks possessed an increased body weight (BW) and decreased cloacal temperature (T^C) compared to controls on PD 37. In addition, TM led to increased BW and lower T^C after both cold and heat stress. Conclusively, our findings suggest that TM has a significant effect on the oxidative function of thermally stressed broilers.

Keywords: broiler; thermal manipulation; antioxidant; heat stress; cold stress

1. Introduction

The term broiler refers to any member of the red junglefowl subspecies, *Gallus gallus domesticus*, that has been reared for the purposes of meat production and consumption [1]. Constituting the largest standing avian population, the broiler has become a vital component of modern human nutrition as a result of the rapid industrialization of the poultry production process [2]. Since the mid-twentieth century, broilers have undergone intensive breeding in order to enhance their growth rates, meat yield, and feed conversion ratios [3]. However, these artificial selection pressures have been largely consumer-driven, focusing solely on improving certain commercially attractive parameters at the expense of immune, metabolic, and skeletal function [4]. As a result, the modern broiler has become increasingly susceptible to the effects of thermal and, in turn, oxidative stresses [5].

Due to impaired metabolic function and expensive energetics, broilers are especially vulnerable to heat stress, which occurs when the broiler is unable to adequately dissipate body heat to the environment [6]. Rising global temperatures have consolidated the threats of heat stress to the development and wellbeing of broiler chickens, and such increases in temperature are exacerbated during the hotter seasons [7]. In addition, broiler heat stress can be caused by certain stages of the poultry production process, especially during their transport from rearing to processing facilities [8]. Broilers subject to heat stress will have a lower body weight due to decreased feed intake, and their innate immune function will be impaired as a result of decreased immune organ weight [9]. In fact, it has been illustrated that heat stress results in oxidative stress in broilers, resulting in a number of adverse metabolic changes [10].

Heat stress is a major cause of oxidative stress in broilers, and oxidative damage deteriorates the appearance, flavor, and nutritional value of broiler meat [11]. Oxidative stress can be defined as the imbalance that occurs when the amount of reactive oxygen species (ROS) in an animal cell exceeds the latter's antioxidant capacity [12]. To prevent oxidative stress, several genes are involved in the maintenance of cellular homeostasis, including NADPH oxidase 4 (*NOX4*), superoxide dismutase (*SOD2*), and catalase [13,14]. Primarily expressed in renal and vascular cells, the *NOX4* gene is constitutively active and codes for an oxygen-sensing enzyme that can also play a role in antimicrobial defense [15–17]. If overexpressed, *NOX4* leads to oxidative stress due to its production of superoxide (O_2^-) radicals and hydrogen peroxide (H_2O_2) molecules [18,19]. To prevent NOX4-associated oxidative stress from occurring, SOD2 and catalase act to dismutate O_2^- and break down H_2O_2, respectively [20].

Unlike heat stress, cold stress in broilers has not been the subject of much research in the context of its relation to oxidative stress. Nonetheless, cold stress has been found to induce oxidative stress and modulate immune function in broilers while also increasing their susceptibility to necrotic enteritis and ascites development [21–25]. Moreover, cold stress was found to affect the thigh muscle of broilers more severely than the breast muscle, and it significantly reduced the feed intake and body weights of broilers but increased their feed conversion ratios [26,27]. As outdoor rearing systems gain more popularity, preventing cold stress will become increasingly costly to the poultry industry, and such costs often fluctuate depending on fuel prices, season, and existing heating systems [28].

To mitigate the damage caused by heat and cold stress, thermal manipulation (TM), which involves embryonic exposure to high or low temperatures, has been found to improve thermotolerance and enhance physiological parameters of broilers [13,29–33]. However, further research needs to be carried out in order to understand the effects of heat- and cold-induced oxidative stress in thermally manipulated broilers. Therefore, the main purpose of the present study was to investigate the effects of both cold and heat stress on the antioxidant defense mechanisms of thermally manipulated broiler chickens.

2. Materials and Methods

Ethical approval for all experimental procedures was obtained from the Animal Care and Use Committee at Jordan University of Science and Technology (approval # 16/3/3/418).

2.1. *Egg Procurement and Incubation*

Fertile Cobb eggs (n = 600) were obtained from local distributors based in Madaba, Jordan. Before incubation, eggs were thoroughly examined, and eggs were excluded if they displayed abnormality or damage (n = 69). The remaining eggs (n = 531) were then randomly divided into two groups, control (n = 266) and thermal manipulation (TM) (n = 265), and incubated in semi-commercial incubators (Masalles S.L., Barcelona, Spain). In the control group, eggs were incubated under standard conditions (37.8 °C and 56% relative humidity (RH)) throughout embryogenesis. In contrast, TM eggs were only incubated under standard conditions from embryonic days (ED) 1 to 9 and 19 to 21, as TM was applied from ED 10 to 18 by incubating the eggs at 39 °C and 65% RH for 18 h/day. On ED 7, candling was performed on each egg in order to exclude infertile and/or nonviable eggs.

2.2. *Hatchery Management*

On hatch day, the hatchability, which is the percentage of fertile eggs that hatch, was calculated according to the following equation: hatchability = (number of hatched chicks/total number of incubated eggs) × 100. Chicks were left in the incubator to dry for the first 24 h of their post-hatch life, after which they were transported to a special area designated for the field experiments. On post-hatch days (PD) 1 and 37, the cloacal temperatures (T^C) and body weights (BW) were recorded, and the number of chicks that died within the whole field experimental period was noted. Dead chickens were histopathologically examined, but no significant obvious findings were reported. Before exposure to thermal stress, chicks were randomly distributed into their coops in groups of ten. In the first week, the temperature of the enclosures was kept at 33 ± 1 °C and was steadily reduced to 24 °C by the end of the third week. The RH during the rearing period was maintained within a range of 45%–52%. Water and appropriate feed were supplied to the chicks ad libitum during the whole field experiment period. On PD 8 and 20, chicks were vaccinated against Newcastle disease, and, on PD 15, the chicks were vaccinated against infectious bursal disease. The overall experimental design is illustrated in Figure 1.

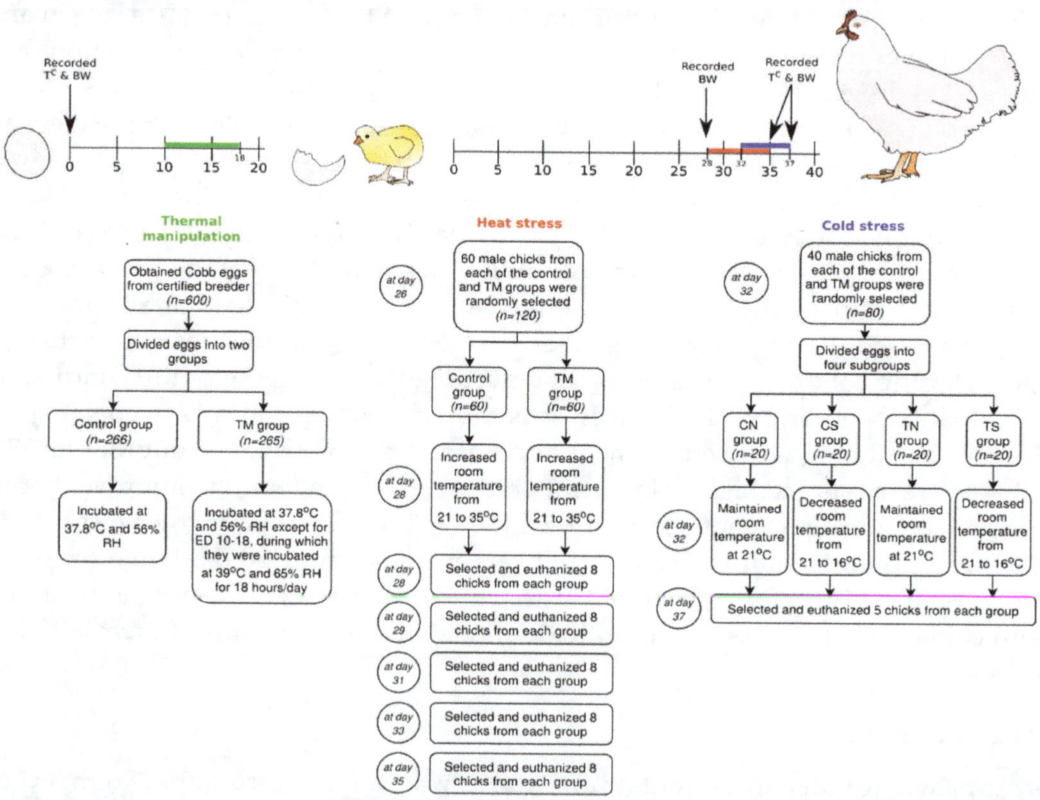

Figure 1. Experimental design showing the three main phases: thermal manipulation, heat stress, and cold stress.

2.3. Experiment 1: Post-Hatch Heat Exposure

On PD 26, male chicks (n = 60) were randomly selected from each of the control and TM groups to be transported to the experimental room for the induction of heat stress. On PD 28, heat stress was induced by raising the temperature of the experimental room to 35 °C and 45%–52% RH until PD 35. During this period, male chicks (n = 60) from each of the control and TM groups were subject to normal conditions (not shown in Figure 1). The experimental and rearing rooms were located on the same floor in order to mitigate transport stress. After 0, 1, 3, 5, and 7 days of heat exposure, chicks (n = 8) were randomly chosen from the control and TM groups. The T^C and BW of the chicks were recorded, after which they were euthanized in order to collect hepatic and splenic organs. Samples were snap-frozen on-site using liquid nitrogen, transferred to the laboratory, and stored at −80 °C.

2.4. Experiment 2: Post-Hatch Cold Exposure

On PD 32, chicks (n = 40) from each of the two incubation groups (control group and TM group) were randomly chosen and subdivided into four subgroups: control exposed to cold stress (CS), TM exposed to cold stress (TS), control exposed to normal conditions (CN) and TM exposed to normal conditions (TN). Cold stress was achieved by lowering the room temperature to 16 °C and 45%–52% RH from PD 32 to 37. At PD 37, BW and T^C were recorded for chicks (n = 5) from each subgroup, and a number of chicks (n = 5) were humanely euthanized in order to collect the liver, spleen, heart, and breast muscle organs. Samples were snap-frozen on-site using liquid nitrogen, transferred to the laboratory, and stored at −80 °C.

2.5. cDNA Synthesis

The Direct-Zol™ RNA MiniPrep (Zymo Research, Irvine, CA, USA) was utilized alongside TRI Reagent® (Zymo Research, Irvine, CA, USA) in order to isolate total RNA from all the collected samples. The Biotek PowerWave XS2 Spectrophotometer (BioTek Instruments, Inc., Winooski, VT, USA) was employed to determine the quantity and quality of the samples, after which 2 µg of total RNA from each sample were inputted into the Superscript III cDNA Synthesis Kit (Invitrogen, Carlsbad, CA, USA) to synthesize cDNA.

2.6. Primer Design and Relative mRNA Quantitation Analysis by Real-Time RT-PCR

The primer sequences that were used for real-time RT-PCR analysis are listed in Table 1. Primers were taken from previous reports [34] and were designed using the PrimerQuest tool on the Integrated DNA Technologies website (Coralville, IA, USA) (https://eu.idtdna.com/pages) and the Nucleotide database on the NCBI (Bethesda, MA, USA) website (https://www.ncbi.nlm.nih.gov/nucleotide/). The QuantiFast SYBR® Green PCR Kit (Qiagen, Hilden, Germany) was utilized on a Rotor-Gene Q MDx 5 plex instrument (Qiagen, USA) according to the manufacturer's protocol. For the internal control, fold changes in gene expression were normalized against the 28S ribosomal RNA. Single target amplification specificity was ensured by the melting curve, and relative quantitation was calculated automatically by the software on the Rotor-Gene Q MDx 5 plex instrument.

Table 1. Primer sequences used for real-time RT-PCR analysis.

Gene	Forward (5′ to 3′)	Reverse (5′ to 3′)
NOX4	CCAGACCAACTTAGAGGAACAC	TCTGGGAAAGGCTCAGTAGTA
SOD2	CTGACCTGCCTTACGACTATG	CGCCTCTTTGTATTTCTCCTCT
Catalase	GAAGCAGAGAGGTTCCCATTTA	CATACGCCATCTGTTCTACCTC
28S rRNA	CCTGAATCCCGAGGTTAACTATT	GAGGTGCGGCTTATCATCTATC

2.7. Statistical Analysis

IBM SPSS Statistics v23.0 (IBM, USA) was used for all statistical analyses performed in the current study. The chi-squared test was used to analyze hatchability and mortality rates. T^C, BW, and the fold changes in mRNA levels of the catalase, *NOX4*, and *SOD2* genes are portrayed as means ± SD. An independent t-test compared between the control and TM groups with respect to several parameters at each time interval (PD 1, 3, 5, 7, 9, 11, 13, 15, 19, 22, 25, 28, 30, 33 and 35). Within the treatment group itself, two-way ANOVA was also used to compare between different parameters at specific time intervals after thermal stress. Statistical significance for parametric differences was set at 0.05.

3. Results

3.1. Effect of Thermal Manipulation (TM) on Hatchability and Physiological Parameters of Broiler Chicks

No significant effect was observed in either the mortality (control = 1.7; TM = 1.7) or the hatchability (control = 85.71; TM = 83.02) rates between the control and TM groups. However, TM led to significantly lower cloacal temperatures (T^C) on PD 1 and 37 and to higher body weights (BW) on PD 37. However, no significant change was observed in hatchling BW (Table 2).

Table 2. Effects of embryonic thermal manipulation (TM) on post-hatch body weight (BW) and cloacal temperature (T^C) of broiler chickens.

	Post-Hatch Day	Control	TM
T^C (°C)	1	39.63 ± 0.24 ^{a}	39.48 ± 0.23 ^{b}
	37	39.05 ± 0.24 ^{a}	38.38 ± 0.22 ^{b}
BW (g)	1	44.2 ± 3.8 ^{a}	42.7 ± 2.8 ^{a}
	37	2302.8 ± 79.7 ^{a}	2440 ± 82.5 ^{b}

^{a,b} within the same row, means ± SD with non-identical superscripts are significantly different.

3.2. Effect of Post-Hatch Heat Stress on Physiological Parameters of Thermally Manipulated Broilers

Table 3 illustrates the effects of heat stress for 7 days (PD 28 to 35) on T^C, BW, and BW gain in the controls and TM broiler chickens. TM significantly decreased the mortality rate during post-hatch heat exposure (control = 12%; TM = 8%). Moreover, heat stress significantly increased the T^C in both groups, but the T^C of controls was significantly higher compared to TM chicks. On day 0 (PD 28) of heat stress, the BW of the TM group was significantly higher than that in controls. Similarly, the BW of controls was significantly lower compared to TM chicks on day 7 (PD 35) of heat stress, but the subgroups exposed to heat stress possessed significantly lower BW and BW gain compared to those exposed to normal conditions.

Table 3. Effects of post-hatch heat stress for 7 days (post-hatch day (PD) 28 to 35) on cloacal temperature (T^C), body weight (BW), and BW gain in broiler chickens subjected to embryonic thermal manipulation and controls.

	Normal Conditions (21 °C; RH 45%–52%)		Heat Stress (35 °C; RH 45%–52%)	
	Control	TM	Control	TM
T^C (°C)	39.65 ± 0.28 ^{a}	39.08 ± 0.21 ^{b}	41.35 ± 0.24 ^{c}	40.15 ± 0.26 ^{d}
BW (g)				
Day 0 (PD 28)	1373.3 ± 51.3 ^{a}	1675.7 ± 83.8 ^{b}	1456.7 ± 82.8 ^{a}	1704 ± 74.4 ^{b}
Day 7 (PD 35)	1847.9 ± 108.1 ^{a}	2108.8 ± 95.8 ^{b}	1645 ± 40.6 ^{c}	1930 ± 50.2 ^{d}
BW gain (g)	474.6 ± 70.9 ^{a}	433 ± 39.1 ^{a}	188.3 ± 47.3 ^{b}	226 ± 34.7 ^{b}

$^{a–d}$ within the same row, means ± SD with non-identical superscripts are significantly different.

3.3. Effect of Post-Hatch Heat Stress on Antioxidant Enzyme mRNA Levels in Thermally Manipulated Broilers

Figure 2 represents the effects of heat stress on the hepatic and splenic mRNA levels of certain antioxidant enzymes in broiler chicks subjected to embryonic TM. Tables S1 and S2 includes the mRNA levels of the same antioxidant genes for broiler chicks (TM and controls) not exposed to heat stress during the same timeframe.

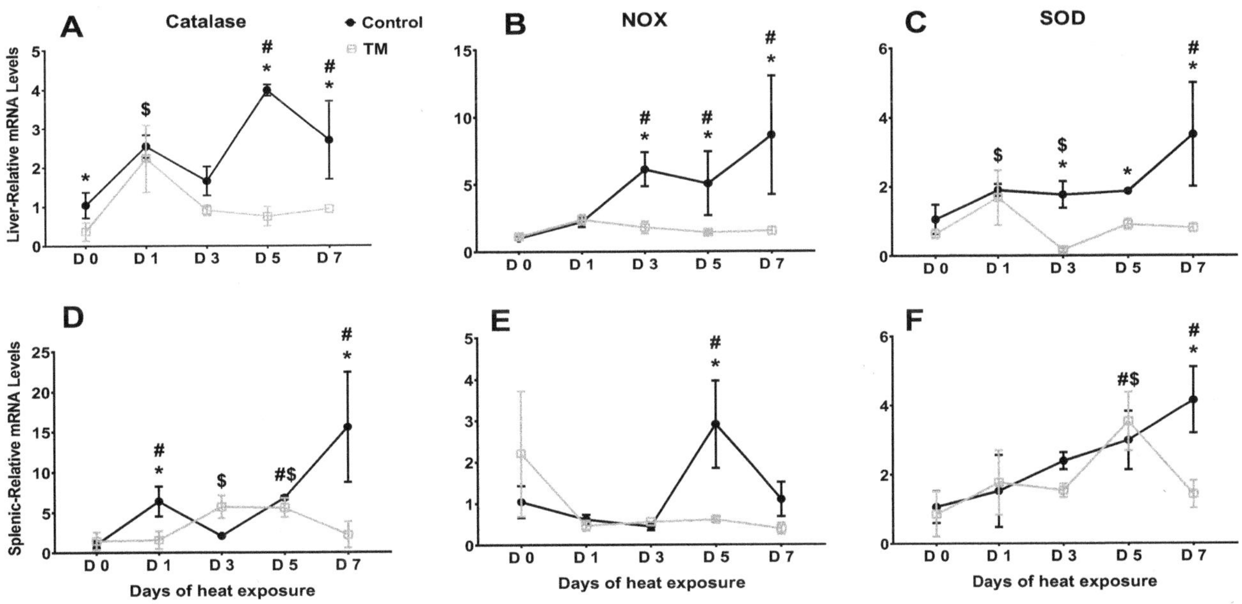

Figure 2. Effect of post-hatch heat stress for 7 days (PD 28 to 35) on the mRNA levels of catalase, *NOX4*, and *SOD2* in the liver (**A–C**) and spleen (**D–F**) of TM broiler chicks (n = 5). * within the same day, means ± SD of TM and control chicks are significantly different. # within the control group, means ± SD of non-identical days differ significantly. $ within the TM group, means ± SD of non-identical days differ significantly.

Catalase. On day 0 (PD 28) of heat stress, TM led to significantly lower catalase mRNA levels in the liver. In the control group, the hepatic mRNA levels of catalase were significantly higher after 5 (PD 33) and 7 (PD 35) days of heat stress compared to day 0, while, in the TM group, the level was significantly higher only after 1 day (PD 29) of heat exposure. The hepatic catalase mRNA level was significantly lower in TM chicks compared to controls after 5 (PD 33) and 7 (PD 35) days of heat stress.

The splenic mRNA level of catalase was not significantly different between TM and control chicks on day 0 (PD 28) of heat stress. However, the level was significantly lower in TM chicks compared to controls after 1 (PD 29) and 7 (PD 35) days of heat stress. Within the control group, the splenic mRNA level of catalase was significantly higher after 1 (PD 29), 5 (PD 33), and 7 (PD 35) days of heat exposure compared to day 0 (PD 28), whereas, in the TM group, the splenic mRNA level of catalase was significantly higher after 3 (PD 31) and 5 (PD 33) days (vs. day 0 (PD 28)).

NOX4. In the liver, the mRNA level of *NOX4* was not significantly different between the TM and control groups on day 0 (PD 28) of heat stress. In contrast, the *NOX4* mRNA level was significantly lower in TM chicks compared to controls after 3 (PD 31), 5 (PD 33), and 7 (PD 35) days of heat stress. Within the control group, the mRNA level was significantly increased after 3 (PD 31), 5 (PD 33), and 7 (PD 35) days of heat stress (vs. day 0 (PD 28)), but, in the TM group, the level did not significantly change during heat stress compared to day 0 (PD 28).

Similarly, the splenic mRNA level of *NOX4* was not significantly different between TM and control chicks on day 0 (PD 28) of heat stress. However, the level was significantly lower in the TM group compared to controls after 5 days (PD 33) of heat stress. Within the control group, the mRNA level of *NOX4* was significantly increased after 5 days (PD 33) of heat exposure in comparison with day 0 (PD 28), while in the TM group, the level did not significantly change during heat exposure in comparison with day 0 (PD 28).

SOD2. The liver mRNA level of *SOD2* was not significantly different between the TM and control groups on day 0 (PD 28) of heat stress. However, *SOD2* levels were significantly lower in TM chicks compared to controls after 3 (PD 31), 5 (PD 33), and 7 (PD 35) days of heat stress. Within the control group, the hepatic mRNA level of *SOD2* was significantly higher after 7 days (PD 35) of heat stress compared to day 0 (PD 28), while, in the TM group, the level significantly increased only after 1 day (PD 29) of heat exposure (vs. day 0 (PD 28)).

The splenic mRNA level of *SOD2* did not significantly differ between the TM and control groups on day 0 (PD 28) of heat stress. Contrastingly, the splenic level was significantly lower in TM chicks compared to controls after 7 days (PD 35) of heat exposure. Within the control group, the splenic mRNA level of *SOD2* was significantly higher after 7 days (PD 35) of heat stress compared to day 0 (PD 28), whereas, in the TM group, the level was significantly higher only after 5 days (PD 33) of heat exposure (vs. day 0 (PD 35)).

3.4. Effect of Post-Hatch Cold Stress on Physiological Parameters of Thermally Manipulated Broilers

Table 4 represents the effects of cold stress for 5 days (PD 32 to 37) on T^C, BW, and BW gain in thermally manipulated broiler chickens and controls. Application of TM significantly decreased the mortality rate during post-hatch exposure to cold stress (control = 5%; TM = 0). In contrast, cold stress did not significantly affect T^C, but, in both the TC and TN subgroups, controls exhibited significantly higher T^C compared to TM chicks. On day 0 (PD 32) of cold exposure, there was no significant change was observed in BW between the control and TM groups. After 5 days (PD 37) of cold stress, the BW of controls was significantly lower in comparison with control chicks exposed to cold stress. Furthermore, cold stress significantly decreased the BW gain in both the control and TM chicks, although the weight gain was significantly lower in controls compared to TM chicks.

Table 4. Effect of post-hatch cold stress for 5 days (post-hatch day (PD) 32 to 37) on cloacal temperature (T^C), body weight (BW), and body weight gain in broiler chickens subjected to embryonic thermal manipulation and controls.

	Normal Conditions (21 °C; RH 45%–52%)		**Cold Stress (16 °C; RH 45%–52%)**	
	Control (CN)	**TM (TN)**	**Control (CS)**	**TM (TS)**
T^C (°C)	39.18 ± 0.35 ^{a}	38.5 ± 0.34 ^{b}	39.3 ± 0.2 ^{a}	38.93 ± 0.32 ^{ab}
BW (g)				
Day 0 (PD 32)	1717.9 ± 137.5 ^{a}	1834 ± 112.8 ^{a}	1720 ± 147.5 ^{a}	1845.5 ± 119.9 ^{a}
Day 5 (PD 37)	2244.3 ± 134.4 ^{a}	2281 ± 101.9 ^{a}	1993.1 ± 131.3 ^{b}	2179 ± 134.8 ^{a}
BW gain (g)	526.4 ± 41.1 ^{a}	447 ± 42.2 ^{b}	273.1 ± 23.9 ^{c}	333.5 ± 53.2 ^{d}

$^{a–d}$ within the same row, means ± SD with non-identical superscripts are significantly different.

3.5. Effect of Post-Hatch Cold stress on mRNA Levels of Antioxidant Enzymes in Thermally Manipulated Broilers

Figure 3 represents the effects of cold stress on the mRNA levels of antioxidant enzymes in the liver, spleen heart and breast muscle of broiler chickens subjected to embryonic thermal manipulation.

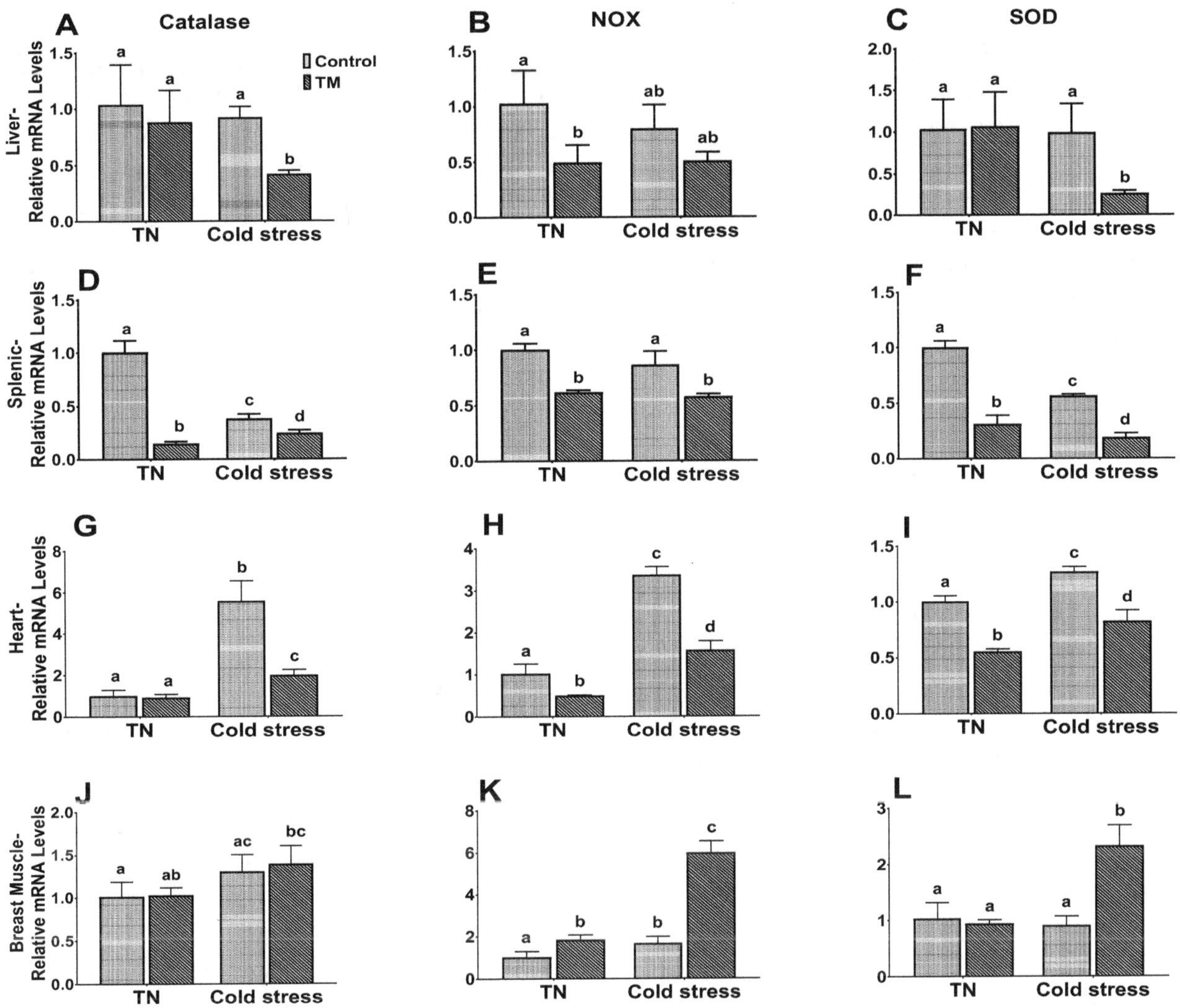

Figure 3. Effect of post-hatch cold stress for 5 days (PD 32 to 37) on the mRNA levels of catalase, *NOX4*, and *SOD2* in the liver (**A**–**C**), spleen (**D**–**F**), heart (**G**–**I**), and breast muscle (**J**–**L**) in TM broiler chickens (n = 5). $^{a–d}$ means ± SD with non-identical superscripts are significantly different.

Catalase. TM did not significantly change the cardiac, hepatic, and muscular mRNA levels of catalase in chicks kept under normal environmental temperatures. However, TM significantly decreased the catalase mRNA level in the spleen. Regarding those chicks exposed to cold stress, the TM group possessed a significantly lower mRNA level of catalase in the liver, spleen, and heart compared to controls.

NOX4. In the chicks of the TN subgroup, TM chicks possessed significantly lower splenic, hepatic, and cardiac mRNA levels of *NOX4* compared to controls. Despite this, muscular NOX4 mRNA levels were significantly higher in the TM chicks. Similar results were observed in the chicks exposed to cold stress.

SOD2. No significant changes were seen in the hepatic and muscular *SOD2* mRNA levels between the TM and control groups exposed to normal conditions. However, the splenic and cardiac levels of *SOD2* mRNA were significantly higher in controls compared to TM chicks. After cold exposure, the cardiac, hepatic, and splenic mRNA levels of *SOD2* were significantly higher in controls compared to TM chicks, but the level in breast muscle was significantly higher in the TM group.

4. Discussion

Oxidative damage is caused by excess reactive oxygen species (ROS), such as superoxide (O_2^-) and hydrogen peroxide (H_2O_2), which are a necessary product of aerobic metabolism [35]. Heat stress is a major cause of oxidative damage in poultry, and it is associated with a modulation in the expression of antioxidant genes, including catalase, *NOX4*, and *SOD2* [10,13]. Thermal manipulation (TM) has often been suggested as a viable method of improving the acquisition of thermotolerance in heat-stressed broilers [31,36–38]. However, the effects of TM and subsequent heat challenge on broiler antioxidant capacity has not been extensively explored. Similarly, a dearth of information exists with regard to the effects of cold stress on broiler gene expression, especially within the context antioxidant gene expression. The objective of the present study was two-fold: it aimed to ascertain the effects of embryonic TM on broilers under conditions of post-hatch heat stress as well as cold stress.

During heat stress, the behavior of broilers is altered as they attempt to decrease their body temperature (T^C), resulting in myriad negative effects on performance [39]. In the current study, TM was found to result in significantly lower T^C on post-hatch days (PD) 1 and 37 and higher body weights (BW) on PD 37 compared to controls. Correspondingly, it has often been reported that TM treatments significantly increased broiler BW [37,40,41] and improved their abilities to regulate their T^C in periods of heat challenge [31,32,42]. Lower T^C during heat stress also improved feed conversion ratios in TM broilers, and it has been suggested that the lower T^C in TM broilers is due to slower metabolic rates as a result of the TM treatment [43].

With regard to post-hatch heat stress, our findings show that TM chickens had significantly decreased mortality rates and BT as well as increased BW compared to controls. Heat stress has been extensively reported to affect broiler physiological parameters [8,44,45]. On a similar note, cold-stressed TM chickens had significantly lower mortality rates than cold-stressed controls. Previously, TM has been found to reduce the mortality rates of broilers during heat challenge [46,47]. Contrastingly, one study reported that heat-stressed TM broilers experienced higher mortality rates than their control counterparts [48]. These differences in findings may be attributed to the fact that there is no one single type of TM treatment, and different studies employ different periods and conditions of TM.

The catalase enzyme is found in the majority of aerobic organisms as well as in some obligate anaerobes [49]. Catalase is responsible for the breakdown of hydrogen peroxide (H_2O_2) into oxygen and water, thereby preventing oxidative damage from occurring in a cell [50]. In the present study, catalase expression was significantly modulated in heat- and cold-stressed TM and control chickens. In fact, heat stress resulted in decreased hepatic and splenic catalase expression in TM chickens compared to controls, while cold stress led to significantly lower cardiac, hepatic, and splenic catalase expression levels in the TM group. Compared to controls, heat-stressed TM chickens were previously reported to exhibit decreased catalase mRNA levels [13]. Moreover, broilers were found to exhibit higher levels of catalase activity during acute heat stress, but this antioxidant capacity decreased with age [51]. In female broilers, cardiac catalase activity was reduced after cold stimulation [52].

To maintain homeostasis, the NOX4 enzyme is heavily involved in the oxygen-sensing process, the latter of which causes it to generate significant amounts of ROS [17]. Additionally, *NOX4* over-expression is often associated with oxidative stress in a number of different organs [18,53,54]. In avian muscle cells, ROS production during heat stress and subsequent oxidative damage has been tentatively attributed to *NOX4* up-regulation [55]. In the present study, hepatic and splenic *NOX4* expression levels were significantly lower in heat-stressed TM chickens compared to controls. Similarly, after cold stress, TM chickens exhibited decreased cardiac, hepatic, and splenic but increased muscular *NOX4* expression than that in controls. Hepatic *NOX4* mRNA expression was previously reported to be lower in TM chickens exposed to heat stress compared to controls [13]. In cultured avian cells, heat stress was found to upregulated *NOX4* mRNA expression [55].

The SOD2 enzyme functions to transform the superoxide (O_2^-) radical into hydrogen peroxide and water, and it plays an important cytoprotective role against oxidative stress [56]. Our findings indicate that both heat and cold exposure led to generally decreased *SOD2* expression in several organs. Compared to controls, heat-stressed TM chickens displayed lower hepatic and splenic *SOD2* expression levels, while cold-stressed TM chickens showed decreased cardiac, hepatic, and splenic *SOD2* expression. Like *NOX4*, however, muscular *SOD2* expression levels were higher in cold-stressed TM chickens compared to their control counterparts. A previous study found that hepatic *SOD2* expression and enzymatic activity were decreased in TM chickens exposed to heat stress [13]. In contrast, another study found that *SOD* mRNA levels in two broiler strains (Cobb and Hubbard) were unaffected by heat stress [57]. Additionally, *SOD2* levels remained unchanged in avian cell cultures exposed to heat stress [55]. The present findings may suggest that lower levels of oxidative *NOX4* expression may lead to lower expression of the anti-oxidative catalase and *SOD2* genes.

Interestingly, mRNA expression levels of the catalase, *NOX4*, and *SOD2* genes in the breast muscle differed from those in the heart, liver, and spleen in cold-stressed TM chickens. Such inter-organ variation in gene expression is to be expected, as expression varies to a larger degree between organs of a single species than between different species [58]. However, in broilers, the breast muscle in particular has been subject to rapid changes in size and conformation over the past few decades due to the artificial selection pressures applied by the commercial poultry industry [59]. This has resulted in a number of abnormalities and myopathies of the breast muscle that is estimated to affect up to 90% of broilers worldwide [60–62]. In fact, broiler breast muscle cells were suggested to constantly undergo hypoxic stress, as the transcriptional profiles of non-stressed broiler breast muscle and heat-stressed layer breast muscle were similar [63].

A number of strengths can be found in the current study. All samples were taken from male Cobb chicks in order to reduce inter-strain and inter-sex genetic variation. Moreover, any non-experimental stress was minimized by ensuring that the rearing and experimental rooms were in close proximity to one another. However, there are some limitations of the present study. Firstly, the effect of TM on the developmental parameters of broiler embryos was not investigated, requiring future research. Secondly, the oxidation levels of lipids, proteins, and DNA in different tissues must still be measured in order to ascertain the final balance of catalase, *NOX4*, and *SOD2* expression. Lastly, the exact impact of TM on embryonic mortality was not considered, which mandates future lines of research in this context.

5. Conclusions

Our findings indicate that TM at 39 °C and 65% RH for 18 h/day from days 10 to 18 of embryonic development might result in positive long-lasting effects on broiler antioxidant capacity. Future research should focus on the effects of TM and subsequent thermal challenge on various types of broiler muscle, as the expression dynamics of the breast muscle was found to differ from those of other organs.

Author Contributions: Conceptualization, K.M.M.S., A.H.T. and M.B.A.-Z.; methodology, K.M.M.S.; software, K.M.M.S. and M.B.A.-Z.; validation K.M.M.S. and M.B.A.-Z.; formal analysis, K.M.M.S. and M.B.A.-Z.; investigation, K.M.M.S.; resources, M.B.A.-Z.; data curation, K.M.M.S. and M.B.A.-Z.; writing—original draft preparation, K.M.M.S. and A.H.T.; writing—review and editing, K.M.M.S., A.H.T. and M.B.A.-Z.; visualization, K.M.M.S., A.H.T. and M.B.A.-Z.; supervision, M.B.A.-Z.; project administration, M.B.A.-Z. and K.M.M.S.; funding acquisition, M.B.A.-Z. All authors have read and agreed to the published version of the manuscript.

Acknowledgments: The authors would like to thank Eng. Ibrahim Alsukhni for his excellent technical assistance and valuable comments.

References

1. McKay, J.C.; Barton, N.F.; Koerhuis, A.N.M.; McAdam, J. The challenge of genetic change in the broiler chicken. *BSAP Occas. Publ.* **2000**, *27*, 1–7. [CrossRef]
2. Bennett, C.E.; Thomas, R.; Williams, M.; Zalasiewicz, J.; Edgeworth, M.; Miller, H.; Coles, B.; Foster, A.; Burton, E.J.; Marume, U. The broiler chicken as a signal of a human reconfigured biosphere. *R. Soc. Open Sci.* **2018**, *5*, 180325. [CrossRef] [PubMed]
3. Tallentire, C.W.; Leinonen, I.; Kyriazakis, I. Breeding for efficiency in the broiler chicken: A review. *Agron. Sustain. Dev.* **2016**, *36*, 66. [CrossRef]

4. Zuidhof, M.J.; Schneider, B.L.; Carney, V.L.; Korver, D.R.; Robinson, F.E. Growth, efficiency, and yield of commercial broilers from 1957, 1978, and 2005. *Poult. Sci.* **2014**, *93*, 2970–2982. [CrossRef] [PubMed]
5. Zaboli, G.; Huang, X.; Feng, X.; Ahn, D.U. How can heat stress affect chicken meat quality? A review. *Poult. Sci.* **2019**, *98*, 1551–1556. [CrossRef] [PubMed]
6. Tickle, P.G.; Hutchinson, J.R.; Codd, J.R. Energy allocation and behaviour in the growing broiler chicken. *Sci. Rep.* **2018**, *8*, 4562. [CrossRef]
7. Nyoni, N.M.B.; Grab, S.; Archer, E.R.M. Heat stress and chickens: Climate risk effects on rural poultry farming in low-income countries. *Clim. Dev.* **2019**, *11*, 83–90. [CrossRef]
8. Lara, L.J.; Rostagno, M.H. Impact of heat stress on poultry production. *Animals* **2013**, *3*, 356–369. [CrossRef]
9. Mishra, B.; Jha, R. Oxidative stress in the poultry gut: Potential challenges and interventions. *Front. Vet. Sci.* **2019**, *6*, 60. [CrossRef]
10. Akbarian, A.; Michiels, J.; Degroote, J.; Majdeddin, M.; Golian, A.; De Smet, S. Association between heat stress and oxidative stress in poultry; mitochondrial dysfunction and dietary interventions with phytochemicals. *J. Anim. Sci. Biotechnol.* **2016**, *7*, 37. [CrossRef]
11. Fellenberg, M.A.; Speisky, H. Antioxidants: Their effects on broiler oxidative stress and its meat oxidative stability. *World's Poult. Sci. J.* **2006**, *62*, 53–70. [CrossRef]
12. Betteridge, D.J. What is oxidative stress? In *Metabolism: Clinical and Experimental*; W.B. Saunders: Philadelphia, PA, USA, 2000; Volume 49, pp. 3–8.
13. Al-Zghoul, M.B.; Sukker, H.; Ababneh, M.M. Effect of thermal manipulation of broilers embryos on the response to heat-induced oxidative stress. *Poult. Sci.* **2019**, *98*, 991–1001. [CrossRef]
14. Nita, M.; Grzybowski, A. The role of the reactive oxygen species and oxidative stress in the pathomechanism of the age-related ocular diseases and other pathologies of the anterior and posterior eye segments in adults. *Oxid. Med. Cell. Longev.* **2016**, *2016*, 3164734. [CrossRef] [PubMed]
15. Kim, J.H.; Lee, J.; Bae, S.J.; Kim, Y.; Park, B.J.; Choi, J.W.; Kwon, J.; Cha, G.H.; Yoo, H.J.; Jo, E.K.; et al. NADPH oxidase 4 is required for the generation of macrophage migration inhibitory factor and host defense against Toxoplasma gondii infection. *Sci. Rep.* **2017**, *7*, 6361. [CrossRef] [PubMed]
16. Chen, F.; Haigh, S.; Barman, S.; Fulton, D.J.R. From form to function: The role of Nox4 in the cardiovascular system. *Front. Physiol.* **2012**, *3*, 412. [CrossRef]
17. Schröder, K.; Zhang, M.; Benkhoff, S.; Mieth, A.; Pliquett, R.; Kosowski, J.; Kruse, C.; Luedike, P.; Michaelis, U.R.; Weissmann, N.; et al. Nox4 Is a protective reactive oxygen species generating vascular NADPH oxidase. *Circ. Res.* **2012**, *110*, 1217–1225. [CrossRef]
18. Kuroda, J.; Ago, T.; Matsushima, S.; Zhai, P.; Schneider, M.D.; Sadoshima, J. NADPH oxidase 4 (Nox4) is a major source of oxidative stress in the failing heart. *Proc. Natl. Acad. Sci. USA* **2010**, *107*, 15565–15570. [CrossRef]
19. Nisimoto, Y.; Diebold, B.A.; Cosentino-Gomes, D.; Lambeth, J.D.; Lambeth, J.D. Nox4: A hydrogen peroxide-generating oxygen sensor. *Biochemistry* **2014**, *53*, 5111–5120. [CrossRef]
20. Ighodaro, O.M.; Akinloye, O.A. First line defence antioxidants-superoxide dismutase (SOD), catalase (CAT) and glutathione peroxidase (GPX): Their fundamental role in the entire antioxidant defence grid. *Alex. J. Med.* **2018**, *54*, 287–293. [CrossRef]
21. Zhao, F.Q.; Zhang, Z.W.; Qu, J.P.; Yao, H.D.; Li, M.; Li, S.; Xu, S.W. Cold stress induces antioxidants and Hsps in chicken immune organs. *Cell Stress Chaperones* **2014**, *19*, 635–648. [CrossRef]
22. Zhang, Z.W.; Lv, Z.H.; Li, J.L.; Li, S.; Xu, S.W.; Wang, X.L. Effects of cold stress on nitric oxide in duodenum of chicks. *Poult. Sci.* **2011**, *90*, 1555–1561. [CrossRef] [PubMed]
23. Surai, P.F.; Kochish, I.I.; Fisinin, V.I.; Kidd, M.T. Antioxidant defence systems and oxidative stress in poultry biology: An update. *Antioxidants* **2019**, *8*, 235. [CrossRef] [PubMed]
24. Baghbanzadeh, A.; Decuypere, E. Ascites syndrome in broilers: Physiological and nutritional perspectives. *Avian Pathol.* **2008**, *37*, 117–126. [CrossRef] [PubMed]
25. Tsiouris, V. Poultry management: A useful tool for the control of necrotic enteritis in poultry. *Avian Pathol.* **2016**, *45*, 323–325. [CrossRef] [PubMed]
26. Dadgar, S.; Crowe, T.G.; Classen, H.L.; Watts, J.M.; Shand, P.J. Broiler chicken thigh and breast muscle responses to cold stress during simulated transport before slaughter. *Poult. Sci.* **2012**, *91*, 1454–1464. [CrossRef] [PubMed]

27. Olfati, A.; Mojtahedin, A.; Sadeghi, T.; Akbari, M.; Martínez-Pastor, F. Comparison of growth performance and immune responses of broiler chicks reared under heat stress, cold stress and thermoneutral conditions. *Span. J. Agric. Res.* **2018**, *16*. [CrossRef]
28. Tsiouris, V.; Georgopoulou, I.; Batzios, C.; Pappaioannou, N.; Ducatelle, R.; Fortomaris, P. The effect of cold stress on the pathogenesis of necrotic enteritis in broiler chicks. *Avian Pathol.* **2015**, *44*, 430–435. [CrossRef]
29. Yalcin, S.; Siegel, P. Exposure to cold or heat during incubation on developmental stability of broiler embryos. *Poult. Sci.* **2003**, *82*, 1388–1392. [CrossRef]
30. Yahav, S.; Rath, R.S.; Shinder, D. The effect of thermal manipulations during embryogenesis of broiler chicks (*Gallus domesticus*) on hatchability, body weight and thermoregulation after hatch. *J. Therm. Biol.* **2004**, *29*, 245–250. [CrossRef]
31. Piestun, Y.; Shinder, D.; Ruzal, M.; Halevy, O.; Brake, J.; Yahav, S. Thermal manipulations during broiler embryogenesis: Effect on the acquisition of thermotolerance. *Poult. Sci.* **2008**, *87*, 1516–1525. [CrossRef]
32. Piestun, Y.; Shinder, D.; Ruzal, M.; Halevy, O.; Yahav, S. The effect of thermal manipulations during the development of the thyroid and adrenal axes on in-hatch and post-hatch thermoregulation. *J. Therm. Biol.* **2008**, *33*, 413–418. [CrossRef]
33. Al-Zghoul, M.B.; Saleh, K.M.; Ababneh, M.M.K. Effects of pre-hatch thermal manipulation and post-hatch acute heat stress on the mRNA expression of interleukin-6 and genes involved in its induction pathways in 2 broiler chicken breeds. *Poult. Sci.* **2019**, *98*, 1805–1819. [CrossRef] [PubMed]
34. Al-Zghoul, M.B.; Alliftawi, A.R.S.; Saleh, K.M.M.; Jaradat, Z.W. Expression of digestive enzyme and intestinal transporter genes during chronic heat stress in the thermally manipulated broiler chicken. *Poult. Sci.* **2019**, *98*, 4113–4122. [CrossRef] [PubMed]
35. Cooper-Mullin, C.; McWilliams, S.R. The role of the antioxidant system during intense endurance exercise: Lessons from migrating birds. *J. Exp. Biol.* **2016**, *219*, 3684–3695. [CrossRef] [PubMed]
36. Saleh, K.M.M.; Al-Zghoul, M.B. Effect of acute heat stress on the mrna levels of cytokines in broiler chickens subjected to embryonic thermal manipulation. *Animals* **2019**, *9*, 499. [CrossRef] [PubMed]
37. Al-Zghoul, M.B.; El-Bahr, S.M. Thermal manipulation of the broilers embryos: Expression of muscle markers genes and weights of body and internal organs during embryonic and post-hatch days. *BMC Vet. Res.* **2019**, *15*, 166. [CrossRef]
38. Zaboli, G.-R.; Rahimi, S.; Shariatmadari, F.; Torshizi, M.A.K.; Baghbanzadeh, A.; Mehri, M. Thermal manipulation during Pre and Post-Hatch on thermotolerance of male broiler chickens exposed to chronic heat stress. *Poult. Sci.* **2017**, *96*, 478–485. [CrossRef]
39. Mack, L.A.; Felver-Gant, J.N.; Dennis, R.L.; Cheng, H.W. Genetic variations alter production and behavioral responses following heat stress in 2 strains of laying hens. *Poult. Sci.* **2013**, *92*, 285–294. [CrossRef]
40. Loyau, T.; Berri, C.; Bedrani, L.; Métayer-Coustard, S.; Praud, C.; Duclos, M.J.; Tesseraud, S.; Rideau, N.; Everaert, N.; Yahav, S.; et al. Thermal manipulation of the embryo modifies the physiology and body composition of broiler chickens reared in floor pens without affecting breast meat processing quality1. *J. Anim. Sci.* **2013**, *91*, 3674–3685. [CrossRef]
41. Piestun, Y.; Druyan, S.; Brake, J.; Yahav, S. Thermal manipulations during broiler incubation alter performance of broilers to 70 days of age. *Poult. Sci.* **2013**, *92*, 1155–1163. [CrossRef]
42. Yahav, S.; Collin, A.; Shinder, D.; Picard, M. Thermal manipulations during broiler chick embryogenesis: Effects of timing and temperature. *Poult. Sci.* **2004**, *83*, 1959–1963. [CrossRef] [PubMed]
43. Piestun, Y.; Halevy, O.; Shinder, D.; Ruzal, M.; Druyan, S.; Yahav, S. Thermal manipulations during broiler embryogenesis improves post-hatch performance under hot conditions. *J. Therm. Biol.* **2011**, *36*, 469–474. [CrossRef]
44. Altan, Ö.; Pabuçcuoğlu, A.; Altan, A.; Konyalioğlu, S.; Bayraktar, H. Effect of heat stress on oxidative stress, lipid peroxidation and some stress parameters in broilers. *Br. Poult. Sci.* **2003**, *44*, 545–550. [CrossRef] [PubMed]
45. Lin, H.; Decuypere, E.; Buyse, J. Acute heat stress induces oxidative stress in broiler chickens. *Comp. Biochem. Physiol. Part A Mol. Integr. Physiol.* **2006**, *144*, 11–17. [CrossRef]
46. Günal, M. The effects of early-age thermal manipulation and daily short-term fasting on performance and body temperatures in broiler exposed to heat stress. *J. Anim. Physiol. Anim. Nutr.* **2012**, *97*, 854–860. [CrossRef]

47. Loyau, T.; Métayer-Coustard, S.; Berri, C.; Crochet, S.; Cailleau-Audouin, E.; Sannier, M.; Chartrin, P.; Praud, C.; Hennequet-Antier, C.; Rideau, N.; et al. Thermal manipulation during embryogenesis has long-term effects on muscle and liver metabolism in fast-growing chickens. *PLoS ONE* **2014**, *9*, e105339. [CrossRef]
48. Collin, A.; Berri, C.; Tesseraud, S.; Rodon, F.E.R.; Skiba-Cassy, S.; Crochet, S.; Duclos, M.J.; Rideau, N.; Tona, K.; Buyse, J.; et al. Effects of thermal manipulation during early and late embryogenesis on thermotolerance and breast muscle characteristics in broiler chickens. *Poult. Sci.* **2007**, *86*, 795–800. [CrossRef]
49. Zamocky, M.; Furtmüller, P.G.; Obinger, C. Evolution of catalases from bacteria to humans. *Antioxid. Redox Signal.* **2008**, *10*, 1527–1547. [CrossRef] [PubMed]
50. Chelikani, P.; Fita, I.; Loewen, P.C. Diversity of structures and properties among catalases. *Cell. Mol. Life Sci.* **2004**, *61*, 192–208. [CrossRef]
51. Del Vesco, A.P.; Khatlab, A.S.; Goes, E.S.R.; Utsunomiya, K.S.; Vieira, J.S.; Oliveira Neto, A.R.; Gasparino, E. Age-related oxidative stress and antioxidant capacity in heat-stressed broilers. *Animal* **2017**, *11*, 1783–1790. [CrossRef]
52. Wei, H.; Zhang, R.; Su, Y.; Bi, Y.; Li, X.; Zhang, X.; Li, J.; Bao, J. Effects of acute cold stress after long-term cold stimulation on antioxidant status, heat shock proteins, inflammation and immune cytokines in broiler heart. *Front. Physiol.* **2018**, *9*, 1589. [CrossRef] [PubMed]
53. Jeong, B.Y.; Lee, H.Y.; Park, C.G.; Kang, J.; Yu, S.-L.; Choi, D.; Han, S.-Y.; Park, M.H.; Cho, S.; Lee, S.Y.; et al. Oxidative stress caused by activation of NADPH oxidase 4 promotes contrast-induced acute kidney injury. *PLoS ONE* **2018**, *13*, e0191034. [CrossRef] [PubMed]
54. Vendrov, A.E.; Vendrov, K.C.; Smith, A.; Yuan, J.; Sumida, A.; Robidoux, J.; Runge, M.S.; Madamanchi, N.R. NOX4 NADPH oxidase-dependent mitochondrial oxidative stress in aging-associated cardiovascular disease. *Antioxid. Redox Signal.* **2015**, *23*, 1389–1409. [CrossRef] [PubMed]
55. Kikusato, M.; Yoshida, H.; Furukawa, K.; Toyomizu, M. Effect of heat stress-induced production of mitochondrial reactive oxygen species on NADPH oxidase and heme oxygenase-1 mRNA levels in avian muscle cells. *J. Therm. Biol.* **2015**, *52*, 8–13. [CrossRef] [PubMed]
56. Velarde, M.C.; Flynn, J.M.; Day, N.U.; Melov, S.; Campisi, J. Mitochondrial oxidative stress caused by Sod2 deficiency promotes cellular senescence and aging phenotypes in the skin. *Aging Albany. NY* **2012**, *4*, 3–12. [CrossRef] [PubMed]
57. Rimoldi, S.; Lasagna, E.; Sarti, F.M.; Marelli, S.P.; Cozzi, M.C.; Bernardini, G.; Terova, G. Expression profile of six stress-related genes and productive performances of fast and slow growing broiler strains reared under heat stress conditions. *Meta Gene* **2015**, *6*, 17–25. [CrossRef]
58. Breschi, A.; Djebali, S.; Gillis, J.; Pervouchine, D.D.; Dobin, A.; Davis, C.A.; Gingeras, T.R.; Guigó, R. Gene-specific patterns of expression variation across organs and species. *Genome Biol.* **2016**, *17*, 151. [CrossRef]
59. Scheuermann, G.N.; Bilgili, S.F.; Hess, J.B.; Mulvaney, D.R. Breast muscle development in commercial broiler chickens. *Poult. Sci.* **2003**, *82*, 1648–1658. [CrossRef]
60. Kuttappan, V.A.; Hargis, B.M.; Owens, C.M. White striping and woody breast myopathies in the modern poultry industry: A review. *Poult. Sci.* **2016**, *95*, 2724–2733. [CrossRef]
61. Huang, X.; Ahn, D.U. The incidence of muscle abnormalities in broiler breast meat—A review. *Korean J. Food Sci. Anim. Resour.* **2018**, *38*, 835–850. [CrossRef]
62. Kawasaki, T.; Iwasaki, T.; Yamada, M.; Yoshida, T.; Watanabe, T. Rapid growth rate results in remarkably hardened breast in broilers during the middle stage of rearing: A biochemical and histopathological study. *PLoS ONE* **2018**, *13*, e0193307. [CrossRef] [PubMed]
63. Zahoor, I.; De Koning, D.J.; Hocking, P.M. Transcriptional profile of breast muscle in heat stressed layers is similar to that of broiler chickens at control temperature. *Genet. Sel. Evol.* **2017**, *49*, 69. [CrossRef] [PubMed]

8

The Role of Innate Immune Response and Microbiome in Resilience of Dairy Cattle to Disease: The Mastitis Model

Valerio Bronzo [1,†], Vincenzo Lopreiato [2,†], Federica Riva [1], Massimo Amadori [3,*], Giulio Curone [1], Maria Filippa Addis [1], Paola Cremonesi [4], Paolo Moroni [1,5], Erminio Trevisi [2] and Bianca Castiglioni [4]

1 Dipartimento di Medicina Veterinaria, Università degli Studi di Milano, 26900 Lodi, Italy; valerio.bronzo@unimi.it (V.B.); federica.riva@unimi.it (F.R.); giulio.curone@unimi.it (G.C.); filippa.addis@unimi.it (M.F.A.); pm389@cornell.edu (P.M.)

2 Dipartimento di Scienze animali, Alimentazione e Nutrizione, Facoltà di Agraria, Scienze Alimentari e Ambientali, Università Cattolica del Sacro Cuore, 29122 Piacenza, Italy; vincenzo.lopreiato@unicatt.it (V.L.); erminio.trevisi@unicatt.it (E.T.)

3 Rete Nazionale di Immunologia Veterinaria, 25125 Brescia, Italy

4 Institute of Biology and Biotechnology in Agriculture, National Research Council (CNR), 26900 Lodi, Italy; paola.cremonesi@ibba.cnr.it (P.C.); bianca.castiglioni@ibba.cnr.it (B.C.)

5 Quality Milk Production Services, Animal Health Diagnostic Center, Cornell University, 240 Farrier Road, Ithaca, NY 14850, USA

* Correspondence: m_amadori@fastwebnet.it;

† These authors contributed equally to this work.

Simple Summary: A major concern for the development of livestock activities is represented by the gradual reduction of antibiotic usage in farm animals, which may disturb the fragile balance between animal health and production. Therefore, it is necessary to maintain the immunocompetence of farm animals within the structure of this new trend toward reduced drug usage. High-yielding dairy cattle often experience more disease prevalence associated with short life expectancy and reduced environmental fitness. These signs of immunosuppression can be linked to metabolic changes observed around calving, which confirms the crucial link between immunity and milk production levels. The immunocompetence of these animals should be re-appraised and new disease control strategies should be based on creating a more efficient immune system. This review summarizes the dairy cow's metabolic response to stress and what role the innate immune system and microbiome play. The review also discusses how new approaches to animal health based on specific intervention at dry-off and in the first weeks after calving are needed as the relevant stressors are pivotal to disease occurrence.

Abstract: Animal health is affected by many factors such as metabolic stress, the immune system, and epidemiological features that interconnect. The immune system has evolved along with the phylogenetic evolution as a highly refined sensing and response system, poised to react against diverse infectious and non-infectious stressors for better survival and adaptation. It is now known that high genetic merit for milk yield is correlated with a defective control of the inflammatory response, underlying the occurrence of several production diseases. This is evident in the mastitis model where high-yielding dairy cows show high disease prevalence of the mammary gland with reduced effectiveness of the innate immune system and poor control over the inflammatory response to microbial agents. There is growing evidence of epigenetic effects on innate immunity genes underlying the response to common microbial agents. The aforementioned agents, along with other non-infectious stressors, can give rise to abnormal activation of the innate immune system, underlying serious disease conditions, and affecting milk yield. Furthermore, the microbiome also plays a role in shaping immune functions and disease resistance as a whole. Accordingly, proper modulation of the microbiome can be pivotal to successful disease control strategies. These strategies can benefit from a fundamental re-appraisal of native cattle breeds as models of disease resistance based on successful coping of both infectious and non-infectious stressors.

Keywords: dairy cattle diseases; innate immune system; metabolic stress; microbiome

1. Introduction

In the last decade, ensuring animal health and welfare with the progressive reduction of drug usage has become a key issue for farmers as well as consumers worldwide. Dairy cattle diseases cause morbidity, mortality, and often decreased profitability for farmers, but antibiotics are now used more responsibly for treatment and control of these diseases [1,2]. Due to the known difficulties in developing novel antibiotic classes, the prudent use of the same products must be targeted. Public concerns have been raised regarding animal disease control, how animals for human consumption are treated with drugs, and the environment in which these animals are raised.

Alternative methods for preventing animal diseases are needed. One idea is through the modulation of the immune system. It has been documented that it is rare for every animal exposed to the same infection to develop symptoms that are clinical; furthermore, different breeds exhibit different traits related to disease [3–6]. It is difficult to explain why some animals in the same group develop varying degrees of the same illness. Genetics, the immune system, management, age, and other factors influence the health of an animal [7,8]. More variables play a role in animal health, making it difficult to pinpoint any single factor (Figure 1).

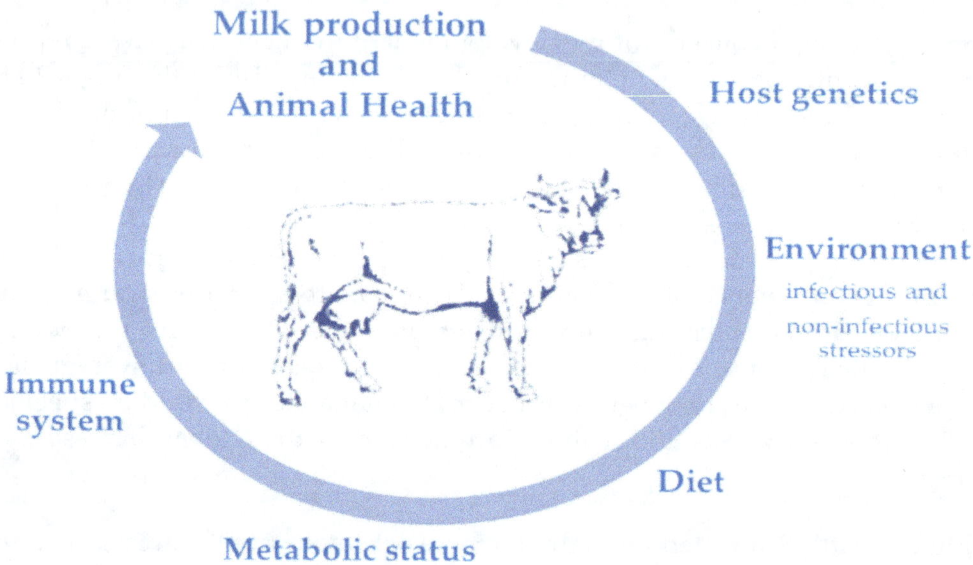

Figure 1. Milk production and animal health are influenced by and correlated to many factors such as genetics, environment stressors, diet, metabolic *status*, and the immunological system that all interact.

During the periparturient period, dairy cows undergo a number of metabolic-, endocrine-, physiologic-, and immune-related changes, rendering cows more susceptible to disease and less efficient. Health problems occurring before and after calving lead to severe negative effects on the productive efficiency of lactating cows. Reductions in the cow's production and increased mortality rates are associated with periparturient health disorders. The costs of antimicrobial drugs, vaccines, labor, and preventive measures must be taken into consideration. During this period, immune system efficiency together with good liver functionality as well as the capability of cows to minimize the gap between nutrient intake (increasing dry matter intake)and nutrient output (milk production) determines the disease resistance capability of the animal [9]. The most important roles of the immune system are to prevent microbial diffusion and to reduce or eliminate infections.

2. Immunocompetence of High Genetic Merit Dairy Cattle and Disease Control Strategies

The immune system has developed along with the phylogenetic evolution as a refined sensing and response system, aimed at neutralizing all the possible noxa affecting or potentially affecting the host's homeostasis [10]. The system has evolved from the recognition of conserved patterns of microbial pathogens to having great potential for recognizing fine specificities of microbial agents. Adaptive immunity rose with phylogenesis approximately 500 million years ago in jawed fish and proceeded to mammals as a result of selective pressures derived from the increased complexity of organs and apparata [11]. As a result, mammals avail themselves of innate immune mechanisms to deal with a plethora of infectious and non-infectious stressors. Adaptive mechanisms (antibodies and antigen-specific T lymphocytes) are used whenever the primary non-adaptive mechanisms fail to control a challenge to homeostasis [12].

Ruminants are no exception to this general rule. Domestication of ruminants began some 10,000 years ago [13] and has since played a vital part in the economic and social advancement of mankind. It can be argued that domestication was an advantage to ruminants in terms of easier access to feeding resources and protection against climatic challenges [14]. The relationship with mankind became complex with the advent of intensive farming and genetic selection for higher production levels. This relationship gave rise to a substantial worsening of animal welfare, and the historical relationship between domestication and welfare has become a bell-shaped dose-response curve [14]. We must find credible solutions to the major problem of ethics and the sustainability of farming activities. These solutions must take into consideration the diverging needs of environmental constraints and high production levels brought about by the increasing world population and its growing demand for animal products.

In this conceptual framework, a major concern for the development of farming activities is represented by the gradual reduction of antibiotic usage in farm animals, which may disturb the fragile balance between animal health and production. It is necessary to stimulate the immunocompetence of farm animals within the structure of this new trend toward reduced drug usage. High-yielding dairy cattle often experience high disease prevalence associated with short life expectancy [15]. Most importantly, they show distinct signs of reduced environmental fitness, shown as coping poorly with both infectious and non-infectious stressors, as observed, e.g., in the hot summer season of 2003 [16]. The immunocompetence of these animals should be re-evaluated and new disease control strategies should be based on increasing the efficiency of the immune system.

2.1. *The Concept of Immunocompetence*

Immunocompetence is the ability of the body to produce a normal immune response following exposure to an antigen. This process involves complex genetic traits [17]. To produce an effective immune response, different cells and genes are necessary along with the ability of innate and adaptive immunities to coordinate. Danger describes the force that dictates the reaction profile of the immune system [18] for both infectious and non-infectious stressors [10]. Microbial infections entail some overlapping signals triggered by both PAMPs (pathogen-associated molecular patterns) and DAMPs (damage-associated molecular patterns). Within this operational framework, the innate immune system begins to destroy the stressors affecting the host's homeostasis. Innate immunity must not cause substantial tissue damage as a result of a disproportionate inflammatory response. If pathogens persist after the innate response, adaptive immunity is induced to control the ongoing infection. The B and T cell receptor activity directed against specific antigens is the main component of immunocompetence. Innate immunity also plays an important part in the recruitment and orientation of receptor responses. These are used sparingly by the host as the response of secondary antibodies and immunological memory benefits represent high energetic cost [19]. Immunocompetence depends on factors such as a diet with adequate protein, energy, and multiple micronutrients. Immunocompetence presents sexual dimorphism where females present a general increased immunoreactivity compared to males [20]. Sexual dimorphism is due to genetic differences (several immune genes are in the X chromosome) and hormonal selective pressure. To achieve good reproductive fitness, females are selected to have a long life span due to a stronger immune system, whereas males need to maximize sexual mating early in life without investing in the immune system [21]. The immunocompetence of an individual undergoes some changes during the lifespan. Calves can adequately react to environmental pathogens through the transfer of colostrum immunoglobulins. Subsequent immunodeficiency or immune-compromised status in calfhood can occur following infections, drug treatments, and prolonged environmental stressful conditions. It is possible to enhance the immune response with three different general approaches: vaccination, passive immunization, and immunomodulation.

Evidence of reduced immunocompetence of high-yielding dairy cattle derives from epidemiological data and experimental studies [22–24]. As for the epidemiological data, the dramatic improvement of milk quality in terms of somatic cell counts was paired with an impressive increase in the milk yield of Holstein cows [25,26]. The impact of these performances on animal welfare and health has been considerable. In this respect, as the genetic ability to produce milk increases, more cows develop production diseases; the associations between increased milk production and increased risk of production diseases, as well as reduced fertility, are clearly documented, but less is known about the biological mechanisms behind these relationships [22]. Cows alive in the North-Eastern part of the USA at 48 months of age decreased from 80% in 1957 to 13% in 2002; on the same farms and in the same time period, the mean calving interval increased from 13 to 15.5 months [22]. As for experimental studies, high-yielding dairy cattle showed distinct signs of immunosuppression, which can be linked to the dramatic metabolic changes observed around calving [23,24]. Metabolic stresses associated with lactation influence the composition of peripheral blood mononuclear cell populations, as opposed to cows submitted to mastectomy [27], which confirms the crucial link between immunity and milk production levels.

2.2. *Metabolic Stress and the Innate Immune System*

Innate and adaptive immune mechanisms are complementary and synergistic. This operational framework has been jeopardized by genetic selection for high milk yield, which led to reduced serum concentrations of lysozyme compared with the other cattle breeds [28]. Lysozyme plays a fundamental antimicrobial role and is part of important regulatory circuits of the inflammatory response [29]. Metabolic priority for offspring survival demands the maintenance of milk yield to the detriment of other functions [30] as the fetus and placenta have the same priority during pregnancy as the brain and Coagulase-negative Staphylococci (CNS) [12]. The high levels of milk yield exceed the potential of dry matter intake and the subsequent negative energy balance gives rise to metabolic stress, shown as a disequilibrium in the homeostasis of a living organism as a result of anomalous utilization of nutrients [31]. The unsatisfactory profiles of the immune response in high-yielding dairy cattle can be either primary (i.e., associated with the genetic selection for high milk/fat/protein yields), or secondary to metabolic stress (Figure 2). Two main signaling pathways monitor nutrient availability, control metabolic stress responses, and exert a central role in modulating innate immunity: the mTOR-(mammalian target of rapamycin) and eIF2α (eukaryotic initiation factor-2α)-dependent signal transduction cascades [31]. The most important regulators of mTOR and eIF2α are cellular energy status (ATP/AMP ratio), amino acid availability, oxygen tension, and oxidative stress. A direct link between metabolism and innate immunity is the binding of free fatty acids to Toll-like Receptors (TLR) 4, which is implicated in the development of inflammation in states of hyperlipidemia; the subsequent cascade of signaling events is very similar to that observed after exposure to microbial stressors [32].

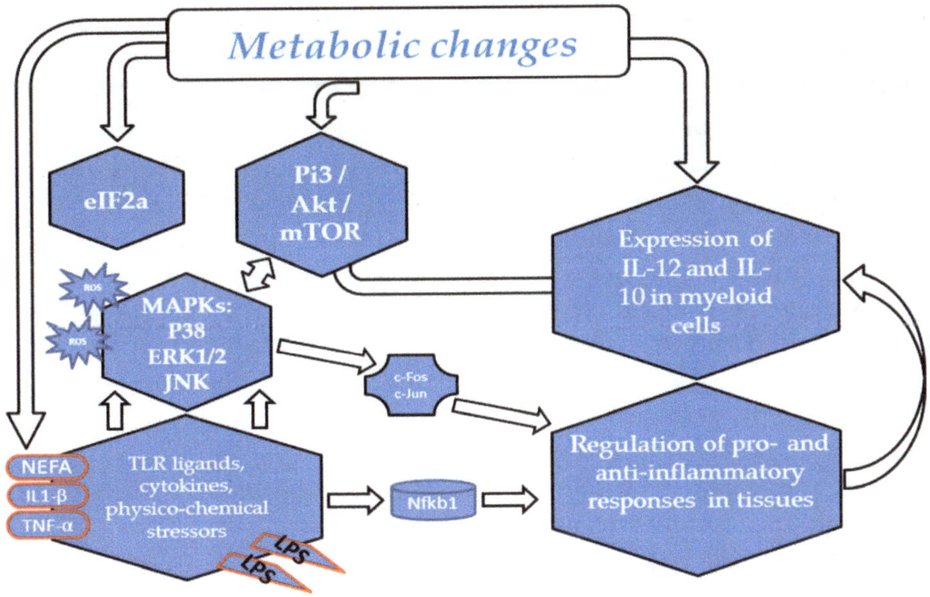

Figure 2. Metabolic stress is perceived by the innate immune system. The Pi3/Akt/mTOR- and eIF2α-dependent signal transduction cascades are the main signaling pathways monitoring nutrient availability and controlling metabolic stress responses. Toll-like receptors (TLRs) are expressed on innate immune cells, such as neutrophils, macrophages, and dendritic cells, and respond to the membrane components of Gram-positive or Gram-negative bacteria and to saturated free fatty acids mainly included in the NEFA (Non-esterified Fatty Acid) that are released by adipose tissue during status of negative energy balance. TLRs provoke rapid activation of innate immunity by inducing production of proinflammatory cytokines and upregulation of costimulatory molecules by both MAPK activation, which in turn activates c-Fos and c-Jun, and NF-kappa B activation through a MyD88-independent pathway. In addition, interleukin-1β (IL1-β) and tumor necrosis factor alpha (TNF-α), as critical cytokines, can induce a wide range of intracellular signal pathways as well as inflammation and immunity as nearly all cells express the respective receptors.

Metabolic stress in the framework of Negative Energy Balance (NEB) should be seen as a crucial element underlying the occurrence of diverse disease conditions of dairy cows. In this respect, the roles of the p38a MAPK/mTOR and Pi3/Akt/mTOR signaling pathways are pivotal to regulating the balance between pro and anti-inflammatory cytokines in tissues in response to environmental stress [33]. This confirms the central role of the innate immune system in response to environmental stressors. Additionally, the potent regulatory actions of the immune system might be conveniently exploited in the future toward vaccines for metabolic diseases, like type 2 diabetes mellitus [34], which is reminiscent of insulin resistance in dairy cows.

2.3. *The Influence of the Microbiome on the Immune System of Dairy Cattle*

The microbiome contributes to the architecture and function of tissues, influences the host energy metabolism, and plays an important role in the balance between health and disease. The microbiota and its metabolites are crucial in the maintenance of host homeostasis [35]. At the beginning of the host's life, the composition of the microbiota evolves into a healthy and viable community that strengthens itself and the host. Early development disturbances such as antibiotics, infections, or poor feed may lead to greater disease susceptibility [36].

Next-generation sequencing has enabled several groups to investigate microbiome influences on disease development. Bovine microbial communities have been described across many anatomical sites [37–40], including the mammary gland [41–43] and the uterus [44–47]. The composition of the bovine microbiome can affect the health [48–50] and performance of animals [51]. In ruminants such as dairy cows, the intestinal community of calves changes rapidly after birth and constantly during the first 12 weeks of life. Bacteroides–Prevotella and Clostridium coccoides–Eubacterium rectale species dominate the calf microbiota in this period [52]. After weaning, the microbiota must also compensate for the change in diet. This is a critical period when several events may affect the microbiota and health of the animal. During weaning Bacteroidetes decreased (remaining the dominant phyla) while Proteobacteria and Firmicutes increased [38]. These changes in microbial community composition, in part, are due to host physiological changes but are also likely due to the introduction of solid feeds because diet is a large driver of microbial community composition and modulation [38]. Weaning in dairy calves elicited an immune response in the lower gastrointestinal tract, but adding solid feed in addition to milk replacer resulted in changes to the immune response as well as gut bacteria [53]. Increased solid feed resulted in an increased total amount of bacteria present in the gastrointestinal tract. Weaning age and method of weaning can also change rumen or gastrointestinal tract microbiome establishment and community structure [54]. Weaning strategies can influence the ability of a calf to adapt to the dietary shift and can influence the severity of production losses. The effects of various feeding strategies and age as determining factors in the extent of microbial shifts in the rumen and feces during weaning still need to be studied.

Studies indicate that bovine gut microbiome can change immune responses [55]. These changes may be through direct and indirect mechanisms, such as through bacterial secretion of antimicrobial compounds or through influencing the expression of genes underlying host mucosal immune responses [56]. While much research on commensal microbes modulating host immune responses exists, studies investigating pathogen and pathobiont impact on host health are few [55,57]. The process of antimicrobial resistance is a relevant public health issue and, although antimicrobial use in human medicine arguably contributes to antimicrobial resistance much more than corresponding use in the livestock sector, it is important that farms proactively apply principles of prudent and judicious use of antimicrobials [58]. Farm animals and humans alike are threatened by this development. To promote early life wellness, pre- and probiotics are used to establish and restore microbiota health. Several studies demonstrated that probiotics and prebiotics achieved a positive balance in the gastrointestinal microbiota of cattle [59]. The functional interactions between gut microbes and relationships between microbes and host cells have yet to be fully investigated. Other pre-existent factors may play a crucial role, including host genetics, environmental conditions, and the resident, established microbiota [36].

3. Immunocompetence in Bovine Mastitis

Immunocompetence in the mammary gland is the outcome of a complex, coordinated network of anatomical, humoral, and cellular factors that are both specific and non-specific [60]. Immunocompetence can vary during lactation, showing depression in the peripartum period due to the hormonal and metabolic stress of calving and milk production [61]. The teat duct epithelium produces keratin that physically traps bacteria and blocks their migration to the mammary cistern. Keratin also has antimicrobial activity due to some bacteriostatic fatty acids (lauric, myristic, palmitoleic, and linoleic), as well as fibrous proteins that bind and damage the microorganism cell wall [62]. The duct epithelium can also modulate the expression of Pathogen Recognition Receptors (PRRs), such as Toll-like Receptors (TLRs), that after binding to PAMPs lead to the expression of inflammatory genes, and the release of cytokines (IL-1beta, TNF-alpha, IL-8) and acute phase proteins (haptoglobin, HP) but also antimicrobial peptides (pentraxin 3 PTX3, lipopolysaccharide-binding protein LBP) [6,63,64]. The mammary gland displays both innate and adaptive immune mechanisms that collaborate to defend the tissue against microbial invasions. The innate immune system is able to recognize the pathogens through TLRs and trigger an inflammatory response to kill them by phagocytosis (facilitated by the expression of surface receptors for Ig and complement proteins), or expression of antimicrobial molecules (lactoferrin, transferrin, lysozyme, defensins, cathelicidin, myeloperoxidases, complement system). Neutrophils respond with the up-regulation of adhesion molecules (L-selectin and beta2-integrin) to reach the damaged tissue [65]. Macrophages can perform phagocytosis, similar to neutrophils, but also act as antigen-presenting cells by exposing to lymphocytes the microbial antigens associated with Major Histocompatibility Complex MHC class II [66]. In the mammary gland of dairy cattle, the prevalence of lymphocyte populations (Th1, Th2, Th17, Treg, T cytotoxic, gamma-delta T cells, B cells) varies during lactation and the role of lymphocytes and natural killer cells is not fully understood under both health and disease conditions [67–69]. The main lymphocyte subset found in the bovine mammary gland is gamma-delta T cells [70]. During the peripartum period, lymphocytes assume a regulatory or suppressor phenotype, whereas at mid-lactation they shift to a cytotoxic phenotype and produce Interferon IFN-gamma [71]. In general, lymphocytes of the mammary gland are less responsive compared to the circulating ones; this could be partly due to a lower efficiency in antigen presentation in this area [61,67]. B cells do not change in number during the lactation stages [65]. B cells of the mammary gland serve as antigen-presenting cells but can also differentiate to plasma cells that produce antibodies (Ig) of four main isotypes: immunoglobulin G (IgG)1, IgG2, IgA, and IgM [72]. The concentrations of Ig in milk vary greatly during lactation. The activation of Th cells induces the expression of different cytokine repertoires that in turn influences the activity of T cytotoxic, B cells, macrophages, neutrophils, and Natural Killer NK cells [72]. The contribution to the immune response of mammary epithelial cells (MEC) is particularly important. MEC express PRRs; once they recognize microbial components, they can activate an innate immune response by expressing pro-inflammatory mediators (IL-1beta, TNF-alpha, IL-6, IL-8, acute phase proteins) and antimicrobial molecules (defensins, cathelicidin, calprotectin) [73]. Depending on the cytokine pattern in the inflamed mammary microenvironment, different responses can be started: Th1 (favoring cell-mediated responses), Th2 (favoring humoral responses), or Th17 (favoring activation and functions of granulocytes). This polarization drives the expression of specific molecules with different biological effects [74].

Decreased immunocompetence in the mammary gland, for instance in the peripartum period, predisposes cows to develop mastitis. In order to ameliorate the immune reactivity of the mammary gland, different strategies have been investigated. Diets can be fortified with minerals and micronutrients. These potentiate the activity of immune cells (such as Se and Vit E) and act as antioxidants (Vit A, Zn, Cu) to protect against the toxic effects of Reactive Oxygen Species (ROS) [75,76]. Another strategy consists in the administration of recombinant cytokines; for example, Granulocyte-Colony Stimulating Factor (G-CSF) results efficacious in the recruitment and differentiation from bone marrow reserves of a high number of polymorphonuclear leukocyte (PMN), as well as in the enhancement of their action at calving, which underlies a major reduction of mastitis prevalence [77]. Finally, vaccines were developed to prevent the insurgence of new infections and reduce the tissue damage induced by pathogens. The controversial results of different types of vaccines have cast doubts on this strategy [78]. It can be argued that merely using vaccines shows poor efficacy, which suggests their association with sanitary measures such as milking hygiene, teat dipping, confinement, and culling of chronically infected cows [79].

3.1. *Epigenetics and Trained Immunity: Implications for the Control of Mastitis*

Recently, evidence demonstrated that the innate immune system has the capability to develop "memory", once attributed only to adaptive immunity. Innate immune memory is known as "trained immunity". Studies show that the innate immune system can modify its response after the first encounter with both infectious and non-infectious stressors [80]. This is reminiscent of the cross-protection observed following different pathogen infections, described previously [81]. The peculiarities of trained immunity consist of the involvement of specific cell types (monocytes, macrophages, NK cells, innate lymphoid cells, ILC) and in epigenetic mechanisms that induce long-lasting adaptation. As a result, these cells remain highly responsive versus non-specific insults after the first recognition of a stressor [80]. In trained immunity, innate immune cells undergo epigenetic re-arrangement, leading to gene- or locus-specific changes in their chromatin profiles after a previous stimulation [80]. The major epigenetic mechanism active in trained immunity is histone modification with chromatin reconfiguration but other processes such as DNA methylation, modulation of microRNA, and long noncoding RNA expression seem to play a role [82]. This provides a transcriptional profile that modifies signaling and metabolism of innate immune cells [80]. Evidence of trained immunity is also described in dairy cows. Mammary epithelial cells stimulated with either Lipopolysaccharides (LPS) or Pam2CSK4 (two TLR ligands) develop endotoxin tolerance by epigenetic mechanisms; this response protects mammary tissues by enhancing the expression of beta-defensins and membrane protectors (Serum Amyloid A3 SAA3, Transglutaminase 3 TGM3) and down-regulating the expression of proinflammatory cytokines (TNF-alpha, IL-1beta) at a subsequent challenge [83]. This suggests that priming epithelial mammary cells with PAMPs induces a protective status by dampening exaggerated inflammation and enhancing bactericidal activity in a subsequent infection.

Trained immunity needs to be dissected to better understand its relevant subtended mechanisms. The identification of epigenetic changes increasing immunocompetence should be conducive to a promising mastitis control strategy. Furthermore, trained immunity in the mammary gland could be helpful in the design of efficacious vaccines combining both memory of adaptive immunity and "trained" innate responses.

3.2. *The Milk Microbiome and the Mammary Gland Health*

The bioactive molecules in milk play an integral role in training the immune system of recently born animals. The intestinal equilibrium of newborns is maintained by a synergistic relationship between antimicrobial peptides, lactoferrins, lysozymes immunoglobulins, and oligosaccharides [84,85]. The nutrient-rich ecosystem of milk allows growth of a wide range of microorganisms [41,86]. These microorganisms may contribute to the development of neonate gut microbiota, interact with the immune system, and regulate inflammatory responses and infection susceptibility [87].

Inflammation of the mammary gland, mastitis, is a response to intramammary infection, metabolic disorders, and trauma. Intramammary infection often occurs from the passage of pathogens beyond the teat canal [62], activating immune responses. Several factors can trigger mammary gland defenses against pathogens [88]. Commensal microbiota residing in the udder [41] may govern mastitis susceptibility. Bacteriocins produced by certain non-aureus Staphylococci (NAS) and *Corynebacterium* species colonizing the teat apices and teat canals may inhibit growth of major mastitis pathogens [89]. Within complex ecosystems, ecosystem diversity can increase resiliency against an influx of external species by supporting favorable interactivity [90]. The complexity of microbe to microbe communications concerning the functional properties of the mammary ecosystem are difficult to understand. It is essential to identify those bacterial species in the milk microbiota that contribute to mammary homeostasis and mastitis pathogen susceptibility [91]. While exploring milk microbiota diversity in relation to udder health, studies have shown a connection between dysbiotic microbiota and mastitis incidence [48,92–94]. In clinical *versus* non-clinical milk samples, clinical sample microbiota had reduced richness and evenness [48,93]. Despite these studies, much remains unknown concerning the ability of commensal microbiota to maintain mammary gland balance and modulate mastitis susceptibility. Derakhshani et al. [91] provided new insight into bacterial community composition and structure, which inhabit the mammary gland. This study shows the possible relationship of bacterial taxa with the inflammatory status of the udder. The identification of that possible hub species and candidate foundation taxa were associated with the inflammatory status of the mammary gland and/or future incidences of clinical mastitis.

In conclusion, more research is necessary to understand the interactions between the microbial world and its hosts. The dissection of these relationships may result in new ways to repair microbial community structure in animals that are affected by organism imbalance.

4. Metabolic Response of Dairy Cows to Challenges: Insights into the Transition Period

It has been well established that high yielding dairy cows undergo several challenges throughout the whole gestation-lactation cycle with the most challenging time frame being in the transition period with the onset of lactation. Complex adaptation processes take place to enable the maintenance of the animals' energy and nutrient homeostasis but many cows fail to successfully cope with the genetically imposed burden of meeting the requirements for the metabolically prioritized mammary gland in early lactation [28,95,96]. Metabolic stress produces a series of effects on productive and reproductive performance, on the immune system, and overall, on the well-being of the dairy cows [97]. Production diseases that imply a metabolic response are not necessarily related to performance level. Concerning the early lactation, Bertoni et al. [98] were able to develop a novel and clear interpretation of the relationship between milk production levels and health status. The authors demonstrated that high-yielding dairy cows with the highest milk production in the first month of lactation were characterized by better liver functionality and a less pronounced inflammatory status. Considerable biological variation in metabolic adaptation exists among individual animals, particularly in the period between late gestation and early lactation, which is accompanied by distinct levels of metabolic stress [99]. In this context, the successful adaptation to the lactational challenges relies on the metabolic robustness and the activation of the immune machinery [9], with performance levels that should not become another disturbing element of this adaptation. The period from late pregnancy over the course of calving is accompanied by a significant reduction in feed intake, causing the entrance into mild/severe NEB of dairy cows. The latter is the result of the sudden increase of milk secretion in early lactation, which is not compensated by a sufficient increase in feed intake, resulting in the metabolism and immunity (mainly the innate) being out of balance until the level of feed intake is able to cover the energy output with milk production.

Looking at later lactational stages, metabolic adaptation responses to environmental (heat stress, facilities, overcrowding, etc.) and immunometabolic stressors (acidosis, mastitis, etc.) have less detrimental effect on animal health because of the favorable energy balance and the unimpaired immune system. In this section, we presented an overview of the metabolic adaptations to different lactational stages, focusing on the transition period and on the effect of the negative energy balance (NEB) at mid and late lactation in comparison with the early lactation, all from a metabolic standpoint.

4.1. *A Multifaceted Challenge Called Transition Period*

Drackley [95] argued that the biology underlying the transition to lactation was the "final frontier" in our understanding of the dairy cow. Since that time, a number of relevant in-depth studies uncovered most of the "obscured field" of the transition period with researchers demonstrating that immune cells are directly involved in a surprising array of metabolic functions including the maintenance of gastrointestinal function, control of adipose tissue lipolysis, which in turn determine liver functionality, and regulation of insulin sensitivity in multiple tissues [100–103]. It was also postulated and highlighted that metabolic changes related to energy and calcium supply in support of lactation occurring concurrently impair the innate immune response [9]. The NEB during the transition period explains this reduced immune function, which is also associated with increased concentrations of some blood metabolites as a result of tissue mobilization [96,104]. PMN and lymphocyte functions decrease gradually, starting about 2 weeks before calving, with the lowest efficiencies between the time of calving and 2 days after [104,105]. According to Kehrli et al. [104], the impaired neutrophil function during the periparturient period can be attributed to many of the hormonal and metabolic changes that prepare the mammary gland for lactation. Around this critical period, metabolism shifts from the demands of pregnancy to those of lactation, increasing demands for energy and protein. Together, these metabolic and immunologic challenges during the peripartal period are important factors that limit the ability of most cows to achieve optimal performance and immune-metabolic status [95,106]. Several "exploratory" studies on the immune function during the peripartum period led researchers to investigate potential interventions that might mitigate the immune dysfunction occurring immediately before and after parturition. The focus has been on stimulation of the circulating numbers and possibly the function of neutrophils using the recombinant bovine granulocyte colony-stimulating factor (rbG-CSF) as reported previously [58,107–110]. Treatment with rbG-CSF, starting from approximately a week before parturition with one injection (15 mg of rbG-CSF) and the second within 24 h after parturition, was able to increase neutrophils, basophils, eosinophils, and monocytes count [108–111]. From a molecular point of view, mRNA abundance of most genes involved in the cell adhesion, migration, recognition, antimicrobial activity, and inflammation cascade was increased. This suggested a complete activation of the immune machinery against the critical period post-partum, at least as a first response of leukocytes to transcriptional regulation [110]. Recently, Lopreiato et al. [102], for the first time, have highlighted the effect of rbG-CSF in maintaining stable cytokine levels during the first month after parturition, reflecting greater regulation of neutrophil recruitment, trafficking, and maturation during the inflammatory response, providing evidence of the immunomodulatory action of rbG-CSF around parturition, when dairy cows are highly immune hypo-reactive. A novel outcome reported by Lopreiato et al. [102] was that increasing the release of pro-inflammatory cytokines, interleukin-6 (IL-6) and interleukin-1β (IL-1β), after parturition upon rbG-CSF treatment did not result in increased systemic inflammation, as shown by haptoglobin and ceruloplasmin plasma levels. This latter finding points out that other mechanisms and/or molecules are likely to drive the inflammation after parturition. Plasma concentrations of IL-1β, IL-6, and tumor necrosis factor alpha (TNF-α) have been shown to be 1.5- to five-fold higher prepartum compared to the early lactation period [112]. Further studies should be undertaken to uncover the unknown mechanisms behind this controversial aspect of inflammation within the transition period.

Besides a systemic inflammation, pro-inflammatory cytokines also act on peripheral cells inducing insulin resistance [113,114]. Under these conditions, circulating glucose is prioritized to the non-insulin-dependent glucose transporters that are expressed on immune cells and mammary glands only [115]. The massive glucose requirements of an activated immune system during systemic inflammation could further reduce the energy available for the other tissues, as the mammary gland does not markedly reduce the glucose uptake, aggravating the NEB occurring in early lactation [115]. When NEB occurs, mobilization of body fat and proteins is induced and free fatty acids (FFA) and amino acids are used as gluconeogenic sources by the liver [116]. A severe NEB occurring in the transition period could induce an FFA overload in the liver, inducing the release of beta-hydroxybutyrate (BHB) into the blood following ineffective oxidation of FFA and impaired pivotal functions [95,103,117]. This systemic inflammation is also known to induce the acute-phase response in liver, implying reduced constitutive protein expression (e.g., albumin, lipoproteins, paraoxonase, and retinol-binding protein), counterbalanced by augmented production of positive acute-phase proteins (APP) such as haptoglobin, ceruloplasmin, serum amyloid A, and C-reactive protein [118]. Oxidative stress also occurs during this period and is driven by the imbalance between the production of reactive oxygen metabolites (ROM), reactive nitrogen species (RNS), and the neutralizing capacity of antioxidant mechanisms in tissues and blood, caused by the increased immune response and the metabolic intensification to support lactogenesis [9,88]. When oxidative stress overwhelms cellular antioxidant capacity, ROM induces an inflammatory response. The increase in oxidative stress and inflammation during this period is also negatively associated with a reduction in liver functionality, and measurement of APP can provide a useful tool to assess liver function as well as inflammation [118]. Liver function is often impaired in transition dairy cows. In this context, it is relevant to point out the scenario occurring in the rumen during the transition period. Few studies have investigated the molecular adaptations of ruminal epithelium during the peripartum period [119–123]. These studies revealed the existence of interactions among genes of the immune system and those involved in the preparation for the onset of lactation [119,121,122], as well as the presence of growth factors that seem to be regulated after parturition [120]. The connections among ruminal fermentation, microbiota, the ensuing ruminal epithelium adaptations, and the consequence on systemic responses (e.g., immunometabolism) of the cow remain unclear. Whether microbial metabolism could affect epithelial gene expression via metabolites remains uncertain. The interaction of rumen content and epithelium with the systemic immune response opens a new scenario in the management of forestomaches. The role of saliva and its composition in terms of immune cells and immunogenic molecules should be further investigated as a potential factor of the reduced immunocompetence in dairy cows, mainly in the transition period [64,124]. Secondly, the role of diet appears crucial not only for an accurate formulation (e.g., fermentability of carbohydrates, protein degradability) but also for nutrient imbalance and/or for microbiota composition, which might alter epithelium functions (e.g., increasing its permeability). Several attempts to improve energy intake and thus avoiding detrimental effects especially after parturition have been proposed. Controlling energy intake during the dry period to near calculated requirements leads to transition success, with fewer diseases and disorders than cows fed high-energy diets [125–127], but also greater DMI around parturition [128]. Prolonged over-consumption of energy during the dry period can decrease post-calving DMI, resulting in negative responses of metabolism with higher NEFA and BHB in blood and greater triacylglycerol in the liver after calving [126]. The diet must be formulated to limit energy intake and meet the requirements for protein, minerals, and vitamins. To date, there little knowledge about diet formulation for the immediate postpartum period in order to optimize transition success and consequently reproduction efficiency. Proper dietary formulation in both dry and close-up periods would maintain or enable rumen adaptation to higher grain diets after calving, which in turn reflects a greater level of energy intake and energy utilization.

Further perspectives are created by the opportunity to control rumen microbiomes by the host animal (genotype) as a result of genetic selection [129].

4.2. The Association between Rumen Microbiome, Cattle Production, and Health Traits

The rumen contains trillions of bacteria, protozoa, and methanogenic archaea as major components. A symbiotic relationship exists between a ruminant host and the microbiota where bacteria are provided shelter and nutrients and the host benefits from essential nutrients released by bacterial fermentation activities. Along with beneficial and essential nutrients, bacterial activity may be connected to the release of harmful compounds including bacterial endotoxins.

Recent studies using an omics-based structure have suggested that differences in rumen microbiota are associated with cattle production and health traits, such as feed efficiency [130,131], methane (CH_4) yield [132], milk composition [133], and ruminal acidosis [134]. Manipulating rumen microbiota may improve cattle productivity and health and reduce CH_4 emissions. Transfaunation of ruminal contents is regularly used to enhance rumen function and milk production [135]. Although studies show that ciliated protozoa responsible for plant material digestion may be successfully transferred, there is more resistance within the bacterial community perhaps due to host-specific properties [136,137], suggesting the importance of the host's genetics influence on rumen microbiota. More studies are needed to provide convincing information about associations between host and rumen microbiota.

5. Native Cattle Breeds, an Interesting "Case Study"

An interesting model for the study of the susceptibility to production diseases could be represented by native cattle breeds. These breeds have been part of livestock history until the 21st century when they were abandoned in favor of more productive cosmopolitan breeds (Holstein, Brown Swiss and Jersey) [138–141]. Some native breeds survived, thanks mainly to the efforts of many small traditional farmers residing mainly in rural marginal areas. The intense genetic selection received by the cosmopolitan breeds in order to improve the productive characteristics led them to develop peculiar physiological features, which have likely impaired some immune defense mechanisms, increasing the incidence of metabolic and infectious diseases, and worsening both fertility and longevity [76,142–144]. These phenomena have been studied in Holstein Friesian (HF) cows, the most widespread and highly selected dairy cattle breed. The intense genetic selection of HF for milk production has been associated with relevant physiological dysfunctions, e.g., reduction of the immune competence, severe NEB, inflammatory-like status, oxidative stress, and hypocalcemia [9]. The metabolic pressure caused by the high, energetic requests of the mammary gland combined with the stress resulting from the pregnancy-calving period in the context of severe NEB can lead to serious disruptions of physiological homeostatic balance [103,104]. All these physiological perturbations seem to be less intense in the "lower productive" native breeds. The scientific community is comparing breeds with different selective pressure in order to improve the comprehension of regulatory mechanisms of cattle physiology. The literature is not very extensive and has some limitations (e.g., number of animals, different environments, diet, and management), but important physiological information can be deduced. Mendoca et al. [145] compared HF and Montbéliarde-sired crossbred cows in the peripartum; no differences were found in terms of metabolic and inflammatory (haptoglobin concentration) responses, milk yield and incidence of typical peripartum diseases (retained fetal membranes, metritis, and subclinical endometritis). Despite that, the HF showed more pyrexia events in early lactation (50.0 vs. 31.4%) and a higher incidence of purulent vaginal discharge (44.2 vs. 26.5%) than crossbred cows. Curone et al. [6] compared HF with Rendena cows, an Italian breed native of the Rendena Valley in Northeastern Italy (Trentino), and observed that HF in the postpartum showed a more severe systemic inflammatory response in terms of haptoglobin, total proteins, globulins, and bilirubin, a more severe fat mobilization associated with lower body muscle mass and lower amino acid mobilization. In this study and in that of Cremonesi et al. [146], detailed insights into the milk microbial population of HF and Rendena along the transition period were also provided. The results highlighted the existence of differences in terms of general microbial diversity, taxonomy, and predicted functional profiles. Those differences might also have an impact on their mammary gland health concerning disease and pathogen resistance. These differences seem related to inflammo-metabolic changes occurring around calving, which suggest a possible relationship among these responses and the mechanisms of resistance in the mammary gland.

The local breed Simmental, when compared with HF cows during the transition period, presented a different metabolic adaptation, in terms of different energy, inflammatory, and oxidative pattern responses. Simmental showed a lower value of BHB and higher mobilization of muscle protein (creatinine) [101]. Simmental cows seemed more sensitive to induction of the immune system after calving, with a greater transcript abundance of proinflammatory cytokines and receptor genes, cell migration- and adhesion-related genes [102,110]. Begley et al. [147] showed that, when infected with Candida albicans, Norwegian Red cows have a greater primary antibody-mediated immune response, producing greater concentrations of immunoglobulin G (IgG) compared to HF cows. One of the largest comparative studies was performed by Bieber et al. [148]. They compared the production, fertility, longevity, and health-associated traits of local native and modern breeds of dairy cattle in 4 different European nations: Austria, Switzerland, Poland, and Sweden. They compared Original Braunvieh and Grey Cattle with Braunvieh (Brown Swiss blood >60%) in Switzerland; Grey Cattle with Braunvieh (Brown Swiss blood >50%) in Austria; Polish Black and White, Polish Red and White, and Polish Red with Polish Holstein Friesian in Poland; and Swedish Red with Swedish Holstein in Sweden. Average milk yields were substantially lower for local compared with commercial breeds in all countries. Local breeds showed a longer productive lifetime and a shorter calving interval with a lower insemination index than commercial breeds. Another approach to re-appraise the native breeds is the use of crossbreed cattle. Several studies showed how dairy producers may improve the longevity, robustness, and fertility of cows and the profitability of dairying by crossing pure HF cows with bulls of different native breeds [149–151]. The lower production level of local breeds is partly compensated by advantages in fertility, health status, and longevity. It is important to remember that the breeding goals should balance productivity with functional traits [152], and the choice of appropriate dairy breeds can be regarded as a key factor for successful health management in dairy farming.

6. Conclusions

The immune system has evolved along with the phylogenetic evolution as a highly refined sensing and response system poised to react against diverse infectious and non-infectious stressors for better survival and adaptation. This operational framework is jeopardized when high-yielding dairy cattle are poorly managed. Metabolic priority for offspring survival is affected by the levels of milk yield, exceeding the potential of dry matter intake. Secondly, the subsequent negative energy balance gives rise to metabolic stress, e.g., a disequilibrium in the homeostasis of a living organism as a result of anomalous utilization of nutrients. It can be argued that high genetic merit for milk yield is correlated with a defective control of the inflammatory response underlying the occurrence of several production diseases. This is evident in the mastitis model where high-yielding dairy cows show high disease prevalence in the framework of reduced effectiveness of the innate immune response.

Effective monitoring tools, immunomodulators, and nutraceuticals should be combined with proper farm management and feeding regimes. Specific intervention protocols should be implemented in the first weeks after calving and at dry-off because the relevant stressors are pivotal to disease occurrence and early culling of high-yielding dairy cattle.

Author Contributions: Conceptualization, M.A., P.M., and B.C.; writing—original draft preparation: introduction and conclusion, V.B., metabolic stresses, V.L. and E.T., microbiomes, P.C., M.F.A., and B.C., immune system, M.A. and F.R., bovine mastitis, P.M. and V.B., native cattle breeds, G.C.; writing—review and editing, V.B., V.L., M.A., M.F.A., P.M., and B.C.; supervision, B.C., M.A., and P.M. All authors have read and agreed to the published version of the manuscript.

Acknowledgments: The Authors thank "Romeo ed Enrica Invernizzi foundation" (Milan, Italy) and AGER 2 "FARM-INN" grant 2017-1130 Project for the financial support of the experiments from which data were used in the present review. The authors acknowledge Daryl Van Nydam and Belinda Gross (QMPS, Animal Health Diagnostic Center, Cornell University, Ithaca, NY) and Agnese Moroni (London School of Economics, London, UK) for their valuable revision of the English text.

References

1. Trevisi, E.; Zecconi, A.; Cogrossi, S.; Razzuoli, E.; Grossi, P.; Amadori, M. Strategies for reduced antibiotic usage in dairy cattle farms. *Res. Vet. Sci.* **2014**, *96*, 229–233. [CrossRef] [PubMed]
2. Wemette, M.; Safi, A.G.; Beauvais, W.; Ceres, K.; Shapiro, M.; Moroni, P.; Welcome, F.L.; Ivanek, R. New York State dairy farmers' perceptions of antibiotic use and resistance: A qualitative interview study. *PLoS ONE* **2020**, *15*, e0232937. [CrossRef] [PubMed]
3. Snowder, G.D.; Van Vleck, L.D.; Cundiff, L.V.; Bennett, G.L. Genetic and environmental factors associated with incidence of infectious bovine keratoconjunctivitis in preweaned beef calves. *J. Anim. Sci.* **2005**, *83*, 507–518. [CrossRef] [PubMed]
4. Snowder, G.D.; Van Vleck, L.D.; Cundiff, L.V.; Bennett, G.L. Influence of breed, heterozygosity, and disease incidence on estimates of variance components of respiratory disease in preweaned beef calves. *J. Anim. Sci.* **2005**, *83*, 1247–1261. [CrossRef]
5. Snowder, G.D.; Van Vleck, L.D.; Cundiff, L.V.; Bennett, G.L. Bovine respiratory disease in feedlot cattle: Environmental, genetic, and economic factors. *J. Anim. Sci.* **2006**, *84*, 1999–2008. [CrossRef]
6. Curone, G.; Filipe, J.; Cremonesi, P.; Trevisi, E.; Amadori, M.; Pollera, C.; Castiglioni, B.; Turin, L.; Tedde, V.; Vigo, D.; et al. What we have lost: Mastitis resistance in Holstein Friesians and in a local cattle breed. *Res. Vet. Sci.* **2018**, *116*, 88–98. [CrossRef]
7. Jeon, S.J.; Elzo, M.; DiLorenzo, N.; Lamb, G.C.; Jeong, K.C. Evaluation of animal genetic and physiological factors that affect the prevalence of Escherichia coli O157 in cattle. *PLoS ONE* **2013**, *8*, e55728. [CrossRef]
8. Bishop, S.C.; Woolliams, J.A. Genomics and disease resistance studies in livestock. *Livest. Sci.* **2014**, *166*, 190–198. [CrossRef]
9. Trevisi, E.; Minuti, A. Assessment of the innate immune response in the periparturient cow. *Res. Vet. Sci.* **2018**, *116*, 47–54. [CrossRef]
10. Amadori, M. *The Innate Immune Response to Noninfectious Stressors: Human and Animal Models*; Academic Press: London, UK, 2016.
11. Flajnik, M.F.; Kasahara, M. Origin and evolution of the adaptive immune system: Genetic events and selective pressures. *Nat. Rev. Genet.* **2010**, *11*, 47–59. [CrossRef]
12. Amadori, M.; Stefanon, B.; Sgorlon, S.; Farinacci, M. Immune system response to stress factors. *Ital. J. Anim. Sci.* **2009**, *8*, 287–299. [CrossRef]

13. Vigne, J.D. Early domestication and farming: What should we know or do for a better under-standing? *Anthropozoologica* **2015**, *50*, 123–150. [CrossRef]
14. Mellor, D.J.; Stafford, K.J. Integrating practical, regulatory and ethical strategies for enhancing farm animal welfare. *Aust. Vet. J.* **2001**, *79*, 762–768. [CrossRef] [PubMed]
15. European Commission, DG Health and Food Safety Overview Report: Welfare of Cattle on Dairy Farms. 2017. Available online: http://ec.europa.eu/food/audits-analysis/overview_reports/act_getPDF.cfm?PDF_ID=1139 (accessed on 11 August 2020).
16. Vitali, A.; Felici, A.; Esposito, S.; Bernabucci, U.; Bertocchi, L.; Maresca, C.; Nardone, A.; Lacetera, N. The effect of heat waves on dairy cow mortality. *J. Dairy Sci.* **2015**, *98*, 4572–4579. [CrossRef] [PubMed]
17. Flori, L.; Gao, Y.; Laloë, D.; Lemonnier, G.; Leplat, J.J.; Teillaud, A.; Cossalter, A.M.; Laffitte, J.; Pinton, P.; de Vaureix, C.; et al. Immunity traits in pigs: Substantial genetic variation and limited covariation. *PLoS ONE* **2011**, *6*, e22717. [CrossRef] [PubMed]
18. Matzinger, P. An innate sense of danger. *Ann. N. Y. Acad. Sci.* **2002**, *961*, 341–342. [CrossRef] [PubMed]
19. Martin, L.B., 2nd; Navara, K.J.; Weil, Z.M.; Nelson, R.J. Immunological memory is compromised by food restriction in deer mice Peromyscus maniculatus. *Am. J. Physiol. Regul. Integr. Comp. Physiol.* **2007**, *292*, R316–R320. [CrossRef]
20. Zandman-Goddardab, G.; Peevac, E.; Shoenfeld, Y. Gender and autoimmunity. *Autoimmun. Rev.* **2007**, *6*, 366–372. [CrossRef]
21. Nunn Charles, L.; Lindenfors, P.; Rhiannon Pursall, E.; Rolff, J. On sexual dimorphism in immune function. *Philos. Trans. R. Soc. B Biol. Sci.* **2009**, *364*, 61–69. [CrossRef]
22. Oltenacu, P.; Broom, D. The impact of genetic selection for increased milk yield on the welfare of dairy cows. *Anim. Welf.* **2010**, *19*, 39–49.
23. Lacetera, N.; Scalia, D.; Franci, O.; Bernabucci, U.; Ronchi, B.; Nardone, A. Short communication: Effects of nonesterified fatty acids on lymphocyte function in dairy heifers. *J. Dairy Sci.* **2004**, *87*, 1012–1014. [CrossRef]
24. Lacetera, N.; Scalia, D.; Bernabucci, U.; Ronchi, B.; Pirazzi, D.; Nardone, A. Lymphocyte Functions in Overconditioned Cows Around Parturition. *J. Dairy Sci.* **2005**, *88*, 2010–2016. [CrossRef]
25. Rupp, R.; Boichard, D. Relationship of early first lactation somatic cell count with risk of subsequent first clinical mastitis. *Livest. Prod. Sci.* **2000**, *62*, 169–180. [CrossRef]
26. Hagnestam-Nielsen, C.; Emanuelson, U.; Berglund, B.; Strandberg, E. Relationship between somatic cell count and milk yield in different stages of lactation. *J. Dairy Sci.* **2009**, *92*, 3124–3133. [CrossRef]
27. Kimura, K.; Goff, J.P.; Kehrli, M.E.; Harp, J.A.; Nonnecke, B.J. Effects of mastectomy on composition of peripheral blood mononuclear cell populations in periparturient dairy cows. *J. Dairy Sci.* **2002**, *85*, 1437–1444. [CrossRef]
28. Trevisi, E.; Amadori, M.; Archetti, I.; Lacetera, N.; Bertoni, G. Inflammatory response and acute phase proteins in the transition period of high-yielding dairy cows. In *Acute Phase Protein*, 2nd ed.; Veas, F., Ed.; InTech: Rijeka, Croatia, 2011; pp. 355–380.
29. Trevisi, E.; Amadori, M.; Cogrossi, S.; Razzuoli, E.; Bertoni, G. Metabolic stress and inflammatory re-sponse in high-yielding, periparturient dairy cows. *Res. Vet. Sci.* **2012**, *93*, 695–704. [CrossRef]
30. Bauman, D.E.; Currie, W.B. Partitioning of nutrients during pregnancy and lactation: A review of mechanisms involving homeostasis homeorhesis. *J. Dairy Sci.* **1980**, *63*, 1514–1529. [CrossRef]
31. Lacetera, N. Metabolic stress, Heat Shock Proteins, and Innate Immune Response. In *The Innate Immune Response to Noninfectious Stressors: Human and Animal Models*; Amadori, M., Ed.; Academic Press: London, UK, 2016; pp. 107–131.
32. Song, M.J.; Kim, K.H.; Yoon, J.M.; Kim, J.B. Activation of Toll-like receptor 4 is associated with insulin resistance in adipocytes. *Biochem. Biophys. Res. Commun.* **2006**, *346*, 739–745. [CrossRef]
33. Katholnig, K.; Kaltenecker, C.C.; Hayakawa, H. p38α senses environmental stress to control innate immune responses via mechanistic target of rapamycin. *J. Immunol.* **2013**, *190*, 1519–1527. [CrossRef]
34. Morais, T.; Andrade, S.; Pereira, S.; Monteiro, M. Vaccines for metabolic diseases: Current perspectives. *Vaccine Dev. Ther.* **2014**, *4*, 55–72.
35. Eberl, G. A new vision of immunity: Homeostasis of the superorganism. *Mucosal Immunol.* **2010**, *3*, 450–460. [CrossRef] [PubMed]
36. Sommer, F.; Anderson, J.; Bharti, R.; Raes, J.; Rosenstiel, P. The resilience of the intestinal microbiota influences health and disease. *Nat. Rev. Microbiol.* **2017**, *15*, 630–638. [CrossRef] [PubMed]

37. Jami, E.; Israel, A.; Kotser, A.; Mizrahi, I. Exploring the bovine rumen bacterial community from birth to adulthood. *ISME J.* **2013**, *7*, 1069–1079. [CrossRef]
38. Meale, S.J.; Li, S.; Azevedo, P.; Derakhshani, H.; Plaizier, J.C.; Khafipour, E.; Steele, M.A. Development of ruminal and fecal microbiomes are affected by weaning but not weaning strategy in dairy calves. *Front. Microbiol.* **2016**, *7*, 582. [CrossRef] [PubMed]
39. Dill-McFarland, K.A.; Breaker, J.D.; Suen, G. Microbial succession in the gastrointestinal tract of dairy cows from weeks to first lactation. *Sci. Rep.* **2017**, *7*, 40864. [CrossRef]
40. Yeoman, C.J.; Ishaq, S.L.; Bichi, E.; Olivo, S.K.; Lowe, J.; Aldridge, B.M. Biogeographical Differences in the Influence of Maternal Microbial Sources on the Early Successional Development of the Bovine Neonatal Gastrointestinal tract. *Sci. Rep.* **2018**, *8*, 3197. [CrossRef]
41. Derakhshani, H.; Fehr, K.B.; Sepehri, S.; Francoz, D.; De Buck, J.; Barkema, H.W.; Plaizier, J.C.; Khafipour, E. Invited review: Microbiota of the bovine udder: Contributing factors and potential implications for udder health and mastitis susceptibility. *J. Dairy Sci.* **2018**, *101*, 10605–10625. [CrossRef]
42. Addis, M.F.; Tanca, A.; Uzzau, S.; Oikonomou, G.; Bicalho, R.C.; Moroni, P. The bovine milk microbiota: Insights and perspectives from -omics studies. *Mol. Biosyst.* **2016**, *12*, 2359–2372. [CrossRef]
43. Oikonomou, G.; Addis, M.F.; Chassard, C.; Nader-Macias, M.E.F.; Grant, I.; Delbès, C.; Bogni, C.I.; Le Loir, Y.; Even, S. Milk Microbiota: What Are We Exactly Talking About? *Front. Microbiol.* **2020**, *11*, 60. [CrossRef]
44. Machado, V.S.; Oikonomou, G.; Bicalho, M.L.; Knauer, W.A.; Gilbert, R.; Bicalho, R.C. Investigation of postpartum dairy cows' uterine microbial diversity using metagenomic pyrosequencing of the 16S rRNA gene. *Vet. Microbiol.* **2012**, *159*, 460–469. [CrossRef]
45. Santos, T.M.; Bicalho, R.C. Diversity and succession of bacterial communities in the uterine fluid of postpartum metritic, endometritic and healthy dairy cows. *PLoS ONE* **2012**, *7*, e53048. [CrossRef] [PubMed]
46. Jeon, S.J.; Galvão, K.N. An Advanced Understanding of Uterine Microbial Ecology Associated with Metritis in Dairy Cows. *Genom. Inform.* **2018**, *16*, e21. [CrossRef] [PubMed]
47. Klibs, N.; Galvão, K.N.; Bicalho, R.C.; Jeon, S.J. Symposium review: The uterine microbiome associated with the development of uterine disease in dairy cows. *J. Dairy Sci.* **2019**, *102*, 11786–11797.
48. Oikonomou, G.; Bicalho, M.L.; Meira, E.; Rossi, R.E.; Foditsch, C.; Machado, V.S.; Teixeira, A.G.V.; Santisteban, C.; Schukken, Y.H.; Bicalho, R.C. Microbiota of cow's milk; distinguishing healthy, sub-clinically and clinically diseased quarters. *PLoS ONE* **2014**, *9*, e85904. [CrossRef] [PubMed]
49. Lima, S.F.; Teixeira, A.G.; Higgins, C.H.; Lima, F.S.; Bicalho, R.C. The upper respiratory tract microbiome and its potential role in bovine respiratory disease and otitis media. *Sci. Rep.* **2016**, *6*, 29050. [CrossRef]
50. Zinicola, M.; Lima, F.; Lima, S.; Machado, V.; Gomez, M.; Döpfer, D.; Guard, C.; Bicalho, R. Altered microbiomes in bovine digital dermatitis lesions, and the gut as a pathogen reservoir. *PLoS ONE* **2015**, *10*, e0120504. [CrossRef]
51. Lima, F.S.; Oikonomou, G.; Lima, S.F.; Bicalho, M.L.; Ganda, E.K.; Filho, J.C.; Lorenzo, G.; Trojacanec, P.; Bicalhoa, R. Prepartum and postpartum rumen fluid microbiomes: Characterization and correlation with production traits in dairy cows. *Appl. Environ. Microbiol.* **2015**, *81*, 1327–1337. [CrossRef]
52. Uyeno, Y.; Sekiguchi, Y.; Kamagata, Y. rRNA-based analysis to monitor succession of faecal bacterial communities in Holstein calves. *Lett. Appl. Microbiol.* **2010**, *51*, 570–577. [CrossRef]
53. Malmuthuge, N.; Li, M.; Goonewardene, L.A.; Oba, M.; Guan, L.L. Effect of calf starter feeding on gut microbial diversity and expression of genes involved in host immune responses and tight junctions in dairy calves during weaning transition. *J. Dairy Sci.* **2013**, *96*, 3189–3200. [CrossRef]
54. Meale, S.J.; Li, S.C.; Azevedo, P.; Derakhshani, H.; DeVries, T.J.; Plaizier, J.C.; Steele, M.A.; Khafipour, E. Weaning age influences the severity of gastrointestinal microbiome shifts in dairy calves. *Sci. Rep.* **2017**, *7*, 198. [CrossRef]
55. Taschuk, R.; Griebel, P.J. Commensal microbiome effects on mucosal immune system development in the ruminant gastrointestinal tract. *Anim. Health Res. Rev.* **2012**, *13*, 129–141. [CrossRef] [PubMed]
56. Buffie, C.; Pamer, E. Microbiota-mediated colonization resistance against intestinal pathogens. *Nat. Rev. Immunol.* **2013**, *13*, 790–801. [CrossRef] [PubMed]
57. Ward, P.; Guévremont, E. Comparison of intestinal bacterial populations between two dairy cattle herds colonized or not by *Campylobacter jejuni*. *Foodborne Pathog. Dis.* **2014**, *11*, 966–968. [CrossRef] [PubMed]
58. Van Schyndel, S.J.; Carrier, J.; Bogado Pascottini, O.; LeBlanc, S.J. The effect of pegbovigrastim on circulating neutrophil count in dairy cattle: A randomized controlled trial. *PLoS ONE* **2018**, *13*, e0198701. [CrossRef]

59. Barkema, H.W.; von Keyserlingk, M.A.; Kastelic, J.P.; Lam, T.J.; Luby, C.; Roy, J.P.; LeBlanc, S.J.; Keefe, G.P.; Kelton, D.F. Invited review: Changes in the dairy industry affecting dairy cattle health and welfare. *J. Dairy Sci.* **2015**, *98*, 7426–7445. [CrossRef]
60. Sordillo, L.M.; Shafer-Weaver, K.; De Rosa, D. Immunobiology of the mammary gland. *J. Dairy Sci.* **1997**, *80*, 1851–1865. [CrossRef]
61. Waller, K.P. Mammary Gland Immunology around Parturition. In *Biology of the Mammary Gland*; Springer: New York, NY, USA, 2002; pp. 231–245.
62. Paulrud, C.O. Basic concepts of the bovine teat canal. *Vet. Res. Commun.* **2005**, *29*, 215–245. [CrossRef]
63. Rinaldi, M.; Li, R.W.; Bannerman, D.D.; Daniels, K.M.; Evock-Clover, C.; Silva, M.V.B.; Paape, M.J.; Van Ryssen, B.; Burvenich, C.; Capuco, A.V. A sentinel function for teat tissues in dairy cows: Dominant innate immune response elements define early response to E. coli mastitis. *Funct. Integr. Genom.* **2010**, *10*, 21–38. [CrossRef]
64. Filipe, J.F.S.; Riva, F.; Bani, P.; Trevisi, E.; Amadori, M. Ruminal fluids as substrate for investigating production diseases of small and large ruminant species. *CAB Rev.* **2019**, *14*, 1–12. [CrossRef]
65. Paape, M.J.; Shafer-Weaver, K.; Capuco, A.V.; Van Oostveldt, K.; Burvenich, C. Immune surveil-lance of mammary tissue by phagocytic cells. *Adv. Exp. Med. Biol.* **2000**, *480*, 259–277.
66. Denis, M.; Parlane, N.A.; Lacy-Hulbert, S.J.; Summers, E.L.; Buddle, B.M.; Wedlock, D.N. Bactericidal activity of macrophages against *Streptococcus uberis* is different in mammary gland secretions of lactating and drying off cows. *Vet. Immunol. Immunopathol.* **2006**, *114*, 111–120. [CrossRef] [PubMed]
67. Taylor, B.C.; Dellinger, J.D.; Cullor, J.S.; Stott, J.L. Bovine milk lymphocytes display the phenotype of memory Tcells and are predominantly $CD8^+$. *Cell. Immunol.* **1994**, *156*, 245–253. [CrossRef] [PubMed]
68. Shafer-Weaver, K.A.; Pighetti, G.M.; Sordillo, L.M. Diminished mammary gland lymphocyte functions parallel shifts in trafficking patterns during the postpartum period. *Proc. Soc. Exp. Biol. Med.* **1996**, *212*, 271–279. [CrossRef] [PubMed]
69. Aitken, S.L.; Corl, C.M.; Sordillo, L.M. Immunopathology of mastitis: Insights into disease recognition and resolution. *J. Mammary Gland Biol. Neoplasia* **2011**, *16*, 291–304. [CrossRef] [PubMed]
70. Machugh, N.D.; Mburu, J.K.; Carol, M.J.; Wyatt, C.R.; Orden, J.A.; Davis, W.C. Identification of two distinct subsets of bovine T cells with unique cell surface phenotype and tissue distribution. *Immunology* **1997**, *92*, 340–345. [CrossRef]
71. Hisatsune, T.; Enomoto, A.; Nishijimaetal, K.I. $CD8^+$ suppressor T cell clone capable of inhibiting the antigen-and anti-Tcell receptor-induced proliferation of Th clones without cytolytic activity. *J. Immunol.* **1990**, *145*, 2421–2426.
72. Sordillo, L.M. Mammary Gland Immunobiology and Resistance to Mastitis. *Vet. Clin. N. Am. Food Anim. Pract.* **2018**, *34*, 507–523. [CrossRef]
73. Lahoussa, H.; Moussay, E.; Rainard, P.; Riollet, C. Differential cytokine and chemokine responses of bovine mammary epithelial cells to *Staphylococcus aureus* and *Escherichia coli*. *Cytokine* **2007**, *38*, 12–21. [CrossRef]
74. Brown, W.C.; Rice-Ficht, A.C.; Estes, D.M. Bovine type 1 and type 2 responses. *Vet. Immunol. Immunopath.* **1998**, *63*, 45–55. [CrossRef]
75. Hogan, J.S.; Weiss, W.P.; Smith, K.L. Role of vitamin E and selenium in host defense against mastitis. *J. Dairy Sci.* **1993**, *76*, 2795–2803. [CrossRef]
76. Sordillo, L.M. Nutritional strategies to optimize dairy cattle immunity. *J. Dairy Sci.* **2016**, *99*, 4967–4982. [CrossRef] [PubMed]
77. Canning, P.; Hassfurther, R.; TerHune, T.; Rogers, K.; Abbott, S.; Kolb, D. Efficacy and clinical safety of pegbovigrastim for pre-venting naturally occurring clinical mastitis in periparturient primiparous and multiparous cows on US commercial dairies. *J. Dairy Sci.* **2017**, *100*, 6504–6515. [CrossRef] [PubMed]
78. Scali, F.; Camussone, C.; Calvinho, L.F.; Cipolla, M.; Zecconi, A. Which are important targets in development of *S. aureus* mastitis vaccine? *Res. Vet. Sci.* **2015**, *100*, 88–99. [CrossRef]
79. Ismail, Z.B. Mastitis vaccines in dairy cows: Recent developments and recommendations of application. *Vet. World* **2017**, *10*, 1057–1062. [CrossRef] [PubMed]
80. Netea, M.G.; Quintin, J.; van der Meer, J.W. Trained immunity: A memory for innate host defense. *Cell Host Microbe* **2011**, *9*, 355–361. [CrossRef]
81. Quintin, J.; Cheng, S.C.; van der Meer, J.W.; Netea, M.G. Innate immune memory: Towards a better understanding of host defense mechanisms. *Curr. Opin. Immunol.* **2014**, *29*, 1–7. [CrossRef]

82. Foster, S.L.; Hargreaves, D.C.; Medzhitov, R. Gene-specific control of inflammation by TLR-induced chromatin modifications. *Nature* **2007**, *447*, 972–978. [CrossRef]
83. Gunther, J.; Petzl, W.; Zerbe, H.; Schuberth, H.J.; Seyfert, H.M. TLR ligands, but not modulators of histone modifiers, can induce the complex immune response pattern of endotoxin tolerance in mammary epithelial cells. *Innate Immun.* **2017**, *23*, 155–164. [CrossRef]
84. Gill, H.S.; Doull, F.; Rutherfurd, K.; Cross, M. Immunoregulatory peptides in bovine milk. *Br. J. Nutr.* **2000**, *84*, 111–117. [CrossRef]
85. Newburg, D.S. Innate immunity and human milk. *J. Nutr.* **2005**, *135*, 1308–1312. [CrossRef]
86. Fernandez, L.; Langa, S.; Martin, V.; Maldonado, A.; Jimenez, E.; Martin, R.; Rodriguez, J.M. The human milk microbiota: Origin and potential roles in health and disease. *Pharmacol. Res.* **2013**, *69*, 1–10. [CrossRef] [PubMed]
87. Lee, Y.K.; Mazmanian, S.K. Has the microbiota played a critical role in the evolution of the adaptive immune system? *Science* **2010**, *330*, 1768–1773. [CrossRef] [PubMed]
88. Sordillo, L.M.; Aitken, S.L. Impact of oxidative stress on the health and immune function of dairy cattle. *Vet. Immunol. Immunopathol.* **2009**, *128*, 104–109. [CrossRef] [PubMed]
89. Braem, S.; Abrahamse, E.L.; Duthoo, W.; Notebaert, W. What determines the specificity of conflict adaptation? A review, critical analysis, and proposed synthesis. *Front. Psychol.* **2014**, *5*, 1131. [CrossRef]
90. Hajishengallis, G.; Darveau, R.; Curtis, M. The keystone-pathogen hypothesis. *Nat. Rev. Microbiol.* **2012**, *10*, 717–725. [CrossRef]
91. Derakhshani, H.; Plaizier, J.C.; De Buck, J.; Barkema, H.W.; Khafipour, E. Composition and co-occurrence patterns of the microbiota of different niches of the bovine mammary gland: Potential associations with mastitis susceptibility, udder inflammation, and teat-end hyperkeratosis. *Anim. Microbiome* **2020**, *2*, 11. [CrossRef]
92. Kuehn, J.S.; Gorden, P.J.; Munro, D.; Rong, R.; Dong, Q.; Plummer, P.J.; Wang, C.; Phillips, G.J. Bacterial community profiling of milk samples as a means to understand culture-negative bovine clinical mastitis. *PLoS ONE* **2013**, *8*, e61959. [CrossRef]
93. Ganda, E.K.; Gaeta, N.; Sipka, A.; Pomeroy, B.; Oikonomou, G.; Schukken, Y.H.; Bicalho, R.C. Normal milk microbiome is reestablished following experimental infection with Escherichia coli independent of intramammary antibiotic treatment with a third-generation cephalosporin in bovines. *Microbiome* **2017**, *5*, 74. [CrossRef]
94. Falentin, H.; Rault, L.; Nicolas, A.; Bouchard, D.S.; Lassalas, J.; Lamberton, P.; Aubry, J.M.; Marnet, P.G.; Le Loir, Y.; Even, S. Bovine teat microbiome analysis revealed reduced alpha diversity and significant changes in taxonomic profiles in quarters with a history of mastitis. *Front. Microbiol.* **2016**, *7*, 480. [CrossRef]
95. Drackley, J.K.; Cardoso, F.C. Prepartum and postpartum nutritional management to optimize fertility in high-yielding dairy cows in confined TMR systems. *Animal* **2014**, *8*, 5–14. [CrossRef]
96. Ingvartsen, K.L.; Moyes, K. Nutrition, immune function and health of dairy cattle. *Animal* **2013**, *7*, 112–122. [CrossRef] [PubMed]
97. Drackley, J.K. Biology of Dairy Cows during the Transition Period: The Final Frontier? *J. Dairy Sci.* **1999**, *82*, 2259–2273. [CrossRef]
98. Bertoni, G.; Trevisi, E.; Han, X.; Bionaz, M. Effects of inflammatory conditions on liver activity in puerperium period and consequences for performance in dairy cows. *J. Dairy Sci.* **2008**, *91*, 3300–3310. [CrossRef] [PubMed]
99. Gross, J.J.; Bruckmaier, R.M. Invited review: Metabolic challenges and adaptation during different functional stages of the mammary gland in dairy cows: Perspectives for sustainable milk production. *J. Dairy Sci.* **2019**, *102*, 2828–2843. [CrossRef]
100. Bradford, B.J.; Swartz, T.H. Review: Following the smoke signals: Inflammatory signaling in metabolic homeostasis and homeorhesis in dairy cattle. *Animal* **2020**, *14*, s144–s154. [CrossRef]
101. Lopreiato, V.; Minuti, A.; Trimboli, F.; Britti, D.; Morittu, V.M.; Cappelli, F.P.; Loor, J.J.; Trevisi, E. Immunometabolic status and productive performance differences between periparturient Simmental and Holstein dairy cows in response to pegbovigrastim. *J. Dairy Sci.* **2019**, *102*, 9312–9327. [CrossRef]
102. Lopreiato, V.; Palma, E.; Minuti, A.; Loor, J.J.; Lopreiato, M.; Trimboli, F.; Morittu, V.M.; Spina, A.A.; Britti, D.; Trevisi, E. Pegbovigrastim Treatment around Parturition Enhances Postpartum Immune Response Gene Network Expression of whole Blood Leukocytes in Holstein and Simmental Cows. *Animals* **2020**, *10*, 621. [CrossRef]

103. Alharthi, A.; Zhou, Z.; Lopreiato, V.; Trevisi, E.; Loor, J.J. Body condition score prior to parturition is associated with plasma and adipose tissue biomarkers of lipid metabolism and inflammation in Holstein cows. *J. Anim. Sci. Biotechnol.* **2018**, *9*, 1–12. [CrossRef]
104. Kehrli, M.E.; Nonnecke, B.J.; Roth, J.A. Alterations in bovine neutrophil function during the periparturient period. *Am. J. Vet. Res.* **1989**, *50*, 207–214. [PubMed]
105. Batistel, F.; Arroyo, J.M.; Garces, C.I.M.; Trevisi, E.; Parys, C.; Ballou, M.A.; Cardoso, F.C.; Loor, J.J. Ethyl-cellulose rumen-protected methionine alleviates inflammation and oxidative stress and improves neutrophil function during the periparturient period and early lactation in Holstein dairy cows. *J. Dairy Sci.* **2017**, *101*, 480–490. [CrossRef] [PubMed]
106. Loor, J.J.; Bionaz, M.; Drackley, J.K. Systems Physiology in Dairy Cattle: Nutritional Genomics and Beyond. *Annu. Rev. Anim. Biosci.* **2013**, *1*, 365–392. [CrossRef] [PubMed]
107. McDougall, S.; LeBlanc, S.J.; Heiser, A. Effect of prepartum energy balance on neutrophil function following pegbovigrastim treatment in periparturient cows. *J. Dairy Sci.* **2017**, *100*, 7478–7492. [CrossRef] [PubMed]
108. Heiser, A.; LeBlanc, S.J.; McDougall, S. Pegbovigrastim treatment affects gene expression in neutrophils of pasture-fed, periparturient cows. *J. Dairy Sci.* **2018**, *101*, 8194–8207. [CrossRef] [PubMed]
109. Trimboli, F.; Morittu, V.M.; Di Loria, A.; Minuti, A.; Spina, A.A.; Piccioli-Cappelli, F.; Trevisi, E.; Britti, D.; Lopreiato, V. Effect of Pegbovigrastim on Hematological Profile of Simmental Dairy Cows during the Transition Period. *Anim. J.* **2019**, *9*, 841. [CrossRef]
110. Lopreiato, V.; Minuti, A.; Morittu, V.M.; Britti, D.; Piccioli-Cappelli, F.; Loor, J.J.; Trevisi, E. Short communication: Inflammation, migration, and cell-cell interaction-related gene network expression in leukocytes is enhanced in Simmental compared with Holstein dairy cows after calving. *J. Dairy Sci.* **2020**, *103*, 1908–1913. [CrossRef]
111. Kimura, K.; Goff, J.P.; Canning, P.; Wang, C.; Roth, J.A. Effect of recombinant bovine granulocyte colony-stimulating factor covalently bound to polyethylene glycol injection on neutrophil number and function in periparturient dairy cows. *J. Dairy Sci.* **2014**, *97*, 4842–4851. [CrossRef]
112. Trevisi, E.; Jahan, N.; Bertoni, G.; Ferrari, A.; Minuti, A. Pro-inflammatory cytokine profile in dairy cows: Consequences for new lactation. *Ital. J. Anim. Sci.* **2015**, *14*, 285–292. [CrossRef]
113. Kushibiki, S.; Hodate, K.; Shingu, H.; Ueda, Y.; Shinoda, M.; Mori, Y.; Itoh, T.; Yokomizo, Y. Insulin resistance induced in dairy steers by tumor necrosis factor alpha is partially reversed by 2,4–thiazolidinedione. *Domest. Anim. Endocrinol.* **2001**, *21*, 25–37. [CrossRef]
114. Lopreiato, V.; Hosseini, A.; Rosa, F.; Zhou, Z.; Alharthi, A.; Trevisi, E.; Loor, J.J. Dietary energy level affects adipose depot mass but does not impair in vitro subcutaneous adipose tissue response to short-term insulin and tumor necrosis factor-α challenge in nonlactating, nonpregnant Holstein cows. *J. Dairy Sci.* **2018**, *101*, 10206–10219. [CrossRef]
115. Kvidera, S.K.; Horst, E.A.; Abuajamieh, M.; Mayorga, E.J.; Fernandez, M.V.S.; Baumgard, L.H. Glucose requirements of an activated immune system in lactating Holstein cows. *J. Dairy Sci.* **2017**, *100*, 2360–2374. [CrossRef]
116. Herdt, T.H. Ruminant adaptation to negative energy balance. Influences on the etiology of ketosis and fatty liver. *Vet. Clin. N. Am. Food Anim. Pract.* **2000**, *16*, 215–230. [CrossRef]
117. Minuti, A.; Jahan, N.; Lopreiato, V.; Piccioli-Cappelli, F.; Bomba, L.; Capomaccio, S.; Loor, J.J.; Ajmone-Marsan, P.; Trevisi, E. Evaluation of circulating leukocyte transcriptome and its relationship with immune function and blood markers in dairy cows during the transition period. *Funct. Integr. Genom.* **2020**, *20*, 293–305. [CrossRef] [PubMed]
118. Bertoni, G.; Trevisi, E. Use of the liver activity index and other metabolic variables in the assessment of metabolic health in dairy herds. *Vet. Clin. N. Am. Food Anim. Pract.* **2013**, *29*, 413–431. [CrossRef] [PubMed]
119. Dionissopoulos, L.; AlZahal, O.; Steele, M.A.; Matthews, J.C.; McBride, B.W. Transcriptomic changes in ruminal tissue induced by the periparturient transition in dairy cows. *Am. J. Anim. Vet. Sci.* **2014**, *9*, 36–45. [CrossRef]
120. Steele, M.A.; Schiestel, C.; AlZahal, O.; Dionissopoulos, L.; Laarman, A.H.; Matthews, J.C.; McBride, B.W. The periparturient period is associated with structural and transcriptomic adaptations of rumen papillae in dairy cattle. *J. Dairy Sci.* **2015**, *98*, 2583–2595. [CrossRef]

121. Minuti, A.; Palladino, A.; Khan, M.J.; Alqarni, S.; Agrawal, A.; Piccioli-Capelli, F.; Hidalgo, F.; Cardoso, F.C.; Trevisi, E.; Loor, J.J. Abundance of ruminal bacteria, epithelial gene expression, and systemic biomarkers of metabolism and inflammation are altered during the peripartal period in dairy cows. *J. Dairy Sci.* **2015**, *98*, 8940–8951. [CrossRef]
122. Bach, A.; Guasch, I.; Elcoso, G.; Chaucheyras-Durand, F.; Castex, M.; Fàbregas, F.; Garcia-Fruitos, E.; Aris, A. Changes in gene expression in the rumen and colon epithelia during the dry period through lactation of dairy cows and effects of live yeast supplementation. *J. Dairy Sci.* **2018**, *101*, 2631–2640. [CrossRef]
123. Knoblock, C.E.; Shi, W.; Yoon, I.; Oba, M. Effects of supplementing a *Saccharomyces cerevisiae* fermentation product during the periparturient period on the immune response of dairy cows fed fresh diets differing in starch content. *J. Dairy Sci.* **2019**, *102*, 6199–6209. [CrossRef]
124. Trevisi, E.; Amadori, M.; Riva, F.; Bertoni, G.; Bani, P. Evaluation of innate immune responses in bovine forestomachs. *Res. Vet. Sci.* **2014**, *96*, 69–78. [CrossRef]
125. Dann, H.M.; Morin, D.E.; Bollero, G.A.; Murphy, M.R.; Drackley, J.K. Prepartum intake, postpartum induction of ketosis, and periparturient disorders affect the metabolic status of dairy cows. *J. Dairy Sci.* **2005**, *88*, 3249–3264. [CrossRef]
126. Janovick, N.A.; Boisclair, Y.R.; Drackley, J.K. Prepartum dietary energy intake affects metabolism and health during the periparturient period in primiparous and multiparous Holstein cows. *J. Dairy Sci.* **2011**, *94*, 1385–1400. [CrossRef] [PubMed]
127. Graugnard, D.E.; Bionaz, M.; Trevisi, E.; Moyes, K.M.; Salak-Johnson, J.L.; Wallace, R.L.; Drackley, J.K.; Bertoni, G.; Loor, J.J. Blood immunometabolic indices and polymorphonuclear neutrophil function in peripartum dairy cows are altered by level of dietary energy prepartum. *J. Dairy Sci.* **2012**, *95*, 1749–1750. [CrossRef] [PubMed]
128. Beever, D.E. The impact of controlled nutrition during the dry period on dairy cow health, fertility and performance. *Anim. Reprod. Sci.* **2006**, *96*, 212–226. [CrossRef] [PubMed]
129. John Wallace, R.; Sasson, G.; Garnsworthy, P.C.; Tapio, I.; Gregson, E.; Bani, P.; Huhtanen, P.; Bayat, A.R.; Strozzi, F.; Biscarini, F.; et al. A heritable subset of the core rumen microbiome dictates dairy cow productivity and emissions. *Sci. Adv.* **2019**, *5*, eaav8391. [CrossRef] [PubMed]
130. Shabat, S.K.; Sasson, G.; Doron-Faigenboim, A.; Durman, T.; Yaacoby, S.; Berg Miller, M.E.; White, B.A.; Shterzer, N.; Mizrahi, I. Specific microbiome-dependent mechanisms underlie the energy harvest efficiency of ruminants. *Isme J.* **2016**, *10*, 2958–2972. [CrossRef]
131. Li, F.; Guan, L.L. Metatranscriptomic profiling reveals linkages between the active rumen microbiome and feed efficiency in beef cattle. *Appl. Environ. Microbiol.* **2017**, *83*, e00061-17. [CrossRef]
132. Xue, M.Y.; Sun, H.Z.; Wu, X.H.; Liu, J.X.; Guan, L.L. Multi-omics reveals that the rumen microbiome and its metabolome together with the host metabolome contribute to individualized dairy cow performance. *Microbiome* **2020**, *8*, 64. [CrossRef]
133. Jami, E.; White, B.A.; Mizrahi, I. Potential role of the bovine rumen microbiome in modulating milk composition and feed efficiency. *PLoS ONE* **2014**, *9*, e85423. [CrossRef]
134. McCann, J.C.; Luan, S.; Cardoso, F.C.; Derakhshani, H.; Khafipour, E.; Loor, J.J. Induction of Subacute Ruminal Acidosis Affects the Ruminal Microbiome and Epithelium. *Front. Microbiol.* **2016**, *7*, 701. [CrossRef]
135. DePeters, E.J.; George, L.W. Rumen transfaunation. *Immunol. Lett.* **2014**, *162*, 69–76. [CrossRef]
136. Weimer, P.J.; Stevenson, D.M.; Mantovani, H.C.; Man, S.L.C. Host Specificity of the Ruminal Bacterial Community in the Dairy Cow Following Near-Total Exchange of Ruminal Contents. *J. Dairy Sci.* **2010**, *93*, 5902–5912. [CrossRef] [PubMed]
137. Li, F.; Li, C.; Chen, Y.; Liu, J.; Zhang, C.; Irving, B.; Fitzsimmons, C.; Plastow, G.; Guan, L.L. Host genetics influence the rumen microbiota and heritable rumen microbial features associate with feed efficiency in cattle. *Microbiome* **2019**, *7*, 92. [CrossRef] [PubMed]
138. Rischkowsky, B.; Pilling, D. *The State of the World's Animal Genetic Resources for Food and Agriculture*; Commission on Genetic Resources for Food and Agriculture Food and Agriculture Organization of the United Nations, FAO: Rome, Italy, 2007.
139. Ugarte, E.; Ruiz, R.; Gabia, D.; Beltrán de Heredia, I. Impact of high-yielding foreign breeds on the Spanish dairy sheep industry. *Livest. Prod. Sci.* **2001**, *71*, 3–10. [CrossRef]

140. Zander, K.K.; Signorello, G.; De Salvo, M.; Gandini, G.; Drucker, A.G. Assessing the total economic value of threatened livestock breeds in Italy: Implications for conservation policy. *Ecol. Econ.* **2013**, *93*, 219–229. [CrossRef]
141. Marsoner, T.; Egarter Vigl, L.; Manck, F.; Jaritz, G.; Tappeiner, U.; Tasser, E. Indigenous livestock breeds as indicators for cultural ecosystem services: A spatial analysis within the Alpine Space. *Ecol. Indic.* **2018**, *94*, 55–63. [CrossRef]
142. Ingvartsen, K.L.; Dewhurst, R.J.; Friggens, N.C. On the relationship between lactational performance and health: Is it yield or metabolic imbalance that cause production diseases in dairy cattle? A position paper. *Livest. Prod. Sci.* **2003**, *83*, 277–308. [CrossRef]
143. Knegsel, A. Metabolic adaptation during early lactation: Key to cow health, longevity and a sustainable dairy production chain. *CAB Rev. Perspect. Agric. Vet. Sci. Nutr. Nat. Resour.* **2014**. [CrossRef]
144. Kukučková, V.; Moravčíková, N.; Ferenčaković, M.; Simčič, M.; Mészáros, G.; Sölkner, J.; Trakovická, A.; Kadlečík, O.; Curik, I.; Kasarda, R. Genomic characterization of Pinzgau cattle: Genetic conservation and breeding perspectives. *Conserv. Genet.* **2017**, *18*, 893–910. [CrossRef]
145. Mendonça, L.G.D.; Abade, C.C.; da Silva, E.M.; Litherland, N.B.; Hansen, L.B.; Hansen, W.P.; Chebel, R.C. Comparison of peripartum metabolic status and postpartum health of Holstein and Montbéliarde-sired crossbred dairy cows. *J. Dairy Sci.* **2014**, *97*, 805–818. [CrossRef]
146. Cremonesi, P.; Ceccarani, C.; Curone, G.; Severgnini, M.; Pollera, C.; Bronzo, V.; Riva, F.; Addis, M.F.; Filipe, J.; Amadori, M.; et al. Milk microbiome diversity and bacterial group prevalence in a comparison between healthy Holstein Friesian and Rendena cows. *PLoS ONE* **2018**, *13*, e0205054. [CrossRef]
147. Begley, N.; Buckley, F.; Pierce, K.M.; Fahey, A.G.; Mallard, B.A. Differences in udder health and immune response traits of Holstein-Friesians, Norwegian Reds, and their crosses in second lactation. *J. Dairy Sci.* **2009**, *92*, 749–757. [CrossRef] [PubMed]
148. Bieber, A.; Wallenbeck, A.; Leiber, F.; Fuerst-Waltl, B.; Winckler, C.; Gullstrand, P.; Walczak, J.; Wójcik, P.; Neff, A.S. Production level, fertility, health traits, and longevity in local and commercial dairy breeds under organic production conditions in Austria, Switzerland, Poland, and Sweden. *J. Dairy Sci.* **2019**, *102*, 5330–5341. [CrossRef] [PubMed]
149. Heins, B.J.; Hansen, L.B.; Seykora, A.J. Production of pure Holsteins versus crossbreds of Holstein with Normande, Montbeliarde, and Scandinavian Red. *J. Dairy Sci.* **2006**, *89*, 2799–2804. [CrossRef]
150. Heins, B.J.; Hansen, L.B.; De Vries, A. Survival, lifetime production, and profitability of Normande × Holstein, Montbéliarde × Holstein, and Scandinavian Red × Holstein crossbreds versus pure Holsteins. *J. Dairy Sci.* **2012**, *95*, 1011–1021. [CrossRef]
151. Heins, B.J.; Hansen, L.B.; Seykora, A.J. Fertility and survival of pure Holsteins versus crossbreds of Holstein with Normande, Montbeliarde, Scandinavian red. *J. Dairy Sci.* **2006**, *89*, 4944–4951. [CrossRef]
152. Fuerst-Waltl, B.; Fuerst, C.; Obritzhauser, W.; Egger-Danner, C. Sustainable breeding objectives and possible selection response: Finding the balance between economics and breeders' preferences. *J. Dairy Sci.* **2016**, *99*, 9796–9809. [CrossRef]

9

RNA Sequencing (RNA-Seq) based Transcriptome Analysis in Immune Response of Holstein Cattle to Killed Vaccine against Bovine Viral Diarrhea Virus Type I

Bryan Irvine Lopez [1,†], Kier Gumangan Santiago [2,3,†], Donghui Lee [2], Seungmin Ha [4] and Kangseok Seo [2,*]

1 Division of Animal Genomics and Bioinformatics, National Institute of Animal Science, Rural Development Administration, Wanju 55365, Korea; irvinelopez@korea.kr
2 Department of Animal Science and Technology, Sunchon National University, Suncheon 57922, Korea; santiagokier2015@gmail.com (K.G.S.); a3832737@naver.com (D.L.)
3 Department of Animal Science, College of Agriculture, Central Luzon State University, Science City of Muñoz 3120, Philippines
4 Dairy Science Division, National Institute of Animal Science, Rural Development Administration, Cheonan 31000, Korea; justusha@korea.kr
* Correspondence: sks@sunchon.ac.kr
† These authors contributed equally to this work.

Simple Summary: Due to the undeniable detrimental impact of bovine viral diarrhea virus (BVDV) on cattle worldwide, various preventive approaches are carried out to control the spread of this disease. Among the established preventive approaches, vaccination remains the most widely used cost-effective method of control. Hence, a deeper study into the host immune response to vaccines will further refine the efficacy of these vaccines; the identification of differentially expressed genes (DEGs) related to immune response might bring a long-lasting solution. Thus far, studies showing the genes related to the immune response of cattle to vaccines are still limited. Therefore, this study identified DEGs in animals with high and low sample to positive (S/P) ratio based on the BVDV antibody level, using RNA sequencing (RNA-seq) transcriptome analysis, and functional enrichment analysis in gene ontology (GO) annotations and the Kyoto Encyclopedia of Genes and Genomes (KEGG) pathway. Results revealed that several upregulated and downregulated genes were significantly annotated to antigen processing and presentation (MHC class I), immune response, and interferon-gamma production, indicating the immune response of the animals related to possible shaping of their adaptive immunity against the BVDV type I. Moreover, significant enrichment to various KEGG pathways related to the development of adaptive immunity was observed.

Abstract: Immune response of 107 vaccinated Holstein cattle was initially obtained prior to the ELISA test. Five cattle with high and low bovine viral diarrhea virus (BVDV) type I antibody were identified as the final experimental animals. Blood samples from these animals were then utilized to determine significant differentially expressed genes (DEGs) using the RNA-seq transcriptome analysis and enrichment analysis. Our analysis identified 261 DEGs in cattle identified as experimental animals. Functional enrichment analysis in gene ontology (GO) annotations and Kyoto Encyclopedia of Genes and Genomes (KEGG) pathways revealed the DEGs potentially induced by the inactivated BVDV type I vaccine, and might be responsible for the host immune responses. Our findings suggested that inactivated vaccine induced upregulation of genes involved in different GO annotations, including antigen processing and presentation of peptide antigen (via MHC class I), immune response, and positive regulation of interferon-gamma production. The observed downregulation of other genes involved in immune response might be due to inhibition of toll-like receptors (TLRs) by the upregulation of the Bcl-3 gene. Meanwhile, the result of KEGG pathways revealed that the majority of DEGs were upregulated and enriched to different pathways, including cytokine-cytokine receptor interaction, platelet activation, extracellular matrix (ECM) receptor interaction, hematopoietic cell lineage, and ATP-binding cassette (ABC) transporters. These significant pathways supported our initial findings and are known to play a vital role in shaping adaptive immunity against BVDV type 1. In addition, type 1 diabetes mellitus pathways tended to be significantly enriched. Thus, further studies are needed to investigate the prevalence of type 1 diabetes mellitus in cattle vaccinated with inactivated and live BVDV vaccine.

Keywords: Bovine Viral Diarrhea Virus; RNA-Seq; Transcriptome analysis; Holstein cattle

---

1. Introduction

Bovine viral diarrhea virus (BVDV) is an economically important pathogen of domestic and wild ruminants affecting multiple organ systems, incurring most economic losses due to respiratory diseases, low reproductive performance (due to reduced conception rates), early embryonic deaths, abortion, congenital weak calves, and high costs of control programs [1–4]. BVDV belongs to the genus *Pestivirus* within the family *Flaviviridae*, with two species, namely BVDV1 and BVDV2; both consist of strains, belonging to biotypes non-cytopathogenic or cytopathogenic, based on cell-cultured characteristics [5]. The non-cytopathogenic strain has the ability to cross the maternal placenta, infecting the growing fetus at early gestation (before 150 gestation days) due to the undeveloped immune system and failure of recognizing the virus as foreign [6]. This fetal infection affects fetal development [7], and results in persistently infected born calves, shedding lifelong reservoir of BVDV in the herd, while cytopathic BVDV plays a vital role by superinfecting persistently infected cattle, leading to mucosal disease [5]. In addition, recent studies reported that the immunosuppressive ability of BVDV heightens other viral disease potentiators, particularly the bovine respiratory disease [8–10]. The differences in genotypes and biotypes of BVDV, a wide range of susceptible hosts, the ability to induce persistent infection, and intervene with both innate and adaptive immunity, makes the prevention and control program difficult [4].

To date, modified live viral and inactivated viral vaccines are widely used to prevent the consequences of BVDV infection [11]. However, vaccine efficacy varies, depending on the animal's nutritional status [12], maternal antibody from the dam colostrum [13], and the presence of persistently infected cattle in the herd. Thus far, numerous studies were conducted to improve vaccine efficacy against BVDV, yet still remains prevalent among the cattle herd worldwide.

Numerous studies focusing on the transcriptomic analysis of animals infected with various diseases were carried out. In the study of Li et al. [4], various differentially expressed genes (DEGs) related to goat immune response, including inflammation, defense response, cell locomotion, and cytokine/chemokine-mediated signaling were revealed by transcriptome analysis with samples from BVDV2 artificially infected goat peripheral blood mononuclear cells (PBMCs). Similar methodology was done in the study of Singh et al. [14], where various significant DEGs related to the immune system processes of goat and sheep against bluetongue virus serotype 16 (BTV-16) were revealed, such as NFκB, MAPK, Ras, NOD, RIG, TNF, TLR, JAK-STAT, and VEGF signaling pathways. Meanwhile, comparative transcriptomic analyses between infected and non-infected animals were conducted by Barreto et al. [15], where infected bovine were observed to have massive changes in the expression profiles of keratinocyte, immune system, cell proliferation, and apoptosis genes.

All of these studies used transcriptome analysis and next-generation sequencing (NGS) approach particularly the RNA sequencing (RNA-Seq). RNA sequencing is a developed method that uses deep sequencing technology for transcriptome profiling [16]; aside from providing a comprehensive picture of the transcriptome, it also reveals the activity and mechanism of the molecular structure and explores the biological function of a gene [17]. Furthermore, future works using this technology are considered, such as genetic linkage mapping, quantitative trait analysis, disease-resistant strains, effective vaccines, and therapies development [18].

Although genotyping and RNA sequencing still remain costly, such studies may provide novel insights and solid foundation in improving herd performance through the robustness of animals against viral diseases. However, studies pertaining to the immune responses of the animal to the vaccine were not fully explored. Thus, the objective of this study is to identify differentially expressed genes (DEGs) related to the functional immune response of the host vaccinated with the inactivated BVDV type I vaccine, and to provide insight on how vaccines improve the immunity of animals against diseases.

2. Materials and Methods

2.1. Experimental Animals and Vaccination

A total of 107 vaccinated Holstein Cattle (*Bos taurus)* was used in the study. Multivalent killed vaccine Bar Vac Elite 4-HS (Boehringer Ingelheim Vetmedica, Inc., St Joseph, MO, USA) containing antigen of infectious bovine rhinotracheitis virus, bovine viral diarrhea virus (BVDV, type I), bovine respiratory syncytial virus (BRSV), Myxovirus parainfluenza type 3 (PI3) and *Haemophilus somnus* bacterin were given intramuscularly, as prescribed by the manufacturer.

Blood samples were collected from the jugular vein at 7, 28, and 168 d post-vaccination. Subsequently, blood was allowed to coagulate for 1–2 h at 4 °C and centrifugate for 20 min at room temperature with the relative centrifugal force of 1800 × g. Serum was collected and aliquoted into 1.5 mL tubes and stored below −60 °C until ELISA test.

2.2. Serological Antibody Detection

Competitive ELISA, using VDPro BVDV AB ELISA (Median Diagnostics Inc., Chuncheon, Republic of Korea) was used to assay the antibody responses of each animal against the vaccine. Assaying was performed as per manufacturer protocols. Concisely, the BVDV gp63 antigen was allowed to absorb in the polystyrene plate and bind with antibodies in serum samples. It was competed for corresponding hydrogen peroxide conjugated monoclonal antibodies. The chromogenic change after the addition of 3, 3′, 5, 5′-Tetramethylbenzidine substrate was measured at 450 nm optical density using BioTek ELISA reader and Gen5 2.07 software; results with lower color development signify a higher level of antibody. The optical density (OD) value was measured using a microplate reader set at 405 nm and concentration was valued with the corresponding standard references. The obtained OD value of BVDV type I antibodies were evaluated for the comparative value, related to the positive control value, to get antibodies level in the sample to positive (S/P) ratio form by applying the equation as below.

$$\frac{\text{S}}{\text{P}} = \frac{\text{Sample O.D. value} - \text{Negative Control O.D. value}}{\text{Positive control O.D. value} - \text{Negative Control O.D. value}} \quad (1)$$

The obtained BVDV type I S/P ratio, and other immune-related parameters, such as TNF-alpha, IFN-gamma, IL-17A, IL-1b, IL-4, IL-2, and IL-6 were used as the basis for selecting experimental animals. Among the 107 experimental animals, only ten (10) animals were selected and grouped into two groups, namely the low and high BVDV type I groups; each group had five (5) animals (Figure 1).

2.3. RNA Isolation, Library Preparation, and RNA Sequencing (RNA-seq)

Total RNA was stabilized and isolated from the blood samples (collected after vaccination) of the selected animal groups using Tempus Blood RNA Tube (Applied Biosystems, Seoul, Korea), according to the manufacturer's instructions. RNeasy MinElute Cleanup Kit (Qiagen, Valencia, CA, USA) was used to purify and concentrate the previously isolated RNA. RNA quality based on RNA integrity number (RIN) was determined using Agilent Technologies 2100 Bioanalyzer (Agilent, Santa Clara, CA, USA) with an acceptable RIN value of ≥7. These RNA samples were used to generate RNA-Seq transcriptome libraries, using the TruSeq Stranded Total RNA LT sample preparation kit (Globin) of Illumina (San Diego, CA,

USA). To ensure the quality of prepared libraries, the size of the PCR enriched fragments were verified by checking the template size distribution, by running on Agilent Technologies 2100 Bioanalyzer using a DNA 1000 chip, and were quantified using qPCR according to the Illumina qPCR quantification protocol guide. After a series of quality control and quantification, prepared paired-end libraries for animals with high (test) and low (control) BVDV type I antibody were then sequenced with the Illumina NovaSeq 6000 platform, performed by TNT Research Corporation Limited (Anyang, South Korea).

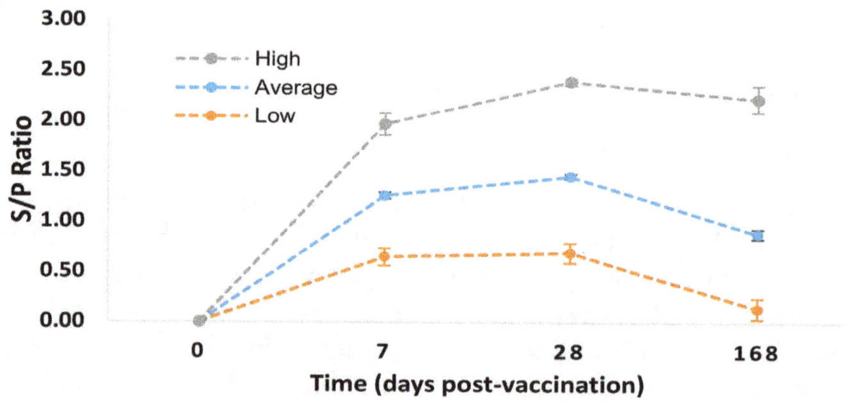

Figure 1. Sample to positive (S/P) ratio of cattle groups identified as high (n = 5), low (n = 5) and average (n = 107) bovine viral diarrhea virus (BVDV) type I antibody level at different time points. The error bars indicate standard error.

2.4. *Reads Trimming, Mapping, and Assembly of Sequenced RNA Reads*

Quality control (QC) of raw paired-end reads were done by trimming reads using Trimmomatic 0.38 (http://www.usadellab.org/cms/?page=trimmomatic). QC included the removal of adapter sequence, contaminant DNA, and low-quality reads with lengths below 36 bp. Clean reads (cDNA) were indexed to reference (*Bos taurus*) cattle genome GCF_002263795.1 ARS-UCD1.2 and were mapped against the reference genome using HISAT2 version 2.1.0 (Bowtie2 aligner) (https://ccb.jhu.edu/software/hisat2/index.shtml). Reference-based aligned read assembly of transcripts was performed using the StringTie 1.3.4d (https://ccb.jhu.edu/software/stringtie/). This allowed the identification of transcript or genes with annotation information in the assembled genome, while genes without annotated information were defined as new transcripts [19]. On the other hand, mapping of each sample without the –e option of StringTie allowed the prediction of novel transcript and novel alternative splicing transcript. The gffcompare program from GFF utilities was used to compare existing annotations and distinguish novel transcript types.

2.5. *Differential Expression Genes (DEGs) Analysis and Clustering*

The identification of DEGs between case and control samples was based on the expression level on each transcript, which was calculated using the fragments per kilobase of exon per million mapped reads (FPKM) method. The DESeq2 package, equipped with fold change and negative binomial (nbinom) Wald test, was used for differential expression analyses. DEGs were identified based on the following parameters: the logarithmic fold change was greater than or equal to 2 ($|fc|>=2$) and nbinom Wald test raw $p < 0.05$. In addition, hierarchical clustering of significant genes was done to determine the similarity level of each sample.

2.6. *Functional Annotation and Enrichment Analysis*

DEGs were based on several functional annotation databases, specifically gene ontology (GO) (http://geneontology.org/) and Kyoto Encyclopedia of Genes and Genomes (KEGG) (http://kegg.jp). Enrichment analysis was performed using the Database for Annotation, Visualization and Integrated Discovery 6.8

(DAVID) tool (http://david.abcc.ncifcrf.gov/) equipped with the modified Fisher's exact test. DEGs with a *p*-value of less than 0.05 were significantly considered enriched in GO terms and KEGG pathways.

3. Results

3.1. Experimental Animals

Table 1 shows the two groups of experimental animals identified in this study, namely, low and high group, based on the level of BVDV type I antibody and level of immune responses, including TNF-alpha, IFN-gamma, IL-17A, IL-1b, IL-4, IL-2, and IL-6. For the earlier group, there were five identified animals namely (ID number), 13064, 13083, 13090, 14010, and 14017, while a similar number of animals belong to the latter group, namely, 14107, 15060, 15071, 15083, and 15094.

3.2. Transcriptome Sequencing Data

An average of 9.0G bp (Table 1) raw data for each sample was obtained from paired-end transcriptome sequencing from the Illumina NovaSeq 6000 platform. Prior to further analysis, raw data were subject to quality control using Trimmomatic version 0.38. The trimmed results show that the total read bases, GC (%), and Q30 (%) of each sample have values ranging from 7.0 G to 11.0 G, 44.86% to 45.99%, and 94.65% to 95.31%, respectively, as shown in Table 1. Trimmed data were mapped against the reference genome (GCF_002263795.1 ARS-UCD1.2) using the HISAT2 program. Obtained mapped reads were then assembled using StringTie-e option version 1.3.4d, which resulted in a total of 100,685 transcripts and 39,127 genes successfully mapped against the reference genome. Thereafter, the removal of low-quality transcripts and genes was done, leaving only 10,000 transcripts and 35,000 genes for differentiation analysis. Furthermore, a total of 1452 novel transcripts, 13,060 novel splicing variants, and 4199 novel genes were identified using the StringTie software.

Table 1. Summary of the mapping information for each sample.

Sample ID	Total Raw Reads	Total Clean Reads	GC (%)	Q30 (%)	No. of Processed Reads	No. of Mapped Reads	No. of Unmapped Reads
13064	1.13E + 10	1.12E + 08	45.52	95.28	1.11E + 08	1.08E + 08	2.32E + 06
13083	9.59E + 09	9.50E + 07	45.73	95.27	9.40E + 07	9.12E + 07	2.74E + 06
13090	9.77E + 09	9.67E + 07	45.22	94.65	9.55E + 07	9.38E + 07	1.70E + 06
14010	8.52E + 09	8.44E + 07	45.00	95.31	8.36E + 07	8.17E + 07	1.82E + 06
14017	9.38E + 09	9.29E + 07	45.99	95.30	9.19E + 07	8.93E + 07	2.55E + 06
14107 *	9.67E + 09	9.58E + 07	45.03	95.22	9.47E + 07	9.27E + 07	2.02E + 06
15060 *	8.31E + 09	8.22E + 07	45.54	95.08	8.13E + 07	7.96E + 07	1.62E + 06
15071 *	9.01E + 09	8.92E + 07	45.87	95.23	8.83E + 07	8.18E + 07	6.37E + 06
15083 *	8.37E + 09	8.29E + 07	44.48	95.19	8.20E + 07	8.02E + 07	1.77E + 06
15094 *	7.42E + 09	7.35E + 07	44.86	94.98	7.26E + 07	7.07E + 07	1.92E + 06

* Animals belongs to high immune responses and BVDV type I antibody group.

3.3. Differentially Expressed Genes

The resulting good quality genes from StringTie software were filtered by excluding genes with at least one zero count, leaving only 45% (16,315 genes) for DEG analysis. Prior to DEG analysis, expression levels between genes of each sample were first normalized using the Relative Log Expression (RLE) normalization method, based on raw read counts (Figure 2).

The analysis of the differently expressed genes (DEGs) were done by comparing the normalized values using the DESeq2 package, equipped with log fold change and nbinom Wald test. A total of 261 genes were considered differentially expressed based on the threshold level (fold change (log2) ≥ 2 and p-value < 0.05) (Figure 3). Results of comparison analysis between animals with high (test) and low (control) BVDV type I antibody groups revealed that 143 genes were classified as up-regulated while the remaining 118 genes were down-regulated (Figure 3).

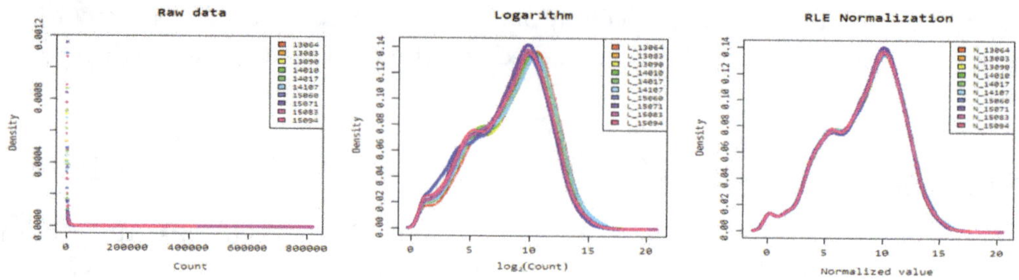

Figure 2. Density plot of normalized data using Relative Log Expression (RLE) normalization method based on read count and log2.

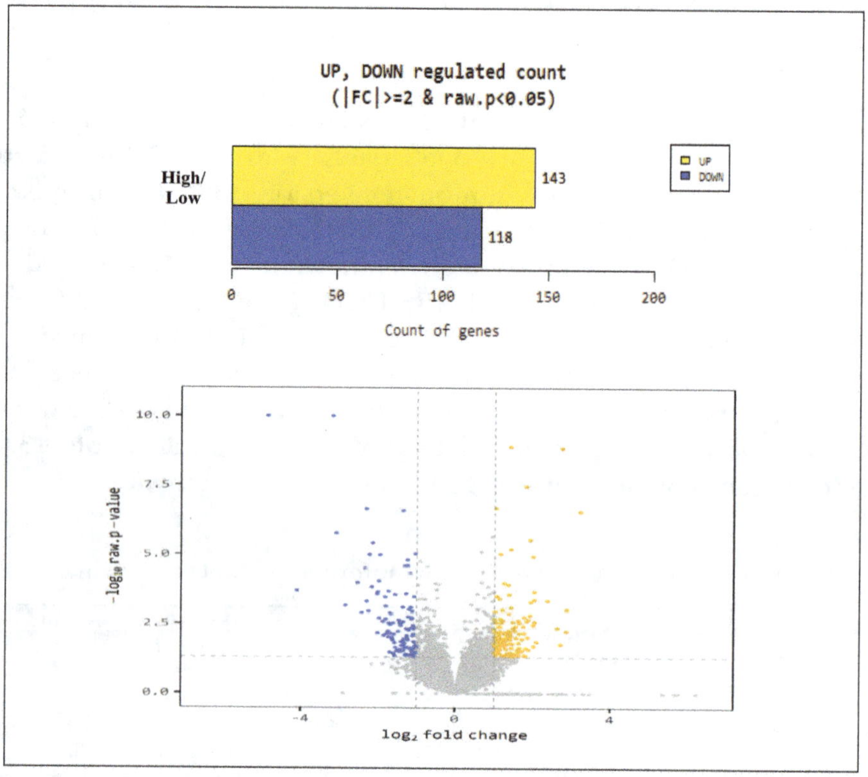

Figure 3. Number of up- and down-regulated genes after comparison of normalized values using the DESeq2 package.

3.4. Functional Enrichment Analysis of Identified DEGs

RNA-seq transcriptome analysis successfully identify a total of 261 DEGs. Several functional annotation databases, such as gene ontology (GO) and KEGG pathway using the Database for Annotation, Visualization and Integrated Discovery 6.8 (DAVID) tool, were used to determine the biological function of these identified DEGs. DAVID gene enrichment analysis revealed 28 significant GO terms throughout the differentiation analysis ($p < 0.05$). However, there were only three GO major categories, namely biological process (GOTERM_BP), cellular component (GOTERM_CC), and molecular function (GOTERM_MF) where the significant DEGs were grouped based on their functionality (Figure 4). In this study, 38 significant DEGs were distributed to top 10 GOTERM_BP, namely antigen processing and presentation of peptide antigen (via MHC class I), immune response, positive regulation of gene expression, negative regulation of gene expression, negative regulation of cell growth, negative regulation of oxidoreductase activity, positive regulation of interferon-gamma production, collagen biosynthetic process, and caveola assembly. In GOTERM_MF, 21 DEGs were distributed into the following top 5 GO terms; calcium ion binding, calcium-dependent cysteine-type endopeptidase activity, SH3 domain binding, superoxide-generating Nicotinamide Adenine Dinucleotide Phosphate (NADPH) oxidase activator activity, and protein complex scaffold.

Meanwhile, 78 DEGs were distributed to the top 7 GOTERM_CC as follows; integral component of membrane, class I protein complex, extracellular region, proteinaceous extracellular matrix, membrane raft, axon and anchored component of the external side of the plasma membrane.

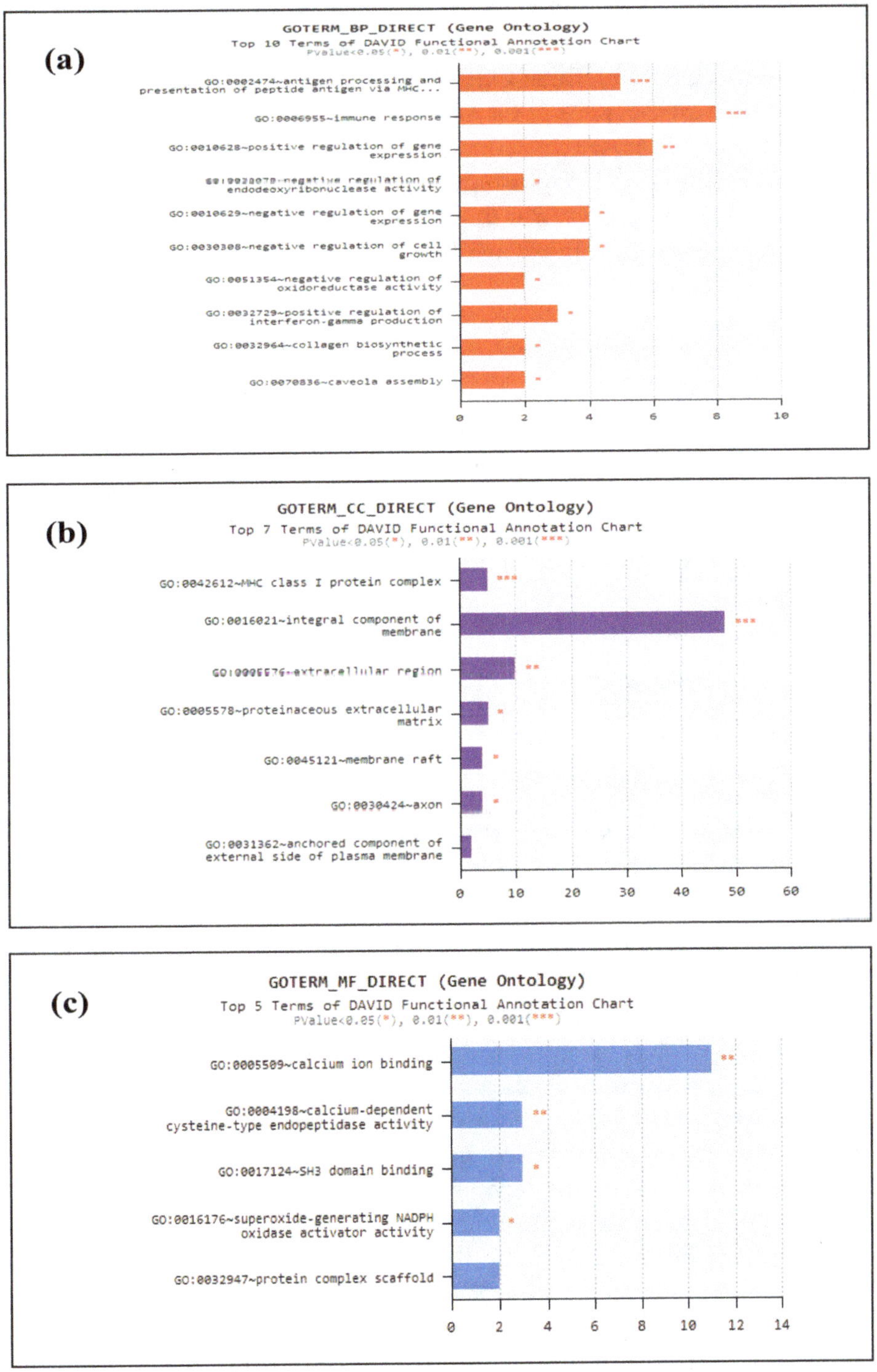

Figure 4. Gene ontology (GO) enrichment analysis of differentially expressed genes (DEGs) in vaccinated cattle, selected based on BVDV type I antibody level **(a)** GOTERM_Biological Process, **(b)** GOTERM_Cellular Component, and **(c)** GOTERM_Molecular Function. GO terms are located on the y-axis and terms with (*) (**) (***) means significant enrichment with a p-value of <0.05, 0.01, and 0.001, respectively.

3.5. KEGG Pathway Enrichment Analysis

To allow deeper understanding of the biological function of significant DEGs, KEGG pathway enrichment analysis was done using DAVID 6.8 tool. Initially, KEGG pathways analysis successfully annotated DEGs into 10 pathways which later reduced into 5 significantly enriched pathways ($P<0.05$) namely; cytokine-cytokine interaction, platelet activation, ECM-receptor interaction, hematopoietic cell lineage, and ABC transporters (Table 2). Cytokine-cytokine interaction pathway involved 2 upregulated (IL18, IL1RAP) and 4 down-regulated DEGs (CCR8, CCL3, IL20RA, TGFB2); hematopoietic cell lineage pathway linked 4 upregulated DEGs (GP5, GP1BA, CD24, GP9); platelet activation pathway with 5 up-regulated DEGs (GP5, P2RX1, MAPK12, GP1BA, GP9); ECM-receptor interaction pathway with 3 up-regulated (GP5, GP1BA, GP9) and 1 down-regulated (ITGB4) DEGs and ABC transporters pathway with 1 upregulated (ABCB11) and 2 downregulated DEGs (LOC100296627, CFTR). Results obtained from GO and KEGG analysis indicated that various DEGs were involved in host immune response to inactivated BVDV Type I vaccine.

Table 2. List of significantly enriched Kyoto Encyclopedia of Genes and Genomes (KEGG) pathways associated with immune response.

	Pathways	ID	DEGs No.	*p*-Value	Up-Regulated Genes	Down-Regulated Genes
1	Platelet activation	bta04611	5	1.34E-02	GP5, P2RX1, GP1BA, GP9	MAPK12
2	Cytokine-cytokine receptor interaction	bta04060	6	2.07E-02	IL18, IL1RAP	CCR8, CCL3, IL20RA,TGFB2
3	ECM-receptor interaction	bta04512	4	2.52E-02	GP5, GP1BA, GP9	ITGB4
4	Hematopoietic cell lineage	bta04640	4	2.91E-02	GP5, GP1BA, CD24, GP9	-
5	ABC transporters	bta02010	3	3.73E-02	ABCB11	LOC100296627, CFTR
6	Type I diabetes mellitus	bta04940	2	5.48E-02	BOLA, PTPRN2	-

ECM—Extra Cellular Matrix, ABC—ATP Binding Cassette

4. Discussion

BVDV infection is undeniably detrimental to bovine raisers by reducing milk yield, and is associated with low reproductive performance and growth retardation, allowing the occurrence of other disease potentiators, premature culling, and a high rate of mortality to young stock [20]. Houe et al. [20] and Carman et al. [21] estimated that national herd could experience economic loss ranging between $10 million and $40 million per million calvings, and $40,000–$100,000 (USD) per herd, respectively. Thus, to prevent such negative effects of BVDV, the development of cost-effective controls, including vaccines and eradication schemes were considered [22]. However, despite effective control programs, BVDV infection remains rampant in most cattle herd worldwide. Evidence reveals that variability of the BVDV strains, cross placental ability of the virus leading to persistent infections, wide spectrum of susceptible hosts, and the ability to interfere both innate and adaptive immunity makes prevention and control, such as vaccination, less effective [4,23].

Recently, similar studies that used next-generation sequencing technology (NGS) purported various DEGs related to animal immune response against viral diseases, providing a deeper understanding of immune responses. Since the development of microarray-based analysis and completion of the Human Genome Project, more advanced sequencing technology has come about, such as RNA-Seq based transcriptome analysis [24]. Compared to DNA microarray-based technology, RNA–Seq provide greater dynamic range by directly revealing sequence identity crucial for annotation quantification of unknown genes and novel transcript isoforms [25,26]. In studies by Li et al., Singh et al., and Barreto et al. [4,14,15], RNA-Seq based transcriptome analyses were used to successfully identify both up- and down-regulated genes related to the host immune response during BVDV, bluetongue virus of sheep and goats, and bovine papillomatosis infection, respectively.

In this study, cattle vaccinated with inactivated multivalent vaccine (BVDV type I, BRSV, Myxovirus parainfluenza type 3 (PI3), *Haemophilus somnus* bacterin) were evaluated days after the last vaccination, to identify and understand changes in gene expressions related to the immune response brought by the vaccine. Specifically, this study examines the only animal with a high and low BVDV type I antibody level; thus, DEGs identified in the transcriptome analysis were highly attributed to the immune response of the animal to inactivated BVDV type I vaccine.

Vaccination is considered an effective tool in preventing and controlling infectious diseases involving the cooperative action of innate and adaptive immunity [27]. Innate immunity plays a key role in triggering adaptive immune response by involving hematopoietic cells, such as macrophages, mast cells, neutrophils, eosinophils, dendritic cells, natural killer cells, and non-hematopoietic cells, such as skin and epithelial linings of the gastrointestinal, genitourinary, and respiratory tract [28]. Meanwhile, adaptive immunity plays its vital role in the immune system as it involves a tightly regulated interaction between antigen -presenting cells and T and B lymphocytes that facilitate pathogen-specific immunologic effector pathways, immunologic memory, and regulation of host immune homeostasis [29].

In this study, functional enrichment analysis revealed upregulated DEGs related to both innate and adaptive immune responses, such as BoLA, IL18, and BCL3. Among identified immune-related genes, the bovine lymphocyte antigen (BoLA) caught the attention of the researcher, as it was directly involved in antigen presentation. The BoLA gene located on chromosomes BTA 23 [30], and generally known as the MHC of cattle, was reported to play an integral role in immune responsiveness and susceptibility to the diseases of the host animal [31]. MHC is a cell surface glycoprotein molecule, having the binding ability to foreign peptides, such as viral proteins, and provides context for the recognition of T-lymphocytes responsible for cell-mediated immunity [32,33]. In studies conducted by Gutierrez et al. [34] and Weigel et al. [35], it was discovered that MHC genes are strongly associated with disease resistance and susceptibility to a wide range of diseases; thus, it can be a natural strategy in controlling infectious diseases, by incorporating it to the selection index and in genetic manipulation techniques.

The IL18 and Bcl-3 gene was also identified, upregulated in this study; IL18 gene play an important role in the T-cell-helper type 1 (Th1) and are involved in the regulation of innate and adaptive immune response by inducing IFN-gamma in natural killer cells (NKC) and T helper (Th1) lymphocytes [36,37]. Primary precursors of IL-18 are expressed in epithelial cells of the body, while the primary sources are macrophages and dendritic cells [38]. In a study conducted on laboratory mice, IL-18 was considered an effective adjuvant by enhancing immunogenicity through its relevant activities, such as activator of NK cells, a strong stimulator of Th1 responses, and other immunoactive cytokines in Th1 cells, monocytes, and NK Cells [38].

Whereas, the BCL3 is a proto-oncogene member of the IkB family, and also reportedly plays an important role in immune responses. In a study by Schwarz et al., it was purported that the Bcl-3 protein interacts specifically with the NFkB subunits (p50 and p52). It was also reported that mice lacking the Bcl-3 gene exhibit normal development and immunoglobin levels, but the humoral immune response was severely affected, and fail to produce antigen-specific antibodies [39]. Further, in the study of Fredericksen et al. [40], it was observed that the BVDV-1 infected Madin-Darby bovine kidney cell line induces immune marker production, such as BCL3, IL-1, IL-8, IL-15, IL-18, Mx-1, IRF-1, and IRF-7 through the NF-kB signaling pathway. Furthermore, Carmody et al. [41] reported that Bcl-3 limits the strength of toll-like receptors (TLRs) that are responsible for triggering inflammatory cytokines production and development of both adaptive and innate immunity through p50 subunit ubiquitination stabilization. Thus, this limitation of TLR responses might be responsible for the downregulation of other DEGs related to inflammatory responses.

Enrichment analysis through KEGG pathways of DEGs was done to understand signal transduction pathways activated and repressed by inactivated antigen (vaccine). Results of KEGG pathway enrichment analysis revealed five (5) significantly enriched pathways, such as platelet activation, cytokine-cytokine receptor interaction, ECM receptor interaction, hematopoietic cell lineage, and ABC transporters. Among identified significant pathways, cytokine-cytokine receptor interaction involved the most number of DEGs. The cytokine-cytokine (c-c) receptor interaction plays a vital role in health during immunological and inflammatory responses to diseases through the synergistic convergence of signaling pathways and divergence of the cytokine signal, which activates another cytokine system [42]. In this study, six (6) significant DEGs under c-c receptor interaction pathways were identified, namely; CCR8, CCL3, IL20RA, TGFB2, IL18, and IL1RAP with only the last two (2) DEGs identified as upregulated (IL18, IL1RAP). Downregulation of other DEGs belonging to c-c receptor interaction and linked to TLR may be attributed to previously reported upregulation of Bcl-3, which limits the duration of TLR responses that control deleterious inflammatory diseases. However, further studies are warranted to fully support this claim.

Another significantly enriched pathway observed in this study is the extracellular matrix (ECM) receptor interaction pathway, which includes four (4) upregulated DEGs, namely, glycoprotein (GpV), GpIba, GpIX, and ITGB4. Briefly, ECM is a non-cellular component found in all tissue and organs, providing cellular constituents its physical framework, and it also plays a vital role in tissue morphogenesis, differentiation, and homeostasis by initiating crucial biochemical and biomechanical signals [43]. Additionally, ECM conveys specific signals to cells resulting in the modulation of basic functions that are important for the early steps of inflammation, particularly the migration of immune cells during tissue inflammation and immune cell differentiation [44]. These functions of ECM are believed to be mediated primarily by integrins under the family of cell surface receptors [45]. In support, Kroll et al. [46] and Englund et al. [47] reported that platelet membranes, such as GpIb and GpIX, when bound to the von Willebrand factor (vWF), would help transmit signals to the platelet that leads to platelet activation and adhesion. Whereas, the platelet glycoprotein (GP) Ib-IX-V complex is responsible for platelet rolling and adhesion to the site of injury [48]. As such, the literature suggests that the upregulation of integrin subunit beta 4 (ITGB4), GpV, GpIba, and GpIX in this study might be involved in the immune-related functions of ECM.

Fascinatingly, enrichment of ECM receptor pathways supported the succeeding enriched pathways, such as the hematopoietic cell lineage and platelet activation pathways. In a study by Klein [49], it was reported that the ECM matrix molecules (collagen, proteoglycans, and glycoproteins) are part of the bone marrow microenvironment that plays a very significant role in promoting hematopoietic cell proliferation and differentiation. Thus, the upregulation of all DEGs under the hematopoietic cell lineage pathway (GP5, GP1BA, CD24, GP9) supports the observed upregulation of some DEGs under the ECM pathway.

On the other hand, the platelet activation pathway, which are believed to be related to ECM glycoprotein, was reported to be triggered during viral antigen-antibody complexes, from which virus-induced platelet activation can modulate platelet count that help shape immune response through their released products that suppressed infection [50]. Under this pathway, there were four identified upregulated DEGs, namely, GP5, P2RX1, GP1BA, and GP9, with only MAPK12 as down-regulated.

Another important enriched pathway is the ATP-binding cassette (ABC) transporter, which purportedly plays a crucial role in adaptive immunity by its ability to shuttle degrade proteasomal products into the endoplasmic reticulum (ER), which then loaded to MHC class I before antigen presentation on the cell surface [51,52]. In the study of Hinz and Tampé [53], it was also reported that transporters associated with antigen processing (TAP) could be challenged with a number of viral factors, which prevent antigen translocation and loading MHC class I in virally infected cells. Thus, this literature suggests that the upregulation of ABCB11 (ABC transporter pathways) previously observed in this study was associated with the development of adaptive immunity against BVDV Type I.

Another interesting pathway that tended to be significantly enriched was the type 1 diabetes mellitus pathway. This information catches the attention of researchers due to a previous report that cattle infected with the BVD-mucosal disease virus can induce insulin-dependent diabetes mellitus [54].

5. Conclusions

The results of this study showed significantly identified DEGs under different immune-related gene ontologies and signaling pathways in response to BVDV type 1 antigen. These observed findings will surely provide assistance by enlightening end-users and other researchers on the changes happening in the animal immune system brought by vaccination. In addition, the potential inclusion of DEGs to animal improvement programs, such as breeding, selection, and genetic manipulation techniques will surely help improve the efficacy of the vaccine. Furthermore, the DEGs, annotation, and pathways identified in this study can be utilized for future studies concerning the immune response of cattle to vaccines.

Author Contributions: Conceptualization, K.S.; Data curation, K.S.; Formal analysis, B.I.L. and D.L.; Methodology, B.I.L., S.H. and K.S.; Project administration, K.S.; Supervision, K.S.; Visualization, S.H. and K.S.; Writing—original draft, K.G.S.; Writing—review & editing, B.I.L. and K.S. All authors have read and agreed to the published version of the manuscript.

References

1. Grooms, D.L. Reproductive consequences of infection with bovine viral diarrhea virus. *Vet. Clin. N. Am-Food A.* **2004**, *20*, 5–19. [CrossRef] [PubMed]
2. Khodakaram-Tafti, A.; Farjanikish, G.H. Persistent bovine viral diarrhea virus (BVDV) infection in cattle herds. *Iran. J. Vet. Res.* **2017**, *18*, 154–163. [CrossRef]
3. Pinior, B.; Firth, C.L.; Richter, V.; Lebl, K.; Trauffler, M.; Dzieciol, M.; Hutter, S.E.; Burgstaller, J.; Obritzhauser, W.; Winter, P.; et al. A systematic review of financial and economic assessments of bovine viral diarrhea virus (BVDV) prevention and mitigation activities worldwide. *Prev. Vet. Med.* **2017**, *137*, 77–92. [CrossRef] [PubMed]
4. Li, W.; Mao, L.; Shu, X.; Liu, R.; Hao, F.; Li, J.; Liu, M.; Yang, L.; Zhang, W.; Sun, M.; et al. Transcriptome analysis reveals differential immune related genes expression in bovine viral diarrhea virus-2 infected goat peripheral blood mononuclear cells (PBMCs). *BMC Genomics* **2019**, *20*. [CrossRef] [PubMed]
5. Brownlie, J.; Clarke, M.C.; Howard, C.J.; Pocock, D.H. Pathogenesis and epidemiology of bovine virus diarrhoea virus infection of cattle. *Ann. Rech. Vet.* **1987**, *18*, 157–166.
6. Hansen, T.R.; Smirnova, N.P.; Van Campen, H.; Shoemaker, M.L.; Ptitsyn, A.A.; Bielefeldt-Ohmann, H. Maternal and fetal response to fetal persistent infection with bovine viral diarrhea virus. *Am. J. Reprod. Immunol.* **2010**, *64*, 295–306. [CrossRef]
7. Smirnova, N.P.; Bielefeldt-Ohmann, H.; Van Campen, H.; Austin, K.J.; Han, H.; Montgomery, D.L.; Shoemaker, M.L.; van Olphen, A.L.; Hansen, T.R. Acute non-cytopathic bovine viral diarrhea virus infection induces pronounced type I interferon response in pregnant cows and fetuses. *Virus Res.* **2008**, *132*, 49–58. [CrossRef]
8. Richer, L.; Marois, P.; Lamontagne, L. Association of bovine viral diarrhea virus with multiple viral infections in bovine respiratory disease outbreaks. *Can. Vet. J.* **1988**, *29*, 713–717.
9. Campbell, J.R. Effect of bovine viral diarrhea virus in the feedlot. *Vet. Clin. North Am. Food Anim. Pract.* **2004**, *20*, 39–50. [CrossRef]
10. Zanella, R.; Casas, E.; Snowder, G.; Neibergs, H.L. Fine mapping of loci on BTA2 and BTA26 associated with bovine viral diarrhea persistent infection and linked with bovine respiratory disease in cattle. *Front. Genet.* **2011**, *2*. [CrossRef]
11. Newcomer, B.W.; Chamorro, M.F.; Walz, P.H. Vaccination of cattle against bovine viral diarrhea virus. *Vet. Microbiol.* **2017**, *206*, 78–83. [CrossRef] [PubMed]
12. Rashid, A.; Rasheed, K.; Akhtar, M. Factors influencing vaccine efficacy - a general review. *J. Anim.Plant. Sci.* **2009**, *19*, 22–25.
13. Niewiesk, S. Maternal antibodies: Clinical significance, mechanism of interference with immune responses, and possible vaccination strategies. *Front. Immunol.* **2014**, *5*, 446. [CrossRef] [PubMed]

14. Singh, A.; Prasad, M.; Mishra, B.; Manjunath, S.; Sahu, A.R.; Bhuvana Priya, G.; Wani, S.A.; Sahoo, A.P.; Kumar, A.; Balodi, S.; et al. Transcriptome analysis reveals common differential and global gene expression profiles in bluetongue virus serotype 16 (BTV-16) infected peripheral blood mononuclear cells (PBMCs) in sheep and goats. *Genomics Data* **2017**, *11*, 62–72. [CrossRef]
15. Barreto, D.M.; Barros, G.S.; Santos, L.A.B.O.; Soares, R.C.; Batista, M.V.A. Comparative transcriptomic analysis of bovine papillomatosis. *BMC Genomics* **2018**, *19*, 949. [CrossRef] [PubMed]
16. Wang, Z.; Gerstein, M.; Snyder, M. RNA-Seq: A revolutionary tool for transcriptomics. *Nat. Rev. Genet.* **2009**, *10*, 57–63. [CrossRef]
17. Zhao, F.R.; Xie, Y.L.; Liu, Z.Z.; Shao, J.J.; Li, S.F.; Zhang, Y.G.; Chang, H.Y. Transcriptomic analysis of porcine PBMCs in response to FMDV infection. *Acta Trop.* **2017**, *173*, 69–75. [CrossRef]
18. Sudhagar, A.; Kumar, G.; El-Matbouli, M. Transcriptome analysis based on RNA-Seq in understanding pathogenic mechanisms of diseases and the immune system of fish: A comprehensive review. *Int. J. Mol. Sci.* **2018**, *19*, 245. [CrossRef]
19. Liu, C.; Liu, Y.; Liang, L.; Cui, S.; Zhang, Y. RNA-Seq based transcriptome analysis during bovine viral diarrhoea virus (BVDV) infection. *BMC Genomics* **2019**, *20*, 774. [CrossRef]
20. Houe, H. Economic impact of BVDV infection in dairies. *Biologicals* **2003**, *31*, 137–143. [CrossRef]
21. Carman, S.; Van Dreumel, T.; Ridpath, J.; Hazlett, M.; Alves, D.; Dubovi, E.; Tremblay, R.; Bolin, S.; Godkin, A.; Anderson, N. Severe acute bovine viral diarrhea in Ontario, 1993–1995. *J. Vet. Diagn. Invest.* **1998**, *10*, 27–35. [CrossRef] [PubMed]
22. Lindberg, A.L.E. Bovine viral Diarrhoea virus infections and its control. A review. *Vet. Q.* **2003**, *25*, 1–16. [CrossRef] [PubMed]
23. Ridpath, J.F. Immunology of BVDV vaccines. *Biologicals* **2013**, *41*, 14–19. [CrossRef] [PubMed]
24. Mutz, K.O.; Heilkenbrinker, A.; Lönne, M.; Walter, J.G.; Stahl, F. Transcriptome analysis using next-generation sequencing. *Curr. Opin. Biotechnol.* **2013**, *24*, 22–30. [CrossRef]
25. Hrdlickova, R.; Toloue, M.; Tian, B. RNA-Seq methods for transcriptome analysis. *Wiley Interdiscip. Rev. RNA* **2017**, *8*, e1364. [CrossRef]
26. Garber, M.; Grabherr, M.G.; Guttman, M.; Trapnell, C. Computational methods for transcriptome annotation and quantification using RNA-seq. *Nat. Methods* **2011**, *8*, 469–477. [CrossRef]
27. Buonaguro, L.; Pulendran, B. Immunogenomics and systems biology of vaccines. *Immunol. Rev.* **2011**, *239*, 197–208. [CrossRef]
28. Kaur, B.P.; Secord, E. Innate Immunity. *Pediatr. Clin. North Am.* **2019**, *66*, 905–911. [CrossRef]
29. Bonilla, F.A.; Oettgen, H.C. Adaptive immunity. *J. Allergy Clin. Immunol.* **2010**, *125*, S33–S40. [CrossRef]
30. Bhushan, B.; Patra, B.N.; Das, P.J.; Dutt, T.; Kumar, P.; Sharma, A.; Umang; Dandapat, S.; Ahlawat, S.P.S. Polymorphism of exon 2-3 of bovine major histocompatibility complex class I BoLa-A gene. *Genet. Molec. Biol.* **2007**. [CrossRef]
31. Untalan, P.M.; Pruett, J.H.; Steelman, C.D. Association of the bovine leukocyte antigen major histocompatibility complex class II DRB3*4401 allele with host resistance to the Lone Star tick, Amblyomma americanum. *Vet. Parasitol.* **2007**, *145*, 190–195. [CrossRef] [PubMed]
32. Zhong, J.F.; Harvey, J.T.; Boothby, J.T. Characterization of a harbor seal class I major histocompatability complex cDNA clone. *Immunogenetics* **1998**, *48*, 422–424. [CrossRef] [PubMed]
33. Janeway, C.A.; Travers, P.; Walport, M.; Al, E. *Principles of innate and adaptive immunity. Immunobiology: The Immune System in Health and Disease*, 5th ed.; Janeway, C., Travers, P., Walport, M., Shlomchik, M., Eds.; Taylor & Francis, Inc.: Abingdon, UK, 2001.
34. Gutiérrez, S.E.; Esteban, E.N.; Lützelschwab, C.M.; Juliarena, M.A. Major Histocompatibility Complex-Associated Resistance to Infectious Diseases: The Case of Bovine Leukemia Virus Infection. In *Trends and Advances in Veterinary Genetics*; Abubakar, M., Ed.; IntechOpen: London, UK, 2017. [CrossRef]
35. Weigel, K.A.; Freeman, A.E.; Kehrli, M.E.; Stear, M.J.; Kelley, D.H. Association of Class I Bovine Lymphocyte Antigen Complex Alleles with Health and Production Traits in Dairy Cattle. *J. Dairy Sci.* **1990**, *73*, 2538–2546. [CrossRef]
36. Wawrocki, S.; Druszczynska, M.; Kowalewicz-Kulbat, M.; Rudnicka, W. Interleukin 18 (IL-18) as a target for immune intervention. *Acta Biochim. Pol.* **2016**, *63*, 59–63. [CrossRef] [PubMed]
37. Nakamura, K.; Okamura, H.; Wada, M.; Nagata, K.; Tamura, T. Endotoxin-induced serum factor that stimulates gamma interferon production. *Infect. Immun.* **1989**, *57*, 590–595. [CrossRef]

38. Dinarello, C.A. Interleukin 1 and interleukin 18 as mediators of inflammation and the aging process. *Am. J. Clin. Nutr.* **2006**, *83*, 447S–455S. [CrossRef]
39. Schwarz, E.M.; Krimpenfort, P.; Berns, A.; Verma, I.M. Immunological defects in mice with a targeted disruption in Bcl-3. *Genes Dev.* **1997**, *11*, 187–197. [CrossRef]
40. Fredericksen, F.; Carrasco, G.; Villalba, M.; Olavarría, V.H. Cytopathic BVDV-1 strain induces immune marker production in bovine cells through the NF-κB signaling pathway. *Mol. Immunol.* **2015**, *68*, 213–222. [CrossRef]
41. Carmody, R.J.; Ruan, Q.; Palmer, S.; Hilliard, B.; Chen, Y.H. Negative regulation of toll-like receptor signaling by NF-κB p50 ubiquitination blockade. *Science* **2007**, *317*, 675–678. [CrossRef]
42. Turrin, N.P.; Plata-Salamán, C.R. Cytokine-cytokine interactions and the brain. *Brain Res. Bull.* **2000**, *51*, 3–8. [CrossRef]
43. Frantz, C.; Stewart, K.M.; Weaver, V.M. The extracellular matrix at a glance. *J. Cell Sci.* **2010**, *123*, 4195–4200. [CrossRef] [PubMed]
44. Sorokin, L. The impact of the extracellular matrix on inflammation. *Nat. Rev. Immunol.* **2010**, *10*, 712–723. [CrossRef] [PubMed]
45. Giancotti, F.G.; Ruoslahti, E. Integrin Signaling. *Science* **1999**, *285*, 1028–1033. [CrossRef] [PubMed]
46. Kroll, M.H.; Harris, T.S.; Moake, J.L.; Handin, R.I.; Schafer, A.I. Von Willebrand factor binding to platelet Gplb initiates signals for platelet activation. *J. Clin. Invest.* **1991**, *88*, 1568–1573. [CrossRef]
47. Englund, G.D.; Bodnar, R.J.; Li, Z.; Ruggeri, Z.M.; Du, X. Regulation of von Willebrand Factor Binding to the Platelet Glycoprotein Ib-IX by a Membrane Skeleton-dependent Inside-out Signal. *J. Biol. Chem.* **2001**, *276*, 16952–16959. [CrossRef]
48. Luo, S.Z.; Mo, X.; Afshar-Kharghan, V.; Srinivasan, S.; López, J.A.; Li, R. Glycoprotein Ibα forms disulfide bonds with 2 glycoprotein Ibβ subunits in the resting platelet. *Blood* **2007**, *109*, 603–609. [CrossRef]
49. Klein, G. The extracellular matrix of the hematopoietic microenvironment. *Experientia* **1995**, *51*, 914–926. [CrossRef]
50. Assinger, A. Platelets and infection - An emerging role of platelets in viral infection. *Front. Immunol.* **2014**, *5*, 649. [CrossRef]
51. Procko, E.; Gaudet, R. Antigen processing and presentation: TAPping into ABC transporters. *Curr. Opin. Immunol.* **2009**, *21*, 84–91. [CrossRef]
52. Seyffer, F.; Tampé, R. ABC transporters in adaptive immunity. *BBA-Gen Subjects* **2015**, *1850*, 449–460. [CrossRef]
53. Hinz, A.; Tampé, R. ABC transporters and immunity: Mechanism of self-defense. *Biochemistry* **2012**, *51*, 4981–4989. [CrossRef] [PubMed]
54. Tajima, M.; Yazawa, T.; Hagiwara, K.; Kurosawa, T.; Takahashi, K. Diabetes Mellitus in Cattle Infected with Bovine Viral Diarrhea Mucosal Disease Virus. *J. Vet. Med.* **1992**, *39*, 616–620. [CrossRef] [PubMed]

10

Influence of Age and Immunostimulation on the Level of Toll-Like Receptor Gene (*TLR3*, *4*, and *7*) Expression in Foals

Anna Migdał [1,*], Łukasz Migdał [1], Maria Oczkowicz [2], Adam Okólski [3] and Anna Chełmońska-Soyta [4,5]

1 Department of Genetics, Animal Breeding and Ethology, Faculty of Animal Sciences, University of Agriculture in Krakow, al. 29 Listopada 46, 31-425 Kraków, Poland; lukasz.migdal@urk.edu.pl
2 Department of Animal Molecular Biology, National Research Institute of Animal Production, Krakowska 1, 32-083 Balice, Poland; maria.oczkowicz@izoo.krakow.pl
3 Institute of Veterinary Science, University Centre of Veterinary Medicine UJ-UR, University of Agriculture in Krakow, al. Mickiewicza 24/28, 30-059 Kraków, Poland; adam.okolski@urk.edu.pl
4 Laboratory of Reproductive Immunology, Hirszfeld Institute of Immunology and Experimental Therapy, Polish Academy of Sciences, Weigla 12 Street, 53-114 Wroclaw, Poland; anna.chelmonska-soyta@hirszfeld.pl
5 Department of Immunology, Pathophysiology and Veterinary Preventive Medicine, Division of Immunology and Veterinary Preventive Medicine, Faculty of Veterinary Medicine, Wroclaw University of Environmental and Life Sciences, Norwida 31 Street, 50-375 Wroclaw, Poland
* Correspondence: anna.migdal@urk.edu.pl;

Simple Summary: Detailed knowledge of the molecular mechanisms of immunoglobulin synthesis appears necessary for a better understanding of foal immunity maturity and its influencing factors. At the same time, it encourages studies regarding the influence of the signaling cascade's proteins on the primary immunological response, which provides an opportunity to develop extremely precise methods of regulating acquired immunity. The results revealed that the expression of the*TLR3* and *TLR4* genes, as well as the levels of immunoglobulins and interleukins, can be modulated by stimulation with the pharmacological agent, and that the expression of the *TLR3* and *TLR4*genes in peripheral blood cells is dependent on age.

Abstract: The aim of this study was to investigate the molecular mechanisms leading to the identification of pathogens by congenital immune receptors in foals up to 60 days of age. The study was conducted on 16 foal Polish Pony Horses (Polish Konik) divided into two study groups: control (n = 9) and experimental (n = 7). Foals from the experimental group received an intramuscular duplicate injection of 5 mL of Biotropina (Biowet) at 35 and 40 days of age. The RNA isolated from venous blood was used to evaluate the expression of the*TLR3*, *TLR4*, and *TLR7* genes using RT-PCR. The results of the experiment demonstrated a statistically significant increase in the level of *TLR3* gene expression and a decrease in the level of*TLR4* gene expression with foal aging. The level of *TLR7* gene expression did not show age dependence. Immunostimulation with Biotropina had a significant impact on the level of the genes' expression for Toll-like receptors. It increased the level of *TLR4* expression and decreased *TLR3* expression. Thus, it was concluded that the expression of the*TLR3* and *TLR4*genes in peripheral blood cells is dependent on age. This experiment demonstrated a strong negative correlation between *TLR3* and *TLR4* gene expression.

Keywords: *TLR3*; *TLR4*; *TLR7*; foals; immunostimulation; gene expression

1. Introduction

Immune response differs in newborn and adult horses. Despite involving similar components, the regulation of immunity and the response to antigens vary. Foals are born with small, non-protective amounts of endogenous serum immunoglobulins (i.e., IgM and IgG) [1]. Immunoglobulin transport is limited due to the structure of the horse placenta (placenta spuria). That is why the suckling of colostrum is essential in the first hours of a foal's life. Immunological outcomes in newborn foals differ as compared to adults and are distinguished by modified cytokine profiles, as well as reduced antibody and T-cell responses [2]. Moreover, foals have a very low level of immunoglobulins in their blood plasma. An innate immune system composed of pre-existing or rapidly induced defenses is critical for newborn foals, while an antigen-specific response requires exposure to pathogens and time for development after birth [3]. The effectiveness of the immunological reaction is controlled by a complexity of direct and indirect mechanisms involving interactions among various cells and cytokine-induced actions. Many different immune cells are involved in maintaining a balanced immune response [4]. Receptors called pathogen recognition receptors (PRRs) represent very important elements found in immune cells. Thanks to their conservative structure, these receptors can recognize signals associated with a variety of pathogens. Pathogen-associated molecular patterns (PAMPs), PRR ligands, are molecules specific to viruses, bacteria, and other microorganisms with evolutionarily conserved structures [5]. Toll-like receptors (TLRs) are the most closely investigated PRRs and are one of the most essential components of immune responses [6,7]. Toll-like receptors play a key role in activating and stimulating innate as well as acquired immunity [8]. Identification of the threat and activation of TLRs triggers an immune response, leading to the elimination of this threat from the organism, which involves two basic reactions, namely, inflammatory, and antiviral. Cells with activated receptors release large amounts of proinflammatory cytokines, chemokines, and defensins, and these released factors initiate the migration and aggregation of immune cells (e.g., leukocytes, macrophages, mast cells, and dendritic cells) at the site of the pathogen invasion [7]. Activated TLRs present on the surface of macrophages lead to increased synthesis of the proinflammatory cytokines IL-1, -6, -8, -12, and TNF-α. In addition, complexes of ligands and TLR4 receptors increase the phagocytic activity of macrophages and stimulate the production of reactive oxygen species (ROIs) and the synthesis of nitric oxide (NO). TLR-activated macrophages enhance the expression of major histocompatibility complexes I and II (MHCI and MHCII), CD80, CD86, and co-stimulators that make immune cells more efficient in displaying T-cell antigens that induce specific immune responses [9,10].

Approximately 20% of foals die before the end of the second month, which brings significant economic and breeding losses [11,12]. This justifies undertaking research into new and novel techniques for stimulation of the immune system. Gaining insight into the behavior of TLRs seems to be necessary for expanding our understanding of the mechanism responsible for the development of foal resistance/immunity, and the identification of determinants for further building it up. In addition, it is also an important element contributing to finding innovative solutions in the fight against infections and new ways to improve the prevention and treatment of infections in animals. The paradox of neonatal vaccination is the need of immediate protection during early days, the perceived limitations of the immune system of neonate foals, and the theory of maternal antibody interference [13]. Studies have shown that the immune system of neonatal foals is also naive and immature relative to juvenile and adult horses [14–17]. Several studies have suggested that basal TLR expression in full-term neonatal blood monocytes is similar to that of adults [18,19]. The TLR-mediated production of cytokines by neonatal monocytes, however, is very different in newborns compared to that of adults [19]. Thus far, little is known about the development of the horse immune system during pre- and postnatal periods, which negatively affects the ability to devise strategies for maintaining and improving foal health. Based on its biological properties, as well as the influence of Toll-like receptors on the immune response traits of farm animals and humans, we hypothesized that gene expression for Toll-like receptors TLR-3, TLR-4, and TLR-7 in foals is dependent on factors such as age and immunostimulation. The aim of this work was to investigate the molecular mechanisms leading to the identification of pathogens by congenital immune receptors in foals up to 60 days of age, including the verification of the hypothesis concerning age-related expression of the*TLR3*, *TLR4*, and *TLR7* genes.

2. Materials and Methods

This experiment was granted permission from the Local Ethics Committee in Kraków (no 37, 30 May 2016).

2.1. Animals and Feeding

Studies were carried out on 16 foals representing Polish Pony horses (Polish Konik). This primitive horse breed is genetically and phenotypically closely related to its wild ancestor, the Tarpan Horse (Eurasian wild horse) [20].

All foals with mares were kept in the same stable in individual boxes (size 2.15 × 3.50 m) on permanent straw bedding at the Experimental Station of the University of Agriculture in Krakow. All animals were clinically healthy throughout the experimental period. Mares of 5–17 years of age and 270–340 kg live body weight were not vaccinated during pregnancy. Foal birth weight was 27–35 kg, and weight loss on the first day of life was <1.5%. The horses had all been used by university students in the teaching program. No horses were used for equestrian purposes. Inclusion criteria consisted of foals born from healthy mares with no placentitis, a normal gestational period, an uneventful birth, and normal physical and neurological examination findings. The foals had to successfully stand and nurse within 2 h of birth and remain clinically healthy during the study period.

Mares were fed ad libitum with hay (*Lolium* 40% and *Trifolium L.* 20%) with the addition of oats in the amount of 1.5 kg/mare/day [21]. Foals were fed only with colostrum and mother's milk ad libitum, without additional supplementation. Water was offered from automatic water drinkers (flow ~ 10 L/min).

2.2. Experimental Design

Two weeks before delivery, birth alarms (Abfohlsystem, Jan Wolters, Steinfeld, Germany) were placed in the labia, and mares were moved to box stalls inside a stable lit with natural light (Figure S1). During the experiment, foals were kept with their mothers in individual boxes, and when leaving the stalls with their mothers for the pasture, they were randomly assigned into the following groups:

- The control group (Group C) (n = 9)—foals without any pharmacological and feed additives that may influence immune system;
- The experimental group (Group E) (n = 7)—foals that were administered an immunostimulating agent.

For the immunostimulation, a commercially available immunostimulator was used in the present study, namely, Biotropine (Biowet Drwalew S.A., Drwalew, Poland), which consists of a mixture of inactivated Gram-positive bacteria, e.g., *Staphylococcus aureus* (74 mg/mL), *Streptococcus zooepidermicus* (24.6 mg/mL), *Streptococcus equi* (24.6 mg/mL), *Streptococcus equisimilis* (24.6 mg/mL), *Streptococcus agalactiae* (24.6 mg/mL), *Streptococcus dysgalactiae* (24.6 mg/mL), *Erysipelothrix insidiosa* (49 mg/mL),and Gram-negative bacteria, e.g., *Escherichia coli* (123 mg/mL) and *Pasteurella multocida* (123 mg/mL) as well as pork spleen extract (10 mg/mL). On days 35 and 40 after birth, the foals from the experimental group received an intramuscular (*m. pectoralis descendens*) injection of 5 mL of Biotropine.

2.3. Blood Sampling and Blood Analysis

Blood samples were collected from foals by jugular venipuncture. Blood samples were obtained from foals up until 60 days of age according to the following scheme: After birth before the first suckling and then on the 1st, 3rd, 5th, 10th, 20th, 30th, 40th, 50th, and 60th days of age. Three milliliters of blood were collected into TEMPUS tubes (Applied Biosystems, Foster City, CA, USA) with RNA stabilizing factor. Samples were stored at −20 °C until further processing. Isolation of RNA was carried out using

TEMPUS SPIN (Ambion, Waltham, MA, USA) according to the manufacturer's protocol (Supplementary File 1). One microgram of RNA was transcribed into cDNA using a High-Capacity cDNA Reverse Transcription Kit (Applied Biosystems, Foster City, CA, USA) according to the manufacturer's protocol.

A "No-RT" (non-reverse transcriptase) control was used for selected RNA samples to analyzed contamination in samples.

Gene expression analyses (Table S2 presents the reaction efficiency of each gene) were performed on an Illumina Eco system (Illumina, San Diego, CA, USA, Country)using TaqMan®MGB (Applied Biosystems, Foster City, CA, USA) probes (Table 1). Every sample was analyzed in triplicate in a final volume of 10 µL (Table S1). Amplification was performed according to the following protocol: polymerase activation at 95 °C (2 min) and 40 cycles at 95 °C for 15 s and 60 °C for 1 min. The *SDHA* and *HPRT* genes were used as housekeeping genes (Table 1).

Table 1. Probes used for amplification of Toll-like receptor (TLR) genes and housekeeping genes.

Gen.	Full Name of the Gene	Access Number GenBank	TaqMan Gene Expression Assay ID	Dye
TLR3	Toll-like receptor 3	NC_009170.2	Ec03467747_m1	FAM
TLR4	Toll-like receptor 4	NC_009168.2	Ec03468993_m1	FAM
TLR7	Toll-like receptor 7	NC_009175.2	Ec03467530_m1	VIC
SDHA	Succinate dehydrogenase complex subunit A	XM_001490889	Ec03470479_m1	VIC
HPRT	Hypoxanthinephosphoribosyl transferase	AY372182.1	Ec03470217_m1	VIC

In addition, an analysis of the blood morphotic parameters was performed (Supplementary File 1).

2.4. *Statistical Analysis*

Data are presented as means ± standard error. The data were analyzed using SAS 9.4 software (SAS Institute Inc., Cary, NC, USA). The Shapiro–Wilk test was considered the best test to check the normality of the distribution of random variables. Because the data did not have a normal distribution, the Kruskal–Wallis test was used with immunostimulation and age as the effects. The degree of association between the parameters was examined using a non-parametric Spearman's rank correlation coefficient. Values ranging from 0.0 to 0.5, from 0.5 to 1.0, from −0.5 to 0.0, and from −1.0 to −0.5 indicate weak positive, strong positive, weak negative, and strong negative correlations, respectively.

3. Results

3.1. *Influence of Age on the Expression of TLR3, 4, and 7 mRNA*

The lowest expression of *TLR3* was observed during delivery (6.20 ± 0.89) (Figure 1—data presented from control group). After delivery, the level of *TLR3* mRNA increased. In the period between delivery and 60 days of age, the level of *TLR3* expression increased by 94.34%. We found a highly statistically significant difference between the age and expression of *TLR3* mRNA ($p > 0.01$), as presented in Table 2. From the 5th day of age, we found statistical differences between samples, with the highest expression level on the 60th day after delivery.

The highest level of *TLR4* mRNA expression was observed during the delivery (18.3 ± 2.6) of newborn foals. From the day of the delivery to 20th day of age, we observed a steady significant decrease of *TLR4* mRNA expression (Figure 1) in the blood of the examined foals. During the subsequent days of observation, the expression of the mRNA of this receptor remained at a similar level. The lowest expression value was observed at the 60th day of age (5.82 ± 0.96) (Table 2). Between the delivery day and the 60th day of age, the expression of mRNA for *TLR4* decreased by 76.89%. Statistical analysis showed highly statistically significant differences between the age of foals and the expression of *TLR4* mRNA ($p < 0.01$).

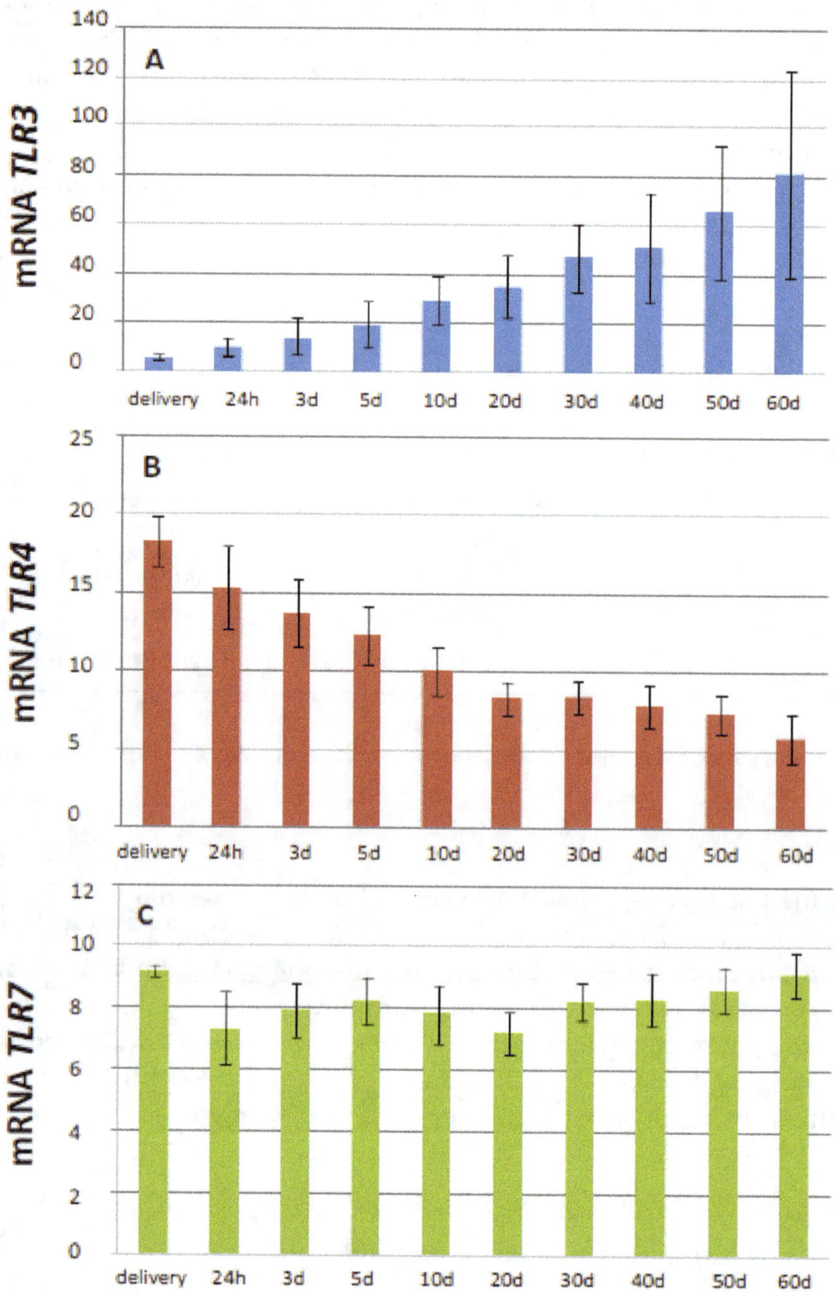

Figure 1. Trends in the change of TLR3 (**A**), TLR4 (**B**), and TLR7 (**C**) expression during foals' growth. Delivery, sample collected at delivery; 24 h, sample collected 24 h after delivery; 3 days, sample collected every 3rd day after delivery; 5 days, sample collected every 5 days after delivery; 10 days, sample collected every 10 days after delivery; 20 days, sample collected every 20 days after delivery; 30 days, sample collected 30 days after delivery; 40 days, sample collected every 40 days after delivery; 50 days, sample collected every 50 days after delivery; 60 days, sample collected 60 days after delivery. The means are reported with their standard errors.

The expression oftheTLR7 gene remained statistically unchanged throughout the experiment (Figure 1). The highest values were observed during the day of delivery (9.20 ± 1.20), while the lowest was observed 20 days after delivery (7.20 ± 0.61). There was no statistically significant correlation between the age and the expression of *TLR7* mRNA ($p > 0.2366$) (Table 2).

Table 2. Expression of *TLR3, TLR4,* and *TLR7* mRNA over the foals' subsequent days of age from the control group (mean ± standard error (SE).

Age	*TLR3*	*TLR4*	*TLR7*
Delivery [1]	6.2 ^{A} ± 0.9 [2]	18.3 ^{A} ± 2.6	9.2 ± 1.2
24 h	9.8 ^{B} ± 1.7	15.3 ^{B} ± 2.2	7.3 ± 0.9
3 days	14.1 ^{A,C} ± 2.1	13.7 ^{C} ± 1.8	7.9 ± 0.8
5 days	19.1 ^{A,B,D} ± 2.2	12.3 ^{A,D} ± 1.5	8.2 ± 0.9
10 days	29.3 ^{A,B,C,E} ± 2.8	10.1 ^{A} ± 1.1	7.8 ± 0.7
20 days	35.1 ^{A,B,C,F} ± 3.1	8.3 ^{A,B} ± 1.1	7.2 ± 0.6
30 days	48.4 ^{A,B,C,D,G} ± 4.9	8.4 ^{A,B} ± 14	8.3 ± 0.9
10 days	53.6 ^{ABCDEF} ± 5.8	7.8 ^{A,B,C} ± 1.2	8.3 ± 0.7
50 days	80.4 ^{ABCDEFG} ± 8.7	7.3 ^{A,B,C} ± 1.5	8.6 ± 0.7
60 days	87.9 ^{A,B,C,D,E,F,G} ± 8.0	5.8 ^{A,B,C,D} ± 0.9	9.2 ± 07

[1] Delivery, sample collected at delivery; 24 h, sample collected 24 h after delivery; 3 days, sample collected 3 days after delivery; 5 days, sample collected 5 days after delivery; 10 days, sample collected 10 days after delivery; 20 days, sample collected 20 days after delivery; 30 days, sample collected 30 days after delivery; 40 days, sample collected 40 days after delivery; 50 days, sample collected 50 days after delivery; 60 days, sample collected 60 days after delivery. [2] Means are reported with their standard errors. Means with same letter in column show highly statistically significant differences ($p < 0.01$).

3.2. *Influence of Stimulation with Biotropina on the Expression of TLR3, 4, and 7 mRNA*

Analysis of changes in the expression of *TLR3* mRNA after the injection of the immunostimulant (Group E) showed a decrease by 41.65% (Table 3), while in the control group (Group C), a dynamic increase in the expression was observed until the last day of observation (116.22 ± 13.93). Highly statistically significant differences were found between immunostimulation and the expression of *TLR3* mRNA.

Table 3. Influence of stimulation with Biotropina on the expression of mRNA for selected Toll-like receptors (*TLR3, TRL4, TLR7*) (mean ± SE).

Age	TLR3		TLR4		TLR7	
	Group C	Group E	Group C	Group E	Group C	Group E
Delivery [1]	8.3 ** ± 1.8 [2]	4.1 ** ± 0.55	19.9 * ± 4.0	13.7 * ± 0.5	12.9 * ± 2.9	7.6 * ± 0.9
24 h	14.7 ** ± 3.8	6.5 ** ± 1.24	17.5 * ± 3.3	11.5 * ± 0.6	10.2 ± 2.1	7.0 ± 0.8
3 days	20.0 ** ± 4.9	8.7 ** ± 2.24	16.7 ** ± 2.4	9.9 ** ± 1.1	9.6 ± 1.7	8.3 ± 1.1
5 days	28.0 ± 2.6	15.1 * ± 1.70	14.5 * ± 1.9	9.7 * ± 1.1	11.4 * ± 2.2	7.4 * ± 0.9
10 days	32.7 ± 3.3	30.1 ± 5.43	10.9 ± 0.7	7.1 ± 1.3	9.7 ± 1.4	7.4 ± 0.6
20 days	36.7 ± 4.6	36.4 ± 4.93	8.0 ± 1.2	7.2 ± 1.5	8.7 ± 1.5	7.0 ± 0.7
30 days	62.2 * ± 9.6	39.6 * ± 7.43	8.2 ± 2.3	7.1 ± 1.9	10.0 ± 2.0	7.1 ± 0.9
40 days	78.2 ** ± 6.8	23.1 ** ± 8.82	6.5 * ± 1.3	10.0 * ± 2.4	9.7 ± 1.6	7.9 ± 0.8
50 days	107.0 ** ± 15.3	26.0 ** ± 9.71	5.5 ± 1.9	6.8 ± 1.9	11.2 * ± 1.2	6.9 * ± 0.9
60 days	116.2 ** ± 13.9	44.6 ** ± 10.20	4.2 ± 1.4	6.5 ± 1.7	11.5 ± 1.2	7.6 ± 0.7

[1] Delivery, sample collected at delivery; 24 h, sample collected 24 h after delivery; 3 days, sample collected 3 days after delivery; 5 days, sample collected 5 days after delivery; 10 days, sample collected 10 days after delivery; 20 days, sample collected 20 days after delivery; 30 days, sample collected 30 days after delivery; 40 days, sample collected 40 days after delivery; 50 days, sample collected 50 days after delivery; 60 days, sample collected 60 days after delivery. [2] Means are reported with their standard errors; Group C, control group; Group E, experimental Biotropina-stimulated group (injection at the 35th and 40th days after delivery). * Means in row/line for receptor show significant differences ($p < 0.05$); ** Means in row/line for receptor show highly statistically significant differences ($p < 0.01$).

The level of *TLR4* mRNA expression at 30 days of age was similar in both groups (Table 3). After Biotropina injection, *TLR4* mRNA expression increased by 41.33% (Group E), while the expression of *TLR4* mRNA in foals from Group C decreased by 20.22%. On the following days after immunostimulation, *TLR4* mRNA expression in the foals from Group E was higher, but we did not find statistically significant differences between groups. Statistical analysis showed statistically significant differences in *TLR4* mRNA expression after immunostimulation.

The initial expression of *TLR7* mRNA before first suckling was higher in Group C. In Group E, the highest level of expression was observed during delivery at 7.57 ± 0.88 (Table 3). In Group C, the expression was higher during the experiment compared to Group E, and we found highly statistically significant differences between groups ($p < 0.001$). No statistically significant differences were found between the expression of *TLR7* mRNA and immunostimulation.

The Spearman's rank correlation test showed a strong negative correlation between the*TLR3* and *TLR4* genes, and lack of correlation between *TLR3* and *TLR7*as well as*TLR4* and *TLR7* (Table 4).

Table 4. Correlations (p-value) of the expression of *TLR3, TLR4,* and *TLR7* mRNA over the subsequent days of age of the foals from the control group.

Gene	Age	*TLR4*	*TLR7*
TLR3	<1 h	−0.160 (0.6273)	0.62857 (0.1631)
	24 h	−0.191 (0.4199)	0.462 (0.1400)
	3 days	−0.100 (0.6726)	0.492 (0.1276)
	5 days	−0.095 (0.6912)	0.328 (0.1582)
	10 days	**−0.350 (0.0299)**	0.567 (0.1917)
	20 days	**−0.582 (0.0071)**	0.423 (0.1634)
	30 days	**−0.04361 (0.0085)**	0.368 (0.1098)
	40 days	**−0.56992 (0.0087)**	**0.472 (0.0355)**
	50 days	**−0.46466 (0.0039)**	**0.76541 (0.0251)**
	60 days	**−0.35338 (0.0026)**	**0.82105 (0.0341)**
TLR4	<1 h		−0.340 (0.1376)
	24 h		−0.385 (0.0936)
	3 days		−0.472 (0.1355)
	5 days		−0.341 (0.1408)
	10 days		−0.191 (0.4199)
	20 days		−0.319 (0.1707)
	30 days		−0.271 (0.2468)
	40 days		−0.53083 (0.1600)
	50 days		**−0.67519 (0.0111)**
	60 days		**−0.360 (0.0116)**

<1 h, sample collected at delivery; 24 h, sample collected 24 h after delivery; 3 days, sample collected 3 days after delivery; 5 days, sample collected 5 days after delivery; 10 days, sample collected 10 days after delivery; 20 days, sample collected 20 days after delivery; 30 days, sample collected 30 days after delivery; 40 days, sample collected 40 days after delivery; 50 days, sample collected 50 days after delivery; 60 days, sample collected 60 days after delivery. Correlations (p-value) bolded show significant differences ($p < 0.05$) while underlined show highly significant differences ($p < 0.01$).

3.3. *Influence of Age and Stimulation with Biotropina on the Level of Blood Morphotic Elements*

Statistical analysis showed (Table 5):

- A significant influence of age on the hematocrit level;
- A highly significant influence of age on the hemoglobin level;
- A significant influence of age on the level of erythrocytes;
- A highly significant influence of age and immunostimulation on the level of leukocytes;
- A highly significant influence of age and immunostimulation on the level of lymphocytes;
- A highly significant influence of immunostimulation on the number of monocytes;
- A significant influence of age and immunostimulation on the number of neutrophils.
- A highly significant influence of immunostimulation, significant influence of age on the number of basophils;
- A highly significant influence of immunostimulation and age on the number of basophils.

Table 5. Level of blood morphotic elements in foals (mean ± SE).

Parameters	Age	<1 h [1]	24 h	3 Days	5 Days	10 Days	20 Days	30 Days	40 Days	50 Days	60 Days
Hematocrit (PCV) %	C	50.00 [2] ± 1.2	43.33 ± 1.2	39.83 ± 1.5	41.11 ± 1.1	41.56 ± 1.9	34.44 ± 1.6	37.33 ± 1.1	36.33 ± 1.3	37.72 ± 1.2	37.56 ± 1.7
	E	50.50 ± 1.2	44.50 ± 1.8	43.67 ± 1.7	39.58 ± 1.5	41.17 ± 0.9	38.20 ± 1.1	39.75 ± 2.9	36.50 ± 1.7	37.25 ± 1.3	37.75 ± 0.9
Hemoglobin (g/dL)	C	15.46 ± 0.7	14.55 ± 0.7	13.26 ± 0.5	13.75 ± 0.7	13.63 ± 0.7	14.57 * ± 1.2	15.11 * ± 0.9	14.85 * ± 1.3	13.30 ± 0.6	13.98 * ± 1.1
	E	13.94 ± 0.9	13.04 ± 1.7	13.50 ± 0.8	12.71 ± 0.6	12.39 ± 0.2	13.03 ± 0.9	11.80 * ± 0.3	11.70 * ± 0.4	12.39 ± 0.5	10.08 * ± 0.3
RBC count (10^6/μL)	C	10.93 ± 0.9	10.62 ± 0.7	9.99 ± 0.6	10.55 ± 0.6	9.53 ± 0.4	10.38 ± 1.3	11.24 ± 1.5	9.98 ± 0.8	10.43 ± 0.8	9.86 ± 0.8
	E	11.50 ± 0.5	10.01 ± 0.3	9.17 ± 0.4	10.24 ± 0.9	9.33 ± 0.8	9.04 ± 0.7	9.59 ± 1.0	9.69 ± 0.7	10.29 ± 0.3	10.22 ± 0.3
WBC count (10^3/μL)	C	7.35 ± 0.8	7.71 ± 0.7	10.35 ± 1.2	9.86 ± 1.0	11.03 ± 0.8	11.30 ± 0.8	12.60 ± 1.0	14.31 ** ± 0.8	14.62 * ± 0.7	13.07 ** ± 0.7
	E	6.25 ± 0.6	8.17 ± 0.5	9.15 ± 0.8	10.64 ± 1.4	12.40 ± 1.1	12.48 ± 0.9	10.91 * ± 1.6	21.75 ** ± 0.5	18.98 * ± 0.4	14.89 ** ± 0.2
Eosinophils (/μL)	C	105 ** ± 2.2	116 ** ± 2.4	72 ** ± 1.5	296 ** ± 6.2	110 ** ± 2.3	226 ** ± 4.7	315 ** ± 6.6	286 ** ± 6.0	292 ** ± 6.1	327 ** ± 6.9
	E	0 ** ± 0.0	16 ** ± 0.3	22 ** ± 0.4	31 ** ± 0.6	37 ** ± 0.7	42 ** ± 0.8	55 ** ± 1.0	206 ** ± 3.7	105 ** ± 1.9	133 ** ± 2.4
Basophils (/μL)	C	44 ± 0.9	39 ± 0.8	31 ± 0.6	99 ± 2.1	55 ± 1.2	113 * ± 2.4	94 * ± 1.9	72 ** ± 1.5	146 ** ± 3.1	196 ** ± 4.1
	E	18 ± 0.3	29 ± 0.5	38 ± 0.7	39 ± 0.7	52 ± 0.9	64 * ± 1.1	75 * ± 1.3	308 ** ± 5.5	205 ** ± 3.7	76 ** ± 1.4
Neutrophils (/μL)	C	4471 * ± 59.5	4488 * ± 59.3	7041 ± 93.4	6903 ± 91.6	5898 * ± 78.3	6104 ± 81.0	7150 * ± 94.9	8583 ± 113.9	8186 ± 108.6	6403 * ± 84.9
	E	5650 ± 50.8	6942 ± 62.5	7374 ± 66.4	7645 ± 68.8	8804 * ± 79.2	7773 ± 69.9	5705 * ± 51.3	9499 * ± 85.5	9109 ± 81.9	7523 ± 67.7
Lymphocytes (/μL)	C	2554 ** ± 35.7	2852 * ± 39.9	3003 * ± 42.0	2465 ± 34.5	4636 ** ± 65.6	4635 * ± 64.9	4945 ** ± 69.2	5150 ** ± 72.1	5701 ** ± 79.8	5880 ** ± 82.3
	E	470 ** ± 4.2	1090 * ± 9.8	1609 ** ± 14.5	2802 ± 25.2	3110 ** ± 28.0	4280 * ± 38.5	4850 ** ± 43.6	10953 ** ± 98.6	9355 ** ± 84.2	7054 ** ± 63.5
Myelocytes (/μL)	C	162 ± 2.3	231 ** ± 3.2	207 * ± 2.9	99 ± 1.4	276 * ± 3.7	226 * ± 3.2	94 ** ± 1.3	215 ** ± 3.0	292 * ± 4.1	261 * ± 3.7
	E	112 ± 1.0	93 **± 0.8	107 *± 0.9	123 ± 1.1	397 * ± 3.6	321 *± 2.9	225 *± 2.0	784 **± 7.1	206 * ± 1.8	104 * ± 0.9

[1] <1, sample collected at delivery; 24 h, sample collected 24 h after delivery; 3 days, sample collected 3 days after delivery; 5 days, sample collected 5 days after delivery; 10 days, sample collected 10 days after delivery; 20 days, sample collected 20 days after delivery; 30 days, sample collected 30 days after delivery; 40 days, sample collected 40 days after delivery; 50 days, sample collected 50 days after delivery; 60 days, sample collected 60 days after delivery. [2] Means are reported with their standard errors. Group C, control group; Group E, experimental Biotropina-stimulated group (injection on the 35th and 40th days after delivery). * Means in row/line for receptor show significant differences ($p < 0.05$); ** means in row/line for receptor show highly statistically significant differences ($p < 0.01$).

4. Discussion

Infectious diseases are common in foals between the first and fifth months of age. Analysis of the concentrations of immune system components during this period in healthy and infected foals may help understand the basics of the maturation of the immune system and also better understand infection mechanisms [22]. To the best of our knowledge, there are very limited reports where weekly collections and the expression of immune-related genes have been performed. Therefore, our results may be interesting for better understanding the changes during the first weeks of a foal's life and the changes it undergoes during this time. Most studies report data from the first 24 h of a foal's life, from the first 42 days, and very often from adult horses. Moreover, most data include thoroughbreds, while we performed our analysis on a primitive horse breed that is known for their adaptation to harsh conditions. While this study was performed on a primitive domestic breed, the results from this study may differ from potential results if performed on selectively breed domestic horses. Flaminio et al. [22] reported that healthy lymphocytes of healthy foals were the lowest at birth and that values increased until the sixth month of age. In our study, we obtained similar results; however, in Polish Pony, lymphocyte counts were higher (Table 5).

4.1. Changes in TLR4 Gene Expression

Because of the increased vulnerability of foals to some pathogens (e.g., *Rhodococcus equi*), it seems reasonable to analyze changes in the expression of the genes that are responsible for the recognition of the conserved constituents of pathogens [23]. In the present study, a highly significant influence of age and stimulation with Biotropina was observed for *TLR4*. Data available in the literature indicate that the influence of age on *TLR4* expression in horses is contradictory. Vendrig et al. [24] found no differences between the expression of *TLR4* in the blood mononuclear cells of foals at 12 h of life or in adult horses. Stimulation with lipopolysaccharides (LPS) resulted in higher *TLR4* mRNA expression in adult horses, while no response to LPS stimulation was found in foals in an in vivo study [24]. In contrast, Tessier et al. [25], having compared *TLR4* mRNA expression in umbilical cord blood and peripheral blood from adult horses, demonstrated higher*TLR4* mRNA expression in umbilical cord blood in response to LPS administration. The influence of age on the expression of *TLR4*was observed by Hansen et al. [26] in horses aged between 5 and 27 years. Higher *TLR4* mRNA levels were found in younger horses, but the decrease in mRNA levels with age were not statistically significant. *TLR4* mRNA levels were higher in blood mononuclear cells compared to the same cells from pulmonary vascular secretions. Osorio et al. [27] and Strong et al. [28] evaluated the expression of the *TLR4* gene in the first weeks of a calf's life, and their results were similar to the one produced in our study. The highest level of*TLR4* gene expression was observed after birth, and a statistically significant decrease in expression was reported during the following days. A similar trend was identified in our study. Yerkovich et al. [29] and Levy et al. [30] showed that the expression of the *TLR4* gene was significantly higher in peripheral blood in premature and full-term infants than in adults, both before and after LPS stimulation [31]. This trend, indicating a decreasing expression of *TLR4* with age, was also found in humans and mice [32,33]. On the other hand, some results illustrate a higher expression of *TLR4* in newborns compared to adults [34] or decreasing expression of *TLR4* after stimulation [35]. The differences in *TLR*4 expression revealed in these studies and in our experiment may be caused by different concentrations of LPS in the stimulation.

4.2. Changes in TLR3 Gene Expression

We found that *TLR3* mRNA levels increased with the age of the foals. Our results are in agreement with other reports about horses and mostly human newborns [25,36–38]. Interestingly, there are reports proving epigenetics control *TLR3* expression mechanisms [36]. As Porras et al. [36] reported in their results from healthy donors, it can be presumed that a low level of *TLR3* in newborns is a developmentally desirable trend. In a mouse model, Zhang et al. [37] reported higher abortion rates linked with higher *TLR3* levels. It was also mentioned that *TLR3* expression was age-dependent, which can be confirmed by our results. As *TLR3* binds double-stranded RNAs (dsRNAs), its decreased level may increase susceptibility to viral infection in young foals. In our study, the lowest level was recorded before the first suckling, which is in agreement with other reports in premature infants [38] and newborns [39,40]. The data presented above, and the results obtained in our study of the *TLR3* gene, may explain the higher incidence of equine herpesvirus-1 (EHV-1) and equine herpesvirus-4 (EHV-4), responsible for massive respiratory tract infections in foals and young horses. A severe course and high mortality due to contracting equine viral arteritis (EVA) in young horses may also be a result of the decreased expression of *TLR3*. Hussey et al. [41] suggested that *TLR3* plays an essential role in recognizing EHV-1 infections. In our study, a decrease in *TLR3* gene expression was observed after stimulation with Biotropina. We analyzed the level of expression in foals up to 60 days of age, but the literature indicates that the immune system of horses develops most intensively until about 90 days of life [42]. Foals have all of the components of an immune system characteristic of adult horses—but many mechanisms of the immune response have yet to mature. The results indicate that activation of horse monocytes by ligands for the *TLR2* and *TLR4* genes increases their expression, but not that of *TLR3*. Additionally, *TLR3* gene expression decreases with the increase of *TLR4* gene expression after the stimulation of monocytes [43].

4.3. Changes in TLR7 Gene Expression

TLR7 is responsible for recognizing guanidine-rich, single-stranded viral RNA (ssRNA) and is an important mediator of the peripheral immune response. Asquith at al. [41] and Slavica at al. [39] observed no effect of age on*TLR7* gene expression in newborns, similar to Talmadge et al. [22] in horses. Belnoue et al. [44] reported significantly higher levels of *TLR7* gene expression in two-week-old foals compared to adult horses. Harrington et al. [9] found neither an age-dependent pattern in the expression of the *TLR7/8* genes, nor did they detect the effect of imidazoquinol R848 stimulation on its expression, despite increasing the levels of IL-6 and IL-8. Our results also did not confirm any relationship between a foal's age and expression of *TLR7*. Until now, little was known about the signaling mechanisms of Toll-like receptors in foals. Identifying the receptors and describing ligands that react with them can provide new insights into immunological responses and can also point to new pathways in the field of therapy and prevention of diseases, particularly infectious ones.

5. Conclusions

In summary, on the basis of the results obtained, it was concluded that the expression of the *TLR3* and *TLR4* genes in peripheral blood cells is dependent on age. The expression of the *TLR3* and *TLR4* genes, as well as the levels of immunoglobulins and interleukins, can be modulated by stimulation with the pharmacological agent Biotropina. This experiment demonstrated a strong negative correlation between *TLR3* and *TLR4* gene expression. Detailed knowledge of the molecular mechanisms of immunoglobulin synthesis appears necessary for a better understanding of foal immunity maturity and its influencing factors. At the same time, this experiment encourages studies regarding the influence of the signaling cascade's proteins on the primary immunological response, providing an opportunity to develop extremely precise methods of regulating acquired immunity. There is still little information about the maturity of a horse's immune system in the pre- and postnatal period, which negatively affects the planning of health protection strategies for foals.

Author Contributions: Conceptualization, A.M., A.O. and A.C.-S.; methodology A.M. and M.O.; collection and analysis of samples, A.M., Ł.M. and A.O.; Data interpretation A.M., Ł.M., M.O. and A.C.-S.; writing A.M. and Ł.M. All authors have read and agreed to the published version of the manuscript.

References

1. Tallmadge, R.; McLaughlin, K.; Secor, E.; Ruano, D.; Matychak, M.; Julia, M.; Flaminio, B.F. Expression of essential Bcell genes and immunoglobulin isotypes suggests active development and gene recombination during equine gestation. *Dev. Comp. Immunol.* **2009**, *33*, 1027–1038. [CrossRef] [PubMed]
2. Perkins, G.A.; Wagner, B. The development of equine immunity: Current knowledge on immunology in the young horse. *Equine Vet. J.* **2015**, *47*, 267–274. [CrossRef]
3. Flamino, M.J.; Rush, B.R.; Davis, E.G.; Hennessy, K.; Shuman, W.; Wilkerson, M.J. Characterization of peripheral blood and pulmonary leukocyte function in healthy foal. *Vet. Immunol. Immunopathol.* **2000**, *73*, 267–285. [CrossRef]
4. Miyara, M.; Sakaguchi, S. Natural regulatory T cells: Mechanisms of suppression. *Trends Mol. Med.* **2007**, *13*, 108–116. [CrossRef] [PubMed]
5. Janeway, C.A., Jr.; Medzhitov, R. Innate immune recognition. *Annu. Rev. Immunol.* **2002**, *20*, 197–216. [CrossRef]
6. Lemaitre, B.; Nicolas, E.; Michaut, L.; Reichhart, J.M.; Hoffmann, J.A. The dorsoventral regulatory gene cassette spätzle/Toll/cactus controls the potent antifungal response in Drosophila adults. *Cell* **1996**, *6*, 973–983. [CrossRef]
7. Medzhitov, R.; Preston-Hurlburt, P.; Janeway, C., Jr. A human homologue of the Drosophila Toll protein signals activation of adaptive immunity. *Nature* **1997**, *388*, 394–397. [CrossRef]
8. Kawai, T.; Akira, S. The role of pattern-recognition receptors in innate immunity: Update on Toll-like receptors. *Nat. Immunol.* **2010**, *11*, 373–384. [CrossRef]
9. Harrington, J.R.; Wilkerson, C.P.; Brake, C.N.; Cohen, N.D. Effects of age and R848 stimulation on expression of Toll-like receptor 8mRNA by foal neutrophils. *Vet. Immunol. Immunopathol.* **2012**, *150*, 10–18. [CrossRef]
10. Hayashi, F.; Means, T.K.; Luster, A.D. Toll-like receptors stimulate human neutrophil function. *Blood* **2003**, *102*, 2660–2669. [CrossRef]
11. Kulisa, M.; Makieła, K.; Długosz, B.; Gaj, M. Thoroughbred foals' mortality causes during first six months of life. PartII. Diseases and injuries. *Roczniki Naukowe Polskiego Towarzystwa Zootechnicznego* **2009**, *5*, 79–84.
12. Haas, S.D.; Bristol, F.; Card, C.E. Risk factors associated with the incidence of foal mortality in a managed mare herd. *Can. Vet. J.* **1996**, *37*, 91–95. [PubMed]
13. Wilson, W.D.; Mihalyi, J.E.; Hussey, S.; Lunn, D.P. Passive transfer of maternal immunoglobulin isotype antibodies against tetanus and influenza and their effect on the response of foals to vaccination. *Equine Vet. J.* **2001**, *33*, 644–650. [CrossRef] [PubMed]
14. Ainsworth, D.M.; Eicker, S.W.; Yeagar, A.E.; Sweeney, C.R.; Viel, L.; Tesarowski, D.; Lavoie, J.P.; Hoffman, A.; Paradis, M.R.; Reed, S.M.; et al. Associations between physical examination, laboratory, and radiographic findings and outcome and subsequent racing performance of foals with *Rhodococcus equi* infection: 115 cases (1984–1992). *J. Am. Vet. Med. Assoc.* **1998**, *213*, 510–515. [PubMed]
15. Breathnach, C.C.; Sturgill-Wright, T.; Stiltner, J.L.; Adams, A.A.; Lunn, D.P.; Horohov, D.W. Foals are interferon gamma-deficient at birth. *Vet. Immunol. Immunopathol.* **2006**, *112*, 199–209. [CrossRef] [PubMed]
16. Boyd, N.K.; Cohen, N.D.; Lim, W.S.; Martens, R.J.; Chaffin, M.K.; Ball, J.M. Temporal changes in cytokine expression of foals during the first month of life. *Vet. Immunol. Immunopathol.* **2003**, *92*, 75–85. [CrossRef]
17. Prescott, J.F.; Nicholson, V.M.; Patterson, M.C.; Zandona Meleiro, M.C.; de Caterino, A.A.; Yager, J.A.; Holmes, M.A. Use of *Rhodococcus equi* virulence-associated protein for immunization of foals against *R. equi* pneumonia. *Am. J. Vet. Res.* **1997**, *58*, 356–359.
18. Fleer, A.; Krediet, T.G. Innate immunity: Toll-like receptors and some more. *Neonatology* **2007**, *92*, 145–157. [CrossRef]
19. Levy, O. Innate immunity of the newborn: Basic mechanisms and clinical correlates. *Nat. Rev. Immunol.* **2007**, *7*, 379–390. [CrossRef]
20. Jaworski, Z. *Tablice Genealogiczne Koników Polskich Genealogical Tables of the Polish Primitive Horse*; Stacja Badawcza Rolnictwa Ekologicznego i Hodowli Zachowawczej Zwierzat PAN: Popielno, Poland, 1997. (In Polish)
21. Hoehler, D. *The Institute for Animal Nutrition and Metabolic Physiology*; Kiel University: Kiel, Germany, 1997.
22. Flaminio, M.; Rush, B.; Shuman, W. Peripheral Blood Lymphocyte Subpopulations and Immunoglobulin Concentrations in Healthy Foals and Foals with *Rhodococcus Equi Pneumonia*. *J. Vet. Intern. Med.* **1999**, *13*, 206–212. [CrossRef]

23. Tallmadge, R.; Wang, M.; Sun, Q.; Felippe, M.J.B. Transcriptome analysis of immune genes in peripheral blood mononuclear cells of young foals and adult horses. *PLoS ONE* **2018**, *13*, e0202646. [CrossRef] [PubMed]
24. Vendrig, J.C.; Coffeng, L.E.; Fink-Gremmels, J. Effects of Separate and Concomitant TLR-2 and TLR-4 Activation in Peripheral Blood Mononuclear Cells of Newborn and Adult Horses. *PLoS ONE* **2013**, *8*, e66897. [CrossRef] [PubMed]
25. Tessier, L.; Bienzle, D.; Williams, L.B.; Koch, T.G. Phenotypic and Immunomodulatory Properties of Equine Cord Blood-Derived Mesenchymal Stromal Cells. *PLoS ONE* **2015**, *10*, e0122954. [CrossRef] [PubMed]
26. Hansen, S.; Baptiste, K.; Fjeldborg, J.; Betancourt, A.; Horohov, D. A comparison of pro-inflammatory cytokine mRNA expression in equine bronchoalveolar lavage (BAL) and peripheral blood. *Vet. Immunol. Immunopathol.* **2014**, *158*, 238–243. [CrossRef]
27. Osorio, J.; Trevisi, E.; Ballou, M.; Bertoni, G.; Drackley, J.; Loor, J. Effect of the level of maternal energy intake prepartum on immune metabolic markers, polymorphonuclear leukocyte function, and neutrophil gene network expression in neonatal Holstein heifer calves. *J. Dairy Sci.* **2013**, *96*, 3573–3587. [CrossRef]
28. Strong, R.; Silva, E.; Cheng, H.; Eicher, S.D. Acute brief heat stress in late gestation alters neonatal calf innate immune functions. *J. Dairy Sci.* **2015**, *98*, 7771–7783. [CrossRef]
29. Yerkovich, S.T.; Wikstrom, M.E.; Suriyaarachchi, D.; Prescott, S.L.; Upham, J.W.; Holt, P.G. Postnatal Development of Monocyte Cytokine Responses to Bacterial Lipopolysaccharide. *Pediatr. Res.* **2007**, *62*, 547–552. [CrossRef]
30. Levy, E.; Xanthou, G.; Petrakou, E.; Zacharioudaki, V.; Tsatsanis, C.; Fotopoulos, S.; Xanthou, M. Distinct Roles of TLR4 and CD14 in LPS-Induced Inflammatory Responses of Neonates. *Pediatr. Res.* **2009**, *66*, 179–184. [CrossRef]
31. Boehmer, E.D.; Goral, J.; Faunce, D.E.; Kovacs, E.J. Age-dependent decrease in Toll-like receptor 4-mediated proinflammatory cytokine production and mitogen-activated protein kinase expression. *J. Leukoc. Biol.* **2003**, *75*, 342–349. [CrossRef]
32. Chelvarajan, R.L.; Collins, S.M.; Van Willigen, J.M.; Bondada, S. The unresponsiveness of aged mice to polysaccharide antigens is a result of a defect in macrophage function. *J. Leukoc. Biol.* **2005**, *77*, 503–512. [CrossRef]
33. Förster-Waldl, E.; Sadeghi, K.; Tamandl, D.; Gerhold, B.; Hallwirth, U.; Meistersinger, K.; Hayde, M.; Prusa, A.R.; Herkner, K.; Boltz-Nitulescu, G.; et al. Monocyte toll-like receptor 4 expression and LPS induced cytokine production increase during gestational aging. *Pediatr. Res.* **2005**, *58*, 121–124. [CrossRef] [PubMed]
34. Levy, O.; Zarember, K.A.; Roy, R.M.; Cywes, C.; Godowski, P.J.; Wessels, M.R. Selective impairment of TLR-mediated innate immunity in human newborns: Neonatal blood plasma reduces monocyte TNF-alpha induction by bacterial lipopeptides, lipopolysaccharide, and imiquimod, but preserves the response to R-848. *J. Immunol.* **2004**, *173*, 4627–4634. [CrossRef] [PubMed]
35. Yan, S.R.; Qing, G.; Byers, D.M.; Stadnyk, A.W.; Al-Hertani, W.; Bortolussi, R. Role of MyD88 in Diminished Tumor Necrosis Factor Alpha Production by Newborn Mononuclear Cells in Response to Lipopolysaccharide. *Infect. Immun.* **2004**, *72*, 1223–1229. [CrossRef]
36. Porrás, A.; Kozar, S.; Russanova, V.; Salpea, P.; Hirai, T.; Sammons, N.; Mittal, P.; Kim, J.Y.; Ozato, K.; Romero, R.; et al. Developmental and epigenetic regulation of the human TLR3 gene. *Mol. Immunol.* **2008**, *46*, 27–36. [CrossRef]
37. Zhang, J.; Wei, H.; Wu, D.; Tian, Z. Toll-like receptor 3 agonist induces impairment of uterine vascular remodeling and fetal losses in CBA × DBA/2 mice. *J. Reprod. Immunol.* **2007**, *74*, 61–67. [CrossRef]
38. Gibbons, D.L.; Haque, S.F.; Silberzahn, T.; Hamilton, K.; Langford, C.; Ellis, P.; Carr, R.; Hayday, A.C. Neonates harbour highly active gamma delta T cells with selective impairments in preterm infants. *Eur. J. Immunol.* **2009**, *39*, 1794–1806. [CrossRef] [PubMed]
39. Pott, J.; Stockinger, S.; Torow, N.; Smoczek, A.; Lindner, C.; McInerney, G.; Bäckhed, F.; Baumann, U.; Pabst, O.; Bleich, A.; et al. Age-Dependent TLR3 Expression of the Intestinal Epithelium Contributes to Rotavirus Susceptibility. *PLoS Pathog.* **2012**, *8*, e1002670. [CrossRef]
40. Slavica, L.; Nordström, I.; Karlsson, M.N.; Valadi, H.; Kacerovsky, M.; Jacobsson, B.; Eriksson, K. TLR3 impairment in human newborns. *J. Leukoc. Biol.* **2013**, *94*, 1003–1011. [CrossRef]
41. Hussey, G.S.; Ashton, L.V.; Quintana, A.M.; Lunn, P.D.; Goehring, L.S.; Annis, K.; Landolt, G. Innate immune responses of airway epithelial cells to infection with Equine herpesvirus-1. *Vet. Microbiol.* **2014**, *170*, 28–38. [CrossRef]

42. Asquith, M.; Haberthur, K.; Brown, M.; Engelmann, F.; Murphy, A.; Al-Mahdi, Z.; Messaoudi, I. Age-dependent changes in innate immune phenotype and function in rhesus macaques (*Macaca mulatta*). *Pathobiol. Aging Age Relat. Dis.* **2012**, *2*, 3331. [CrossRef]
43. Kwon, S.; Vandenplas, M.L.; Figueiredo, M.D.; Salter, C.E.; Andrietti, A.L.; Robertson, T.P.; Moore, J.N.; Hurley, D.J. Differential induction of Toll-like receptor gene expression in equine monocytes activated by Toll-like receptor ligands or TNF-α. *Vet. Immunol. Immunopathol.* **2010**, *138*, 213–217. [CrossRef]
44. Belnoue, E.; Fontannaz, P.; Rochat, A.-F.; Tougne, C.; Bergthaler, A.; Lambert, P.-H.; Pinschewer, D.D.; Siegrist, C.-A. Functional Limitations of Plasmacytoid Dendritic Cells Limit Type I Interferon, T Cell Responses and Virus Control in Early Life. *PLoS ONE* **2013**, *8*, e85302. [CrossRef]

11

Role of the JAK-STAT Pathway in Bovine Mastitis and Milk Production

Muhammad Zahoor Khan [1], Adnan Khan [2], Jianxin Xiao [1], Yulin Ma [1], Jiaying Ma [1], Jian Gao [3] and Zhijun Cao [1,*]

1 State Key Laboratory of Animal Nutrition, Beijing Engineering Technology Research Center of Raw Milk Quality and Safety Control, College of Animal Science and Technology, China Agricultural University, Beijing 100193, China; zahoorkhattak91@163.com (M.Z.K.); dairyxiao@gmail.com (J.X.); ma18810318038@163.com (Y.M.); majiaying@cau.edu.cn (J.M.)

2 Key Laboratory of Animal Genetics, Breeding, and Reproduction, Ministry of Agriculture & National Engineering Laboratory for Animal Breeding, College of Animal Science and Technology, China Agricultural University, Beijing 100193, China; dr.adnan93@cau.edu.cn

3 Department of Clinical Veterinary Medicine, College of Veterinary Medicine, China Agricultural University, Beijing 100193, China; gaojian2016@cau.edu.cn

* Correspondence: caozhijun@cau.edu.cn;

Simple Summary: The cytokine-activated Janus kinase (JAK)—signal transducer and activator of transcription (STAT) pathway has an important role in the regulation of immunity and inflammation. In addition, the signaling of this pathway has been reported to be associated with mammary gland development and milk production. Because of such important functions, the JAK-STAT pathway has been widely targeted in both human and animal diseases as a therapeutic agent. Recently, the *JAK2*, *STATs*, and inhibitors of the JAK-STAT pathway, especially cytokine signaling suppressors (SOCSs), have been reported to be associated with milk production and mastitis-resistance phenotypic traits in dairy cattle. Thus, in the current review, we attempt to overview the development of the JAK-STAT pathway role in bovine mastitis and milk production.

Abstract: The cytokine-activated Janus kinase (JAK)—signal transducer and activator of transcription (STAT) pathway is a sequence of communications between proteins in a cell, and it is associated with various processes such as cell division, apoptosis, mammary gland development, lactation, anti-inflammation, and immunity. The pathway is involved in transferring information from receptors on the cell surface to the cell nucleus, resulting in the regulation of genes through transcription. The Janus kinase 2 (*JAK2*), signal transducer and activator of transcription A and B (STAT5 A & B), STAT1, and cytokine signaling suppressor 3 (*SOCS3*) are the key members of the JAK-STAT pathway. Interestingly, prolactin (Prl) also uses the JAK-STAT pathway to regulate milk production traits in dairy cattle. The activation of *JAK2* and *STATs* genes has a critical role in milk production and mastitis resistance. The upregulation of *SOCS3* in bovine mammary epithelial cells inhibits the activation of *JAK2* and *STATs* genes, which promotes mastitis development and reduces the lactational performance of dairy cattle. In the current review, we highlight the recent development in the knowledge of JAK-STAT, which will enhance our ability to devise therapeutic strategies for bovine mastitis control. Furthermore, the review also explores the role of the JAK-STAT pathway in the regulation of milk production in dairy cattle.

Keywords: bovine mastitis; JAK-STAT pathway; *JAK2*; *STATs*; *SOCS3*; immunity; milk production

1. Introduction

Bovine mastitis is a seriously infectious and contagious disease, which is a massive threat to the dairy industry throughout the globe [1]. Mastitis is the inflammation of the mammary gland, which is characterized by physical, chemical, and microbiological alterations in milk, following pathological changes in udder tissue [2]. Bovine mastitis is described as acute or chronic based on inflammation, redness, and localized heat at the infected area, with more severe symptoms, such as fever, leading to septicemia, and the formation of abscesses [3,4]. There are two types of mastitis: clinical and subclinical mastitis. In most cases, infection with Gram-negative bacteria such as *Escherichia coli* (*E. coli*) can often cause clinical mastitis, and Gram-positive bacteria such as *Staphylococcus aureus* (*S. aureus*) are involved in subclinical mastitis infection [5,6].

Bovine mastitis is considered one of the costly diseases of dairy cattle because of milk losses, treatment costs, and rare death [7,8]. In China, the annual losses of 15–45 billion Chinese Yuan (CNY) have been documented [7], while in the US and India, the dairy industry has experienced losses of 2 billion and 526 million dollars, respectively [9]. In Europe, collectively, the cost due to mastitis has reached 1.55 billion euros per year [10]. This increased frequency was linked to public concerns for animal welfare and has made mastitis the key disease of the dairy sector [11]. In addition, bovine mastitis has a major zoonotic risk, correlated with the shedding of bacteria and their toxins into milk [12].

Mammary epithelial cells are the first line of defense of the mammary gland to invading bacteria. They not only act as physical barriers but also are capable of producing inflammatory mediators. While interacting with invading bacteria, mammary epithelial cells generate multiple inflammatory cytokines [13,14]. Several genes and pathways have been reported to be associated with the regulation of bovine mastitis [15]. It is well known that the innate immune system recognizes the presence of pathogens ligands through a membrane receptor family known as Toll-like receptors (TLRs) [16]. TLRs are pattern recognition receptors (PRRs) on the host cell surface that recognize bacterial-pathogen-associated molecular patterns [17]. Upon activation, TLRs further mediate different important signaling, such as that of the JAK-STAT pathway.

Any disruption in the JAK-STAT pathway may lead to various diseases, including bovine mastitis that compromises the immune system of the host. Furthermore, it has also been documented that *STAT5A* works as a mediator for extracellular prolactin receptors. At the same time, *JAK2* plays a role as a bridge between *STAT5A* and prolactin receptor (PrlR), which is essential for milk production and mammary gland development. Keeping in view the vital role of JAK-STAT signaling in immunity, inflammation, and milk production, the current review paper is designed with aims to summarize the role of the JAK-STAT pathway in bovine mastitis and milk production.

2. General Mechanism of the JAK-STAT Pathway Regulation

There are three main components of the JAK-STAT pathway: receptors, Janus kinases (JAKs), signal transducers, and activators of transcription proteins (*STATs*) [18]. The mammalian JAK family consists of *JAK1*, *JAK2*, *JAK3*, and tyrosine kinase 2 (*TYK2*), which are linked to the cytoplasmic domains of diverse cytokine receptors [19]. Among the seven members of *STATs* (*STAT1*-4, 5a, 5b, and 6) in mammalian cells, *STAT5A* and *STAT5B* show high sequence identity and lie closest in a head-to-head pattern next to *STAT3* [19,20]. The members of the STAT family are involved in cell growth, differentiation, cell survival and apoptosis, and mammary gland development. The cytokines, after attachment with receptors on the cell surface, activate JAKs. The two JAKs come close through receptor oligomerization. Furthermore, these JAKs phosphorylate the receptor complex's intracellular tyrosines, generating the docking sites for STATs. Consequently, the activated *STATs* form hetero- or homodimers, where the Src-homology 2 (SH2) domain of each STAT binds the phosphorylated tyrosine of the opposite STAT, and the dimers then translocate to the cell nucleus to induce transcription of the target genes. JAK-STAT has been revealed to operate downstream of several peptide hormones and cytokines that are necessary for the development of the postnatal and secretory function of the mammary gland [21]. The phosphorylated *STAT5A* and *STAT5B* form homodimers and heterodimers in mammary epithelial cells in order to regulate the process of differentiation, survival, and proliferation through the modification in cellular gene expression [22]. The rapamycin target phosphatidylinositol 3-kinase-protein kinase B/mammalian signaling pathway (PI3K-Akt/mTOR) mediates many cellular processes such as cell proliferation, growth, survival, and metastasis [23], and it is necessary for the development of the mammary gland [24]. A conditional knockout of Akt1 prevents the extensive survival of mammary epithelial cells, which express hyperactive *STAT5*, indicating that the PI3K-Akt/mTOR pathway is a crucial downstream signaling effector of JAK-STAT signaling [25]. To find out the interconnection between different genes and their biological functions in the JAK-STAT pathway, we exploited an online software database for annotation, visualization, and integrated discovery (DAVID; https://david.ncifcrf.gov/) [26], which are summarized in Figure 1.

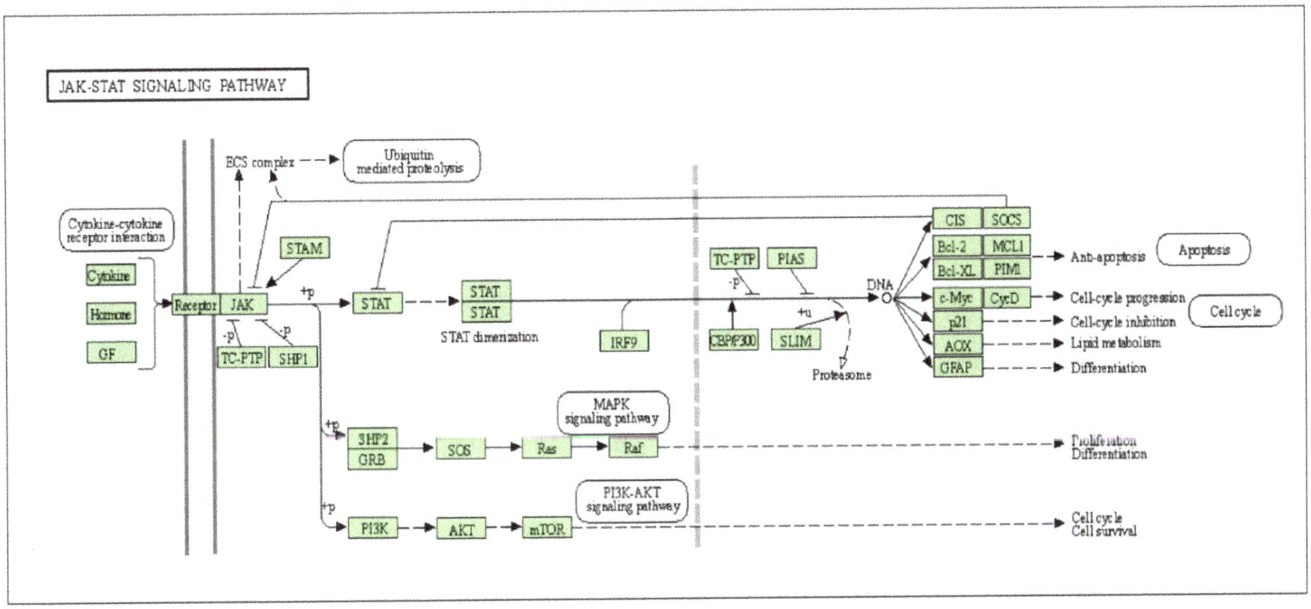

Figure 1. The regulation of the cytokine-activated Janus kinase (JAK)–signal transducer and activator of transcription (STAT) pathway by cytokines, hormones, and growth factors; engagement of the JAK-STAT pathway in the process of differentiation, survival, and proliferation through the modification in cellular gene expression.

STAT5, being the main gene of the JAK-STAT inflammatory signaling pathway, has an essential role in prolactin-induced mammary gland factor and is assumed to be associated with mammary gland development in transgenic mice [27]. Consequently, upon activation, JAK regulates the cellular mechanisms such as cell migration, apoptosis, cell proliferation, and differentiation, which are essential for hematopoietic responses, immune development, mammary gland development, and the lactation process [28]. Cytokines play a vital role in the regulation of the JAK-STAT pathway, which further facilitates immunity and inflammation. Consequently, the JAK-STAT pathway has been widely studied for its critical role in immunity and inflammation [29,30], and evidence indicates that persistent activation of this pathway might lead to many immune- and inflammatory-related diseases [31,32]. Performing a critical role in immunity, cell proliferation, cell differentiation, and inflammation, the JAK-STAT pathway has been widely targeted for therapeutic purposes in several inflammatory diseases [33].

3. The JAK-STAT Pathway Role in Milk Production in Dairy Cattle

The JAK-STAT pathway regulates lactation [34], while PI3K/Akt within the JAK-STAT pathway shows overexpression in lactating cows [35]. Gene deletion analysis in mice has documented an important role of the JAK-STAT signaling pathway in the lactation and development of the mammary gland [36,37]. In the mammary gland, the JAK-STAT pathway, along with *SOCS* signaling, plays a critical role in controlling cytokine signals and has shown an association with mammary gland development and milk production [38]. Moreover, studies have documented the essential role of the JAK-STAT pathway in blood cell differentiation and casein gene regulation during milk production [39,40]. It has been shown that some JAK-STAT-associated proteins are regulated by PrlR, which may establish a balance between growth hormone and milk protein yield [41]. It has been illustrated that by using the JAK-STAT pathway, the lactogenic hormones, through their receptors on cell membranes, regulate milk proteins [42]. Prolactin also uses JAK-STAT signaling and regulates the processes of lactation and reproduction in mammals [43]. It has been documented that a higher concentration of Prl in blood circulation is associated with an increased level of milk production in dairy cattle [44]. During hypothyroidism, a severe decrease in milk production has been documented. Furthermore, it has been found that hypothyroidism decreases the level of prolactin, resulting in lower expression of the JAK-STAT pathway, which is responsible for lower milk production in hypothyroidized rats [45].

3.1. Role of JAKs in Milk Production in Dairy Cattle

JAK2 is the tyrosine kinase responsible for phosphorylation of both PrlR and Stat5, based on tissue culture cell studies. According to one report, in the absence of the *JAK2* gene, mammary epithelium proliferation and differentiation were reduced by 95% around parturition [46]. The endocrine factor prolactin attaches to the PrlRs and causes their dimerization. JAK protein kinases are linked to these receptors and these JAK proteins alter a receptor into a tyrosine kinase receptor. The regulated receptors may specifically phosphorylate inactive *STATs*, which result in dimerization. These dimers are further translocated into the nucleus. The *STATs* attach to the upstream promoter elements of the casein gene and cause their transcription. Growth hormones (GHs) control the growth and development of the mammary gland and regulate milk production and milk protein levels in cattle [41,47]. *STAT5* passes on messages from cytokines and growth factors outside the cell to the nucleus of the mammary gland epithelial cells and thereby mediates the transcription of the gene during pregnancy, lactation, and weaning [48].

It has been consistently reported that the polymorphisms T-C39652459 and T-C39645396, at intron 15 and exon 20, respectively, in the *JAK2* gene, are significantly associated with milk lactose production in dairy cows [49]. Furthermore, the variant *JAK2/RsaI* is involved in the regulation of milk and milk protein and can be considered a milk production marker in dairy cattle [50]. The variants 39630048C/T and 39631175T/C in the *JAK2* gene significantly influence milk fat and milk proteins, respectively, in Chinese Holsteins [51]. PrlR uses *STAT5A* and *JAK2* as mediators to activate the proteins associated with milk production traits [52].

3.2. Role of STATs in Milk Production in Dairy Cattle

STATs are activated by specific ligands, i.e., *STAT5A* is regulated by Prl, while STAT5B regulation is mediated through growth hormones (GHs) [53]. STAT5 is an important intracellular mediator of prolactin signaling and can activate transcription of milk proteins in response to Prl. *STAT5* has been suggested to be candidate marker genes for milk protein yield and composition in dairy cattle [54]. During pregnancy, *STAT5A* and PrlR play essential roles in mammary epithelium proliferation and differentiation [55,56]. Consequently, it has been found that PrlR has a positive impact on lactation performance in cows, possibly due to its involvement in steroid synthesis and cholesterol regulation [57]. During pregnancy and lactation, STAT5A and STAT5B are the essential proteins required for the synthesis of luminal progenitor cells from mammary stem cells and the differentiation of milk-producing alveolar cells [58]. *STAT5A* and *STAT5B* have been linked with the development of the mammary gland during pregnancy [59]. It was previously found that *STATs* promote the mammary gland cells' survival by mediating the promoters of genes essential for milk proteins [34,60]. *STATs* facilitate various peptide hormones and cytokines in targeted cells such as Prl and GH and are linked to milk production. Whey acidic protein (WAP) is expressed in the mammary gland and is associated with the improvement of milk protein. *STAT5* has been considered an important transcription factor that is responsible for the regulations of Prl at 5′ flanking regions of *WAP* [61]. It has been observed that the downregulation of Prl in hypothyroidized rats causes the inhibition of the transcriptional activity of *STAT5.* Consequently, any abnormality in the thyroid gland severely affects milk production efficiency in rats because of the low level of Prl [45]. In addition, GH also regulates the STAT1 gene and its expression has been reported during mammary gland development [62,63]. Furthermore, a study has reported the combination effect of STAT1 with other JAK-STAT signaling members on milk production traits [38]. Keeping in view the important role of *STATs* as a mediator of prolactin signaling, the polymorphisms in these genes were further studied for its role in milk production.

The mutations in the *STAT5A* gene have been reported for their effect on milk yield [64]. Consistently, the *STAT5A/AvaI* polymorphism at position C-T 6853/exon7 was documented to be associated with milk production and could be used as a significant marker for milk improvement [65]. In addition, the *STAT5A/MslI* locus has been found to be correlated with milk yield, milk fat, and protein [65–67]. The polymorphic site A14217G and 17266indelCCT in *STAT5A* have shown significant associations with milk protein percentage and milk yield, respectively [68]. Consequently, Schennink et al. documented that single nucleotide polymorphism (SNP) 9501G>A in *STAT5A* significantly influenced milk fat composition [69]. Khatib et al. noticed that variant 12195T/C in *STAT5A* was significantly linked to a decrease in milk fat and protein percentage in dairy cattle [70]. The variant 31562 T>C in *STAT5B* was reported to be associated with milk yield and milk protein [71]. The association of *CD4* and *STAT5B* with milk traits might be due to their role in the regulation of prolactin-induced mammary gland factor [72]. Moreover, the variant in the STAT 1 gene has been documented to be linked with milk fat, milk protein, and milk yield in dairy cattle [73]. Consequently, the polymorphism STAT1/BspHI has been reported to be associated with milk production traits in Jersey cows [74]. Similarly, Deng et al. reported that SNPs in STAT1 have a significant association with milk production traits and could be a useful addition to the marker-assisted selection for milk production [75].

The above findings reveal that the JAK-STAT pathway plays a central role in the regulation of milk production traits.

4. The JAK-STAT Signaling Role in Bovine Mastitis

As mastitis is an immunity- and inflammatory related disease, scientists have widely targeted the JAK-STAT pathway in bovine mastitis control research. Besides having a critical role in mammary gland development, any abnormal regulation may disturb the normal function of the JAK-STAT pathway, resulting in impairment of mammary gland development and exposure to mammary infections. Buitenhuis et al. found the altered expression of the JAK-STAT pathway in the mammary gland tissue of cows challenged with *E. coli* [76]. It is well known that the JAK-STAT pathway is regulated by IFN, LPS, or growth factors. In its turn, JAK-STAT signaling mediates proinflammatory cytokines. Tiezzi et al. documented the JAK-STAT pathway as a key pathway that regulates clinical mastitis [77]. Recently, it has been reported that cirsimarin (an extract of *Cirsium japonicum* var. ussuriense) treatment suppressed the expression of inflammatory cytokines by downregulating the phosphorylation of the JAK-STAT pathway in the mammary gland. Thus, this substance can be targeted as a therapeutic agent in many inflammatory diseases, including bovine mastitis [78]. It has been shown that 8-methoxypsoralen treatment protects bovine mammary epithelial cells against lipopolysaccharide-induced inflammatory injury by inhibition of the JAK/STAT and NF-κB pathways [79]. JAK-STAT suppression by xanthotoxin resulted in the downregulation of IL-6, nitric oxide (NO), and tumor necrosis factor (TNF-α) induced by LPS in bovine mammary epithelial cells [80]. This mechanism is essential for regulating udder reactions to infection as it controls the chronic accumulation of neutrophils in the bovine mammary gland [81], whereas JAK also serves as a signaling agent for hormones and interleukin receptors [82] and *JAK2* is considered one of the top-rated genes of bovine mastitis tolerance [83].

4.1. Association of *JAK2* Activity with Bovine Mastitis

Any dysfunctions of the JAK-STAT pathway may expose cattle to mastitis because of abnormal activation of the proliferation and apoptosis of cells. From this point of view, it can be expected that mutations in genes involved in the JAK-STAT pathway might be a target in bovine mastitis research. The inflammatory- and immunity-associated diseases are polygenic traits [71], and polymorphisms in immunity-linked genes can regulate the immune responses of the host to pathogens [84]. Two major approaches are dominantly targeted by animal scientists to control mastitis. The first approach is to look for major genes associated with mastitis resistance, while the second one is to target the polymorphisms within genes and their links with mastitis resistance traits.

Many types of mutations in the JAK-STAT pathway have been identified; most of them are related to *JAK2*.

As demonstrated in Table 1, the polymorphism 39630048C/T in *JAK2* is associated with interleukin-17 (IL-17) [85], IL-6, and interferon-gamma (IFN-γ) expression [51]. Furthermore, the SNPs (39652267A/G, 39631175T/C) in the *JAK2* gene have been documented for their significant links with milk somatic cell counts (SCCs), IL-6, and IFN-γ [51,85]. Mutation 39631044G/A in the *JAK2* gene was noticed to be significantly associated with milk somatic cell scores (SCSs) in Chinese Holsteins [85]. Moreover, the polymorphism 39645396C/T in the *JAK2* gene was linked to milk SCCs, IL-6, and IFN-γ [86], while SNP-39631044G/A in *JAK2* was associated with milk SCSs [85]. SCCs and SCSs are widely targeted as early mastitis indicators [7]. Increased SCCs in early lactation can signify the presence of intramammary infection, and, in many countries, the indirect selection against mastitis using milk SCCs is practiced [87]. However, in the early phase of infectivity, the neutrophil and inflammatory cytokine levels increase quicker than milk SCCs [88]. That is why, nowadays, more interest is paid to the increase in cells and cytokine levels in milk and blood, respectively, rather than just the overall SCC, which may provide an early status of udder health [89]. A study showed that inflammatory cytokines (IL-6, IL-17, and IFN-γ, TNF-α) could be used as subclinical mastitis indicators, in addition to SCSs and SCCs [51,86,90]. In addition, it is predicted that the 39645396C/T SNP changes lysine to asparagine [86]. The expression of IL-6 was higher in plasma cell mastitis (PCM), which indicated that the IL-6/STAT3 pathway could play a key role in the pathogenesis of PCM [22,91]. The IL-17 family consists of cytokines that participate in acute and chronic inflammation and provoke the host's defense against microbial organisms [92]. T-helper 17 cells are thought to be a significant source of IL-17A; furthermore, IL-17, producing innate immune cells, activate the fast release of IL-17A [93] in response to pathogens or tissue injury [94].

Table 1. Association of SNPs in *JAK2* with bovine mastitis resistance phenotypic traits.

Gene	Mutation	Reference	Position	Phenotypic Traits	Authors
JAK2	C-T/EXON16	rs210148032	Chr8:39652267	SCC	[51,85]
JAK2	C-T/EXON20	rs110298451	Chr8:39645396	IL-6, IFN-γ, SCC	[51,86]
JAK2	C-T/3′flanking region	rs135128681	Chr8:39630048	IL-6, IFN-γ, SCC	[51,85]
JAK2	T-C/3′flanking region	Novel	Chr8:39631175	IL-6, SCC	[51,85]
JAK2	G-A/3′flanking region	Novel	Chr8:39631044	SCS	[85]
JAK2	5′ upstream	rs379754157	Chr8:39750638	SCC	[49]

IL-17 has been shown to be significantly upregulated in goat milk infected with *E. coli* or *S. aureus* [95]. *IL-17A* production was documented during *S. uberis* mastitis [96], and slightly increased expression was also noticed in the somatic cells of cows infected with *S. aureus* [97]. Furthermore, an in-vitro study illustrated that IL-17A reinforces the ability of mammary epithelial cells (MECs) to resist the consequences produced by *S. aureus* [98]. It has been reported that *IL-17A* and *IL-17F* play a critical role in regulating host–pathogen interactions during the development of mastitis [99]. The SNPs in *IL-17F* and *IL-17A* have been shown to be associated with milk SCCs [90]. Moreover, IL-17 also activates IL-6 with IFN-γ and tumor necrosis factor-alpha (TNF-α) [100]. Usman et al. revealed that

IL-6 is the best indicator of mastitis and can be a target in mastitis control strategies [85]. Altogether, the above-published studies show that IL-17, IL-6, IL-4, IFN-γ, SCS, and SCC are the key indicators of mastitis. The interactions of polymorphisms in *JAK2* with bovine mastitis resistance phenotypic traits (IL-17, IL-6, IL-4, IFN-γ, SCS, and SCC) show that *JAK2* might be considered a useful marker in bovine mastitis resistance strategies.

4.2. Role of STATs in Bovine Mastitis

A variety of cytokines and growth factors activate *STATs*, which are a family of latent transcription factors. During the process of inflammation, *STAT5B* regulates CD4+ T-cells differentiation [101]. STAT1 raised the expression of *SOCS3* and SOCS1 in *S. aureus*-infected mammary epithelial cells [102]. Furthermore, it was reported that upon treatment with JAK inhibitors, the plasma cells in PCM decreased considerably due to the suppression of IL6/STAT/JAK signaling, resulting in the reversion of pathogenesis [91]. Accordingly, it was found that the inflammatory cytokines regulate the JAK-STAT pathway in the mammary gland; in response, the phosphorylation of STAT takes place. The phosphorylated STAT translocates into the nucleus and mediates the production of proinflammatory genes that facilitate mastitis's pathogenesis [78]. It is known that the inflammatory cells are recruited towards the site of infection, in which T-cells, particularly CD4+ cells, are predominantly observed in bovine mastitis [103]. Rivas et al. revealed that *S. aureus*-infected dairy cows showed a remarkable elevation in the level of CD4+ T-cells at the early stage of infection in the mammary gland [104]. Eder's team recently proved that the CD4+T-cell level was higher in dry cows compared to lactating cows. These findings show that a decrease in the level of CD4+ T-cells in lactating dairy might be one of the reasons for susceptibility to infection during this stage [105]. Usman et al. reported a significant association of variant T104010752C in the *CD4* gene with milk SCCs [90]. In the previous study, it was noticed that polymorphisms in *CD4* and *STAT5B* genes are significantly linked with mastitis-resistance phenotypic traits [83]. Furthermore, the polymorphism in *CD4* at locus g.13598C>T showed a significant association with SCS, which is the crucial indicator of mastitis.

The combination geneotype analysis of CD4 g.13598C>T and STAT5b g.31562 T>C is associated with milk SCSs in Chinese Holsteins. Furthermore, it was reported that cows with combination genotypes of CCTT show the highest estimated breeding value (EBV) for SCSs [71]. Another study documented that the silencing of the *CD4* gene through DNA methylation influences the progress of CD4+ T-cells in inflammatory conditions [106]. These findings demonstrate that CD4 protein and CD4+ T-cells play essential roles in host defense during the development of mastitis.

As demonstrated in Table 2, the polymorphism in *STAT5A* (43046497A/C) is associated with IL-6 and also changes the amino acid isoleucine to valine [85]. Similarly, mutation at point 43673888A>G in the *STAT5B* gene was significantly linked to mastitis-resistance phenotypic traits (IL-4 and SCC) [86]. Bochniarz et al. reported the elevated level of IL-6 and decreased level of IL-4 in the milk and serum of cows infected with *S. aureus* [107]. In addition, the polymorphism STAT5A-AvaI was associated with milk SCCs and electrical conductivity (EC) in the milk of mastitic cows [108]. EC in milk is one of the essential indicators of bovine mastitis because of its association with Na and Cl levels, which increase during mastitis. Cai et al. also reported a STAT5A gene through genomewide association studies (GWAS) as a potential candidate marker for bovine mastitis resistance [109]. Based on the above-published findings, we concluded that *STAT5A* and *STAT5B* might be target mastitis-resistance markers in dairy cattle.

Table 2. Association of SNPs in *STAT5A* and *STAT5B* with bovine mastitis resistance phenotypic traits.

Gene	Mutation	Reference	Position	Phenotypic Traits	Authors
STAT5A	A-C/Intron 9	rs109358395	Chr19:43046497	IL-6	[85]
STAT5B	A-G/Intron 4	rs41915686	Chr19:43673888	IL-4, SCC	[86]
STAT5b	T-C/EXON 8		Chr19:31562	SCS	[71]

5. Inhibitors of the JAK-STAT Pathway: Role in Mastitis and Milk Production

The protein inhibitors of activated STAT (PIAS) [110], protein tyrosine phosphatases (PTPs) [111], and cytokine signaling suppressors (SOCSs) [112] are three major classes used by cells to control the JAK-STAT pathway [113]. PIAS proteins are considered important transcriptional coregulators of JAK-STAT signaling because of their significant contribution to the control of gene expression [114]. PIAS proteins restrict the regulation of the JAK-STAT pathway in three ways: (1) by adding a small ubiquitin-like modifier (SUMO) group to STAT and blocking its phosphorylation, (2) by preventing the binding of STAT to DNA [115], and (3) by recruiting histone deacetylase to remove acetyl changes to histones by lowering gene expression [116]. Similarly, PIAS3, a member of the PIAS family, has been identified to inhibit STAT3 signaling after regulation by the cytokine IL-6 [117]. Moreover, PIAS1 could inhibit NF-κB and JAK-STAT activity regulated by cytokine TNF and the LPS endotoxin [110]. PIAS has a major role in cell proliferation [118], cell apoptosis, and the immune response [115]. Protein tyrosine phosphatases (PTPs) are a group of enzymes that remove the phosphate group from the JAK-STAT pathway and prevent the action of signaling [119]. The *STATs* are deactivated by PTPS in both the nucleus and cytoplasm. Src homology phosphatase 2 (SHP-2) is one of the members of PTPs that inactivate STAT5 in the cytoplasm. Similarly, SHP1 prevents the phosphorylation of the JAK-STAT pathway and blocks its further action [120,121]. The general role of JAK-STAT inhibitors has been summarized by recently published reviews in more detail [31,122]. Although the two groups of PTPs and PIAS have essential roles in the regulation of the JAK-STAT pathway, their tasks have not been evaluated in milk production or bovine mastitis to date. Therefore, we have only focused on cytokine signaling suppressors (SOCSs) in our current review.

Some SOCS proteins are triggered by cytokines and pathogenic mediators and, thus, function in a classical negative-feedback loop to impede the transduction of cytokine signals. Consequently, they represent an effective mechanism for the negative regulation of the cytokine-mediated JAK-STAT pathway [123]. The DNA binding of STAT protein regulates the mRNA expression of SOCSs [124]. *SOCS3* can inhibit JAK tyrosine kinase activity directly via its kinase-inhibitory region (KIR), which has been proposed to serve as a pseudosubstrate and is essential for cytokine signal suppression [125]. Undeniably, both a KIR and a KIR-mimetic peptide, classified as the tyrosine kinase inhibitor peptide (TKIP), have been described to inhibit *JAK2*-regulated transcription factor STAT1 phosphorylation [126,127]. The SH2 domain of SOCS can also directly bind to the receptors and prevent the signal from passing to JAK-STAT signaling [128]. Moreover, Kimura et al. revealed that LPS could activate *JAK2* and *STAT5*, which participate in the induction of IL-6, while SOCS1 inhibits this process selectively [129].

The suppression of IL-6 and IFN-γ usually occurs around parturition, which depresses immunity and exposes dairy cattle to mastitis [130]. Normal levels of IL-6 and IFN-γ are necessary for the maintenance of bovine immunity. Moreover, *SOCS3* has been reported to be one of the key inhibitors of IL-6 and IFN-gamma. This evidence shows that *SOCS3* might have a potential role in mastitis development in dairy cattle [131]. Moreover, Fang et al. found that *SOCS3* was significantly upregulated after the mammary gland had been infected with *S. aureus*. The authors further supposed that *SOCS3* could negatively regulate the JAK-STAT pathway, which might be one of the reasons for its critical role in mastitis development [132]. Huang et al. also reported that *SOCS3* is a negative regulator of the JAK-STAT pathway. Furthermore, it was demonstrated that overexpression and inhibition of *SOCS3* brought visible changes in milk protein, which might be due to the action of *SOCS3* on the JAK-STAT pathway [133]. The Huang team further suggested that a low level of *SOCS3* is essential for the regulation of milk synthesis. Similarly, a study reported that *SOCS3* inhibits the induction of Prl and activation of STAT5 [134]. Zahoor et al. found that merTK reduces the inflammatory changes induced by *S. aureus* through *STATs*/SOCS3 signaling [102]. Furthermore, it has been revealed that impaired SOCS1/3 has a crucial role in the susceptibility of mammary epithelial cells to *S. aureus* infections. Additionally, a study reported a polymorphism in SOCS2, which was significantly associated with susceptibility to inflammation of the mammary gland [135]. *SOCS3* also has an inhibitory role in STAT5 regulation, which is one of the strong reasons for their influence on lactational performance in dairy cattle. Further study is highly recommended to find out the specific variants in *SOCS3* that interact with *STAT5* and *JAK2* during mastitis development and milk production in dairy cattle.

6. Conclusions

Altogether, it can be concluded that a delicate equilibrium must be achieved for the effective activation of the JAK/STAT pathway, when the immune system is needed for action against infection, and proper restoration when the infection is diminished. Thus, the JAK-STAT pathway can be considered as a therapeutic option in mastitis control and enhancement of milk production strategies. Furthermore, it is suggested that the interactive mechanism of *SOCS3*, *STATs*, and *JAK2*, *STAT5A*, and *STAT5B* during milk production and mastitis development should be considered in future rodent-knockout research models. It is highly recommended that further polymorphisms in STAT1 and *SOCS3* and their associations with milk production and mastitis resistance traits be found out. Finally, PTPs and PIAS are critical inhibitors of the JAK-STAT pathway, so research on the evaluation of their role in bovine mastitis would be an interesting development.

Author Contributions: Conceptualization, M.Z.K. and Z.C.; writing—original draft preparation, M.Z.K. and A.K.; writing—review and editing, M.Z.K., Y.M., J.G., J.X., J.M., and Z.C. All authors have read and agreed to the published version of the manuscript.

Acknowledgments: We acknowledge the financial support of the National Key Research and Development Program of China (2018YFD0501600). We also acknowledge China Agricultural University, Beijing, China, for providing us an environment of learning. Without this platform, the completion of this work would not have been an easy task.

References

1. Szyda, J.; Mielczarek, M.; Fraęszczak, M.; Minozzi, G.; Williams, J.L.; Wojdak-Maksymiec, K. The genetic background of clinical mastitis in Holstein-Friesian cattle. *Animal* **2019**, *13*, 2156–2163. [CrossRef] [PubMed]
2. Mansor, R.; Mullen, W.; Albalat, A.; Zerefos, P.; Mischak, H.; Barrett, D.C.; Biggs, A.; Eckersall, P.D. A peptidomic approach to biomarker discovery for bovine mastitis. *J. Proteom.* **2013**, *85*, 89–98. [CrossRef] [PubMed]
3. Wang, J.J.; Wei, Z.K.; Zhang, X.; Wang, Y.N.; Fu, Y.H.; Yang, Z.T. Butyrate protects against disruption of the blood-milk barrier and moderates inflammatory responses in a model of mastitis induced by lipopolysaccharide. *Br. J. Pharmacol.* **2017**, *174*, 3811–3822. [CrossRef] [PubMed]
4. Yang, C.; Liu, P.; Wang, S.; Zhao, G.; Zhang, T.; Guo, S.; Jiang, K.F.; Wu, H.C.; Deng, G. Shikonin exerts anti-inflammatory effects in LPS-induced mastitis by inhibiting NF-κB signaling pathway. *Biochem. Biophys. Res. Commun.* **2018**, *505*, 1–6. [CrossRef] [PubMed]
5. Pumipuntu, N.; Kulpeanprasit, S.; Santajit, S.; Tunyong, W.; Kong-ngoen, T.; Hinthong, W.; Indrawattana, N. Screening method for Staphylococcus aureus identification in subclinical bovine mastitis from dairy farms. *Vet. World* **2017**, *10*, 721–726. [CrossRef] [PubMed]
6. Jensen, K.; Günther, J.; Talbot, R.; Petzl, W.; Zerbe, H.; Schuberth, H.J.; Seyfert, H.M.; Glass, E.J. *Escherichia coli*- and *Staphylococcus aureus*-induced mastitis differentially modulate transcriptional responses in neighbouring uninfected bovine mammary gland quarters. *BMC Genom.* **2013**, *14*, 36. [CrossRef]
7. Wang, L.; Yang, F.; Wei, X.J.; Luo, Y.J.; Guo, W.Z.; Zhou, X.Z.; Guo, Z.T. Prevalence and risk factors of subclinical mastitis in lactating cows in Northwest China. *Isr. J. Vet. Med.* **2019**, *74*, 17–22.
8. Seegers, H.; Fourichon, C.; Beaudeau, F. Production effects related to mastitis and mastitis economics in dairy cattle herds. *Vet. Res.* **2003**, *34*, 475–491. [CrossRef] [PubMed]
9. Hamadani, H.; Khan, A.; Banday, M.; Ashraf, I.; Handoo, N.; Shah, A.; Hamadani, A. Bovine Mastitis—A Disease of Serious Concern for Dairy Farmers. *Int. J. Livest. Res.* **2013**, *3*, 42. [CrossRef]

10. Viguier, C.; Arora, S.; Gilmartin, N.; Welbeck, K.; O'Kennedy, R. Mastitis detection: Current trends and future perspectives. Trends Biotechnol. 2009, 27, 486–493. Thompson-Crispi, K.; Atalla, H.; Miglior, F.; Mallard, B.A. Bovine mastitis: Frontiers in immunogenetics. *Front. Immunol.* **2014**, *5*, 1–10.
11. Thompson-Crispi, K.; Atalla, H.; Miglior, F.; Mallard, B.A. Bovine mastitis: Frontiers in immunogenetics. *Front. Immunol.* **2014**, *5*, 1–10. [CrossRef] [PubMed]
12. González, R.N.; Wilson, D.J. Mycoplasmal mastitis in dairy herds. *Vet. Clin. North Am. Food Anim. Pract.* **2003**, *19*, 199–221. [CrossRef]
13. Wellnitz, O.; Bruckmaier, R.M. The innate immune response of the bovine mammary gland to bacterial infection. *Vet. J.* **2012**, *192*, 148–152. [CrossRef] [PubMed]
14. Brenaut, P.; Lefèvre, L.; Rau, A.; Laloë, D.; Pisoni, G.; Moroni, P.; Bevilacqua, C.; Martin, P. Contribution of mammary epithelial cells to the immune response during early stages of a bacterial infection to Staphylococcus aureus. *Vet. Res.* **2014**, *45*. [CrossRef]
15. Segal, S.; Hill, A.V.S. Genetic susceptibility to infectious disease. *Trends Microbiol.* **2003**, *11*, 445–448. [CrossRef]
16. Albiger, B.; Dahlberg, S.; Henriques-Normark, B.; Normark, S. Role of the innate immune system in host defence against bacterial infections: Focus on the Toll-like receptors. *J. Intern. Med.* **2007**, *261*, 511–528. [CrossRef]
17. Bhattarai, D.; Worku, T.; Dad, R.; Rehman, Z.U.; Gong, X.; Zhang, S. Mechanism of pattern recognition receptors (PRRs) and host pathogen interplay in bovine mastitis. *Microb. Pathog.* **2018**, *120*, 64–70. [CrossRef]
18. Brooks, A.J.; Dai, W.; O'Mara, M.L.; Abankwa, D.; Chhabra, Y.; Pelekanos, R.A.; Gardon, O.; Tunny, K.A.; Blucher, K.M.; Morton, C.J.; et al. Mechanism of activation of protein kinase JAK2 by the growth hormone receptor. *Science* **2014**, *344*, 1249783. [CrossRef]
19. Liongue, C.; Ward, A.C. Evolution of the JAK-STAT pathway. *JAKSTAT* **2013**, *2*, e22756. [CrossRef]
20. Liu, X.; Robinson, G.W.; Gouilleux, F.; Groner, B.; Hennighausen, L. Cloning and expression of Stat5 and an additional homologue (Stat5b) involved in prolactin signal transduction in mouse mammary tissue. *Proc. Natl. Acad. Sci. USA* **1995**, *92*, 8831–8835. [CrossRef]
21. Hennighausen, L.; Robinson, W.G. Signaling Pathways in Mammary Gland Development. *Dev. Cell* **2001**, *1*, 467–475. [CrossRef]
22. Furth, P.A.; Nakles, R.E.; Millman, S.; Diaz-Cruz, E.S.; Cabrera, M.C. Signal transducer and activator of transcription 5 as a key signaling pathway in normal mammary gland developmental biology and breast cancer. *Breast Cancer Res.* **2011**, *13*. [CrossRef] [PubMed]
23. Ersahin, T.; Tuncbag, N.; Cetin-Atalay, R. The PI3K/AKT/mTOR interactive pathway. *Mol. Biosyst.* **2015**, *11*, 1946–1954. [CrossRef]
24. Sobolewska, A.; Gajewska, M.; Zarzyńska, J.; Gajkowska, B.; Motyl, T. IGF-I, EGF, and sex steroids regulate autophagy in bovine mammary epithelial cells via the mTOR pathway. *Eur. J. Cell Biol.* **2009**, *88*, 117–130. [CrossRef]
25. Schmidt, J.W.; Wehde, B.L.; Sakamoto, K.; Triplett, A.A.; Anderson, S.M.; Tsichlis, P.N.; Leone, G.; Wagner, K.-U. Stat5 Regulates the Phosphatidylinositol 3-Kinase/Akt1 Pathway during Mammary Gland Development and Tumorigenesis. *Mol. Cell. Biol.* **2014**, *34*, 1363–1377. [CrossRef]
26. Huang, D.W.; Sherman, B.T.; Lempicki, R.A. Systematic and integrative analysis of large gene lists using DAVID bioinformatics resources. *Nat. Protoc.* **2009**, *4*, 44–57. [CrossRef]
27. Vafaizadeh, V.; Klemmt, P.A.B.; Groner, B. Stat5 assumes distinct functions in mammary gland development and mammary tumor formation. *Front. Biosci.* **2012**, *17*, 1232–1250. [CrossRef] [PubMed]
28. Rawlings, J.S.; Rosler, K.M.; Harrison, D.A. The JAK/STAT signaling pathway. *J. Cell Sci.* **2004**, *117*, 1281–1283. [CrossRef]
29. Zhou, G.Y.; Yi, Y.X.; Jin, L.X.; Lin, W.; Fang, P.P.; Lin, X.Z.; Zheng, Y.; Pan, C.W. The protective effect of juglanin on fructose-induced hepatitis by inhibiting inflammation and apoptosis through TLR4 and *JAK2*/STAT3 signaling pathways in fructose-fed rats. *Biomed. Pharmacother.* **2016**, *81*, 318–328. [CrossRef] [PubMed]
30. Zhang, C.; Liu, J.; Yuan, C.; Ji, Q.; Chen, D.; Zhao, H.; Jiang, W.; Ma, K.; Liu, L. *JAK2*/STAT3 is associated with the inflammatory process in periapical granuloma. *Int. J. Clin. Exp. Pathol.* **2019**, *12*, 190–197.
31. Xin, P.; Xu, X.; Deng, C.; Liu, S.; Wang, Y.; Zhou, X.; Ma, H.; Wei, D.; Sun, S. The role of JAK/STAT signaling pathway and its inhibitors in diseases. *Int. Immunopharmacol.* **2020**, *80*, 106210. [CrossRef]

32. Villarino, A.V.; Kanno, Y.; Shea, J.J.O. Mechanism and consequences of JAK/STAT signaling in the immune system. *Nat. Immunol.* **2017**, *18*, 374–384. [CrossRef]
33. Kiu, H.; Nicholson, S.E. Biology and significance of the JAK/STAT signalling pathways. *Growth Factors* **2012**, *30*, 88–106. [CrossRef]
34. Bionaz, M.; Loor, J.J. Gene networks driving bovine mammary protein synthesis during the lactation cycle. *Bioinform. Biol. Insights* **2011**, *5*, 83–98. [CrossRef]
35. Brenaut, P.; Bangera, R.; Bevilacqua, C.; Rebours, E.; Cebo, C.; Martin, P. Validation of RNA isolated from milk fat globules to profile mammary epithelial cell expression during lactation and transcriptional response to a bacterial infection. *J. Dairy Sci.* **2012**, *95*, 6130–6144. [CrossRef]
36. Yamaji, D.; Kang, K.; Robinson, G.W.; Hennighausen, L. Sequential activation of genetic programs in mouse mammary epithelium during pregnancy depends on STAT5A/Bconcentration. *Nucleic Acids Res.* **2013**, *41*, 1622–1636. [CrossRef] [PubMed]
37. Hennighausen, L.; Robinson, G.W.; Wagner, K.U.; Liu, X. Developing a mammary gland is a stat affair. *J. Mammary Gland Biol. Neoplasia* **1997**, *2*, 365–372. [CrossRef]
38. Arun, S.J.; Thomson, P.C.; Sheehy, P.A.; Khatkar, M.S.; Raadsma, H.W.; Williamson, P. Targeted Analysis Reveals an Important Role of JAK-STAT-SOCS Genes for Milk Production Traits in Australian Dairy Cattle. *Front. Genet.* **2015**, *6*, 342. [CrossRef]
39. Briscoe, J.; Guschin, D.; Müller, M. Signal Transduction: Just another signalling pathway. *Curr. Biol.* **1994**, *4*, 1033–1035. [CrossRef]
40. Groner, B.; Gouilleux, F. Prolactin-mediated gene activation in mammary epithelial cells. *Curr. Opin. Genet. Dev.* **1995**, *5*, 587–594. [CrossRef]
41. Sigl, T.; Meyer, H.H.D.; Wiedemann, S. Gene expression analysis of protein synthesis pathways in bovine mammary epithelial cells purified from milk during lactation and short-term restricted feeding. *J. Anim. Physiol. Anim. Nutr.* **2014**, *98*, 84–95. [CrossRef]
42. Tian, Q.; Wang, H.R.; Wang, M.Z.; Wang, C.; Liu, S.M. Lactogenic hormones regulate mammary protein synthesis in bovine mammary epithelial cells via the mTOR and JAK-STAT signal pathways. *Anim. Prod. Sci.* **2016**, *56*, 1803–1809. [CrossRef]
43. Bole-Feysot, C. Prolactin (PRL) and Its Receptor: Actions, Signal Transduction Pathways and Phenotypes Observed in PRL Receptor Knockout Mice. *Endocr. Rev.* **1998**, *19*, 225–268. [CrossRef]
44. Auchtung, T.L.; Rius, A.G.; Kendall, P.E.; McFadden, T.B.; Dahl, G.E. Effects of photoperiod during the dry period on prolactin, prolactin receptor, and milk production of dairy cows. *J. Dairy Sci.* **2005**, *88*, 121–127. [CrossRef]
45. Campo Verde Arboccó, F.; Persia, F.A.; Hapon, M.B.; Jahn, G.A. Hypothyroidism decreases JAK/STAT signaling pathway in lactating rat mammary gland. *Mol. Cell. Endocrinol.* **2017**, *450*, 14–23. [CrossRef]
46. Shillingford, J.M.; Miyoshi, K.; Robinson, G.W.; Grimm, S.L.; Rosen, J.M.; Neubauer, H.; Pfeffer, K.; Hennighausen, L. Jak2 is an essential tyrosine kinase involved in pregnancy-mediated development of mammary secretory epithelium. *Mol. Endocrinol.* **2002**, *16*, 563–570. [CrossRef]
47. Etherton, T.D.; Bauman, D.E. Biology of somatotropin in growth and lactation of domestic animals. *Physiol. Rev.* **1998**, *78*, 745–761. [CrossRef]
48. Liu, X.F.; Li, M.; Li, Q.Z.; Lu, L.M.; Tong, H.L.; Gao, X.J. Stat5a increases lactation of dairy cow mammary gland epithelial cells cultured in vitro. *Vitr. Cell. Dev. Biol. Anim.* **2012**, *48*, 554–561. [CrossRef]
49. Ali, N.; Niaz, S.; Khan, N.U.; Gohar, A.; Khattak, I.; Dong, Y.; Khattak, T.; Ahmad, I.; Wang, Y.; Usman, T. Polymorphisms in JAK2 Gene are Associated with Production Traits and Mastitis Resistance in Dairy Cattle. *Ann. Anim. Sci.* **2019**, *20*, 409–423. [CrossRef]
50. Szewczuk, M. Association of a genetic marker at the bovine Janus kinase 2 locus (*JAK2*/RsaI) with milk production traits of four cattle breeds. *J. Dairy Res.* **2015**, *82*, 287–292. [CrossRef]
51. Khan, M.Z.; Wang, D.; Liu, L.; Usman, T.; Wen, H.; Zhang, R.; Liu, S.; Shi, L.; Mi, S.; Xiao, W.; et al. Significant genetic effects of JAK2 and DGAT1 mutations on milk fat content and mastitis resistance in Holsteins. *J. Dairy Res.* **2019**, *86*, 388–393. [CrossRef] [PubMed]
52. Meredith, B.K.; Kearney, F.J.; Finlay, E.K.; Bradley, D.G.; Fahey, A.G.; Berry, D.P.; Lynn, D.J. Genome-wide associations for milk production and somatic cell score in Holstein-Friesian cattle in Ireland. *BMC Genet.* **2012**, *13*, 21. [CrossRef]

53. Verdier, F.; Rabionet, R.; Gouilleux, F.; Beisenherz-Huss, C.; Varlet, P.; Muller, O.; Mayeux, P.; Lacombe, C.; Gisselbrecht, S.; Chretien, S. A sequence of the CIS gene promoter interacts preferentially with two associated STAT5A dimers: A distinct biochemical difference between STAT5A and STAT5B. *Mol. Cell. Biol.* **1998**, *20*, 389–401. [CrossRef] [PubMed]
54. Bao, B.; Zhang, C.; Fang, X.; Zhang, R.; Gu, C.; Lei, C.; Chen, H. Association between polymorphism in STAT5A gene and milk production traits in chinese holstein cattle. *Anim. Sci. Pap. Rep.* **2010**, *28*, 5–11.
55. Liu, X.; Robinson, G.W.; Wagner, K.U.; Garrett, L.; Wynshaw-Boris, A.; Hennighausen, L. Stat5a is mandatory for adult mammary gland development and lactogenesis. *Genes Dev.* **1997**, *11*, 179–186. [CrossRef]
56. Bionaz, M.; Periasamy, K.; Rodriguez-Zas, S.L.; Everts, R.E.; Lewin, H.A.; Hurley, W.L.; Loor, J.J. Old and new stories: Revelations from functional analysis of the bovine mammary transcriptome during the lactation cycle. *PLoS ONE* **2012**, *7*. [CrossRef]
57. Lacasse, P.; Ollier, S.; Lollivier, V.; Boutinaud, M. New insights into the importance of prolactin in dairy ruminants. *J. Dairy Sci.* **2016**, *99*, 864–874. [CrossRef]
58. Watson, C.J.; Neoh, K. The Stat family of transcription factors have diverse roles in mammary gland development. *Semin. Cell. Dev. Biol.* **2008**, *19*, 401–406. [CrossRef]
59. Teglund, S.; McKay, C.; Schuetz, E.; Van Deursen, J.M.; Stravopodis, D.; Wang, D.; Brown, M.; Bodner, S.; Grosveld, G.; Ihle, J.N. Stat5a and Stat5b proteins have essential and nonessential, or redundant, roles in cytokine responses. *Cell* **1998**, *93*, 841–850. [CrossRef]
60. Dong, B.; Zhao, F.Q. Involvement of the ubiquitous Oct-1 transcription factor in hormonal induction of β-casein gene expression. *Biochem. J.* **2007**, *401*, 57–64. [CrossRef]
61. Ji, M.-R.; Lee, S.I.; Jang, Y.J.; Jeon, M.-H.; Kim, J.S.; Kim, K.W.; Park, J.K.; Yoo, J.G.; Jeon, I.S.; Kwon, D.J.; et al. STAT5 plays a critical role in regulating the 5′-flanking region of the porcine whey acidic protein gene in transgenic mice. *Mol. Reprod. Dev.* **2015**, *82*, 957–966. [CrossRef]
62. Watson, C.J. Stat transcription factors in mammary gland development and tumorigenesis. *J. Mammary Gland Biol. Neoplasia.* **2001**, *6*, 115–127. [CrossRef]
63. Boutinaud, M.; Jammes, H. Growth hormone increases Stat5 and Stat1 expression in lactating goat mammary gland: A specific effect compared to milking frequency. *Domest. Anim. Endocrinol.* **2004**, *27*, 363–378. [CrossRef]
64. Sadeghi, M.; Shahrbabak, M.M.; Mianji, G.R.; Javaremi, A.N. Polymorphism at locus of STAT5A and its association with breeding values of milk production traits in Iranian Holstein bulls. *Livest. Sci.* **2009**, *123*, 97–100. [CrossRef]
65. Selvaggi, M.; Albarella, S.; Dario, C.; Peretti, V.; Ciotola, F. Association of STAT5A Gene Variants with Milk Production Traits in Agerolese Cattle. *Biochem. Genet.* **2017**, *55*, 158–167. [CrossRef] [PubMed]
66. Selvaggi, M.; Dario, C.; Normanno, G.; Celano, G.V.; Dario, M. Genetic polymorphism of STAT5A protein: Relationships with production traits and milk composition in Italian Brown cattle. *J. Dairy Res.* **2009**, *76*, 441–445. [CrossRef]
67. Dario, C.; Selvaggi, M. Study on the STAT5A/AvaI polymorphism in Jersey cows and association with milk production traits. *Mol. Biol. Rep.* **2011**, *38*, 5387–5392. [CrossRef] [PubMed]
68. He, X.; Chu, M.X.; Qiao, L.; He, J.N.; Wang, P.Q.; Feng, T.; Di, R.; Cao, G.L.; Fang, L.; An, Y.F. Polymorphisms of STAT5A gene and their association with milk production traits in Holstein cows. *Mol. Biol. Rep.* **2012**, *39*, 2901–2907. [CrossRef]
69. Schennink, A.; Bovenhuis, H.; Léon-Kloosterziel, K.M.; Van Arendonk, J.A.M.; Visker, M.H.P.W. Effect of polymorphisms in the FASN, OLR1, PPARGC1A, PRL and STAT5A genes on bovine milk-fat composition. *Anim. Genet.* **2009**, *40*, 909–916. [CrossRef]
70. Khatib, H.; Monson, R.L.; Schutzkus, V.; Kohl, D.M.; Rosa, G.J.M.; Rutledge, J.J. Mutations in the STAT5A gene are associated with embryonic survival and milk composition in cattle. *J. Dairy Sci.* **2008**, *91*, 784–793. [CrossRef]
71. He, Y.; Chu, Q.; Ma, P.; Wang, Y.; Zhang, Q.; Sun, D.; Zhang, Y.; Yu, Y.; Zhang, Y. Association of bovine CD4 and STAT5b single nucleotide polymorphisms with somatic cell scores and milk production traits in Chinese Holsteins. *J. Dairy Res.* **2011**, *78*, 242–249. [CrossRef]
72. Li, S.; Rosen, J.M. Nuclear factor I and mammary gland factor (STAT5) play a critical role in regulating rat whey acidic protein gene expression in transgenic mice. *Mol. Cell. Biol.* **1995**, *15*, 2063–2070. [CrossRef]

73. Cobanoglu, O.; Zaitoun, I.; Chang, Y.M.; Shook, G.E.; Khatib, H. Effects of the Signal Transducer and Activator of Transcription 1 (*STAT1*) Gene on Milk Production Traits in Holstein Dairy Cattle. *J. Dairy Sci.* **2006**, *89*, 4433–4437. [CrossRef]
74. Cobanoglu, O.; Zaitoun, I.; Chang, Y.M.; Shook, G.E.; Khatib, H. The Detection of *STAT1* Gene Influencing Milk Related Traits in Turkish Holstein and Jersey Cows. *J. Agric. Sci. Technol. A* **2016**, *6*, 261–269. [CrossRef]
75. Deng, T.X.; Pang, C.Y.; Lu, X.R.; Zhu, P.; Duan, A.Q.; Liang, X.W. Associations between polymorphisms of the STAT1 gene and milk production traits in water buffaloes1. *J. Anim. Sci.* **2016**, *94*, 927–935. [CrossRef]
76. Buitenhuis, B.; Røntved, C.M.; Edwards, S.M.; Ingvartsen, K.L.; Sørensen, P. In depth analysis of genes and pathways of the mammary gland involved in the pathogenesis of bovine *Escherichia coli*-mastitis. *BMC Genom.* **2011**, *12*. [CrossRef]
77. Tiezzi, F.; Parker-Gaddis, K.L.; Cole, J.B.; Clay, J.S.; Maltecca, C. A Genome-Wide Association Study for Clinical Mastitis in First Parity US Holstein Cows Using Single-Step Approach and Genomic Matrix Re-Weighting Procedure. *PLoS ONE* **2015**, *10*, e0114919. [CrossRef] [PubMed]
78. Han, H.S.; Shin, J.S.; Lee, S.B.; Park, J.C.; Lee, K.T. Cirsimarin, a flavone glucoside from the aerial part of Cirsium japonicum var. ussuriense (Regel) Kitam. ex Ohwi, suppresses the JAK/STAT and IRF-3 signaling pathway in LPS-stimulated RAW 264.7 macrophages. *Chem. Biol. Interact.* **2018**, *293*, 38–47. [CrossRef]
79. Li, J.; Yin, P.; Gong, P.; Lv, A.; Zhang, Z.; Liu, F. 8-Methoxypsoralen protects bovine mammary epithelial cells against lipopolysaccharide-induced inflammatory injury via suppressing JAK/STAT and NF-κB pathway. *Microbiol. Immunol.* **2019**, *63*, 427–437. [CrossRef]
80. Lee, S.B.; Lee, W.S.; Shin, J.S.; Jang, D.S.; Lee, K.T. Xanthotoxin suppresses LPS-induced expression of iNOS, COX-2, TNF-α, and IL-6 via AP-1, NF-κB, and JAK-STAT inactivation in RAW 264.7 macrophages. *Int. Immunopharmacol.* **2017**, *49*, 21–29. [CrossRef]
81. Boutet, P.; Boulanger, D.; Gillet, L.; Vanderplasschen, A.; Closset, R.; Bureau, F.; Lekeux, P. Delayed neutrophil apoptosis in bovine subclinical mastitis. *J. Dairy Sci.* **2004**, *87*, 4104–4114. [CrossRef]
82. Moyes, K.M.; Drackley, J.K.; Morin, D.E.; Bionaz, M.; Rodriguez-Zas, S.L.; Everts, R.E.; Lewin, H.A.; Loor, J.J. Gene network and pathway analysis of bovine mammary tissue challenged with Streptococcus uberis reveals induction of cell proliferation and inhibition of PPAR signaling as potential mechanism for the negative relationships between immune response and lipi. *BMC Genom.* **2009**, *10*. [CrossRef]
83. Jiang, L.; Sørensen, P.; Thomsen, B.; Edwards, S.M.; Skarman, A.; Røntved, C.M.; Lund, M.S.; Workman, C.T. Gene prioritization for livestock diseases by data integration. *Physiol. Gen.* **2011**, *44*, 283–330. [CrossRef]
84. Yue, Y.; QiuLing, L.; ZhiHua, J.; JinMing, H.; Lei, Z.; RongLing, L.; JianBin, L.; FangXiong, S.; JiFeng, Z.; ChangFa, W. Three novel single-nucleotide polymorphisms of complement component 4 gene (C4A) in Chinese Holstein cattle and their associations with milk performance traits and CH50. *Vet. Immunol. Immunopathol.* **2012**, *145*, 223–232.
85. Usman, T.; Yu, Y.; Liu, C.; Wang, X.; Zhang, Q.; Wang, Y. Genetic effects of single nucleotide polymorphisms in JAK2 and STAT5A genes on susceptibility of Chinese Holsteins to mastitis. *Mol. Biol. Rep.* **2014**, *41*, 8293–8301. [CrossRef]
86. Usman, T.; Wang, Y.; Liu, C.; Wang, X.; Zhang, Y.; Yu, Y. Association study of single nucleotide polymorphisms in JAK2 and STAT5B genes and their differential mRNA expression with mastitis susceptibility in Chinese Holstein cattle. *Anim. Genet.* **2015**, *46*, 371–380. [CrossRef] [PubMed]
87. Weigel, K.A.; Shook, G.E. Genetic Selection for Mastitis Resistance. *Vet. Clin. N. Am. Food Anim. Pract.* **2018**, *34*, 457–472. [CrossRef]
88. Pilla, R.; Schwarz, D.; König, S.; Piccinini, R. Microscopic differential cell counting to identify inflammatory reactions in dairy cow quarter milk samples. *J. Dairy Sci.* **2012**, *95*, 4410–4420. [CrossRef]
89. Schwarz, D.; Rivas, A.L.; König, S.; Diesterbeck, U.S.; Schlez, K.; Zschöck, M.; Wolter, W.; Czerny, C.P. CD2/CD21 index: A new marker to evaluate udder health in dairy cows. *J. Dairy Sci.* **2013**, *96*, 5106–5119. [CrossRef]
90. Usman, T.; Wang, Y.; Song, M.; Wang, X.; Dong, Y.; Liu, C.; Wang, S.; Zhang, Y.; Xiao, W.; Yu, Y. Novel polymorphisms in bovine CD4 and LAG-3 genes associated with somatic cell counts of clinical mastitis cows. *Genet. Mol. Res.* **2017**, *16*. [CrossRef]
91. Liu, Y.; Zhang, J.; Zhou, Y.H.; Jiang, Y.N.; Zhang, W.; Tang, X.J.; Ren, Y.; Han, S.P.; Liu, P.J.; Xu, J.; et al. IL-6/STAT3 signaling pathway is activated in plasma cell mastitis. *Int. J. Clin. Exp. Pathol.* **2015**, *8*, 12541–12548.

92. Milner, J.D. IL-17 producing cells in host defense and atopy. *Curr. Opin. Immunol.* **2011**, *23*, 784–788. [CrossRef]
93. Cua, D.J.; Tato, C.M. Innate IL-17-producing cells: The sentinels of the immune system. *Nat. Rev. Immunol.* **2010**, *10*, 479–489. [CrossRef]
94. Shibata, K.; Yamada, H.; Hara, H.; Kishihara, K.; Yoshikai, Y. Resident Vδ1 + γδ T Cells Control Early Infiltration of Neutrophils after Escherichia coli Infection via IL-17 Production. *J. Immunol.* **2007**, *178*, 4466–4472. [CrossRef] [PubMed]
95. Jing, X.Q.; Zhao, Y.Q.; Shang, C.C.; Yao, Y.L.; Tian, T.T.; Li, J.; Chen, D.K. Dynamics of cytokines associated with IL-17 producing cells in serum and milk in mastitis of experimental challenging with Staphylococcus aureus and Escherichia coli in dairy goats. *J. Anim. Vet. Adv.* **2012**, *11*, 475–479.
96. Tassi, R.; McNeilly, T.N.; Fitzpatrick, J.L.; Fontaine, M.C.; Reddick, D.; Ramage, C.; Lutton, M.; Schukken, Y.H.; Zadoks, R.N. Strain-specific pathogenicity of putative host-adapted and nonadapted strains of Streptococcus uberis in dairy cattle. *J. Dairy Sci.* **2013**, *96*, 5129–5145. [CrossRef]
97. Tao, W.; Mallard, B. Differentially expressed genes associated with Staphylococcus aureus mastitis of Canadian Holstein cows. *Vet. Immunol. Immunopathol.* **2007**, *120*, 201–211. [CrossRef]
98. Bougarn, S.; Cunha, P.; Gilbert, F.B.; Harmache, A.; Foucras, G.; Rainard, P. Staphylococcal-associated molecular patterns enhance expression of immune defense genes induced by IL-17 in mammary epithelial cells. *Cytokine* **2011**, *56*, 749–759. [CrossRef]
99. Roussel, P.; Cunha, P.; Porcherie, A.; Petzl, W.; Gilbert, F.B.; Riollet, C.; Zerbe, H.; Rainard, P.; Germon, P. Investigating the contribution of IL-17A and IL-17F to the host response during Escherichia coli mastitis. *Vet. Res.* **2015**, *46*. [CrossRef]
100. Ruddy, M.J.; Wong, G.C.; Liu, X.K.; Yamamoto, H.; Kasayama, S.; Kirkwood, K.L.; Gaffen, S.L. Functional Cooperation between Interleukin-17 and Tumor Necrosis Factor-α Is Mediated by CCAAT/Enhancer-binding Protein Family Members. *J. Biol. Chem.* **2004**, *279*, 2559–2567. [CrossRef]
101. Wilson, C.B.; Rowell, E.; Sekimata, M. Epigenetic control of T-helper-cell differentiation. *Nat. Rev. Immunol.* **2009**, *9*, 91–105. [CrossRef]
102. Zahoor, A.; Yang, Y.; Yang, C.; Khan, S.B.; Reix, C.; Anwar, F.; Deng, G. MerTK negatively regulates *Staphylococcus aureus* induced inflammatory response via Toll-like receptor signaling in the mammary gland. *Mol. Immunol.* **2020**, *122*, 1–12. [CrossRef]
103. Mehrzad, J.; Zhao, X. T lymphocyte proliferative capacity and CD4+/CD8+ ratio in primiparous and pluriparous lactating cows. *J. Dairy Res.* **2008**, *75*, 457–465. [CrossRef] [PubMed]
104. Rivas, A.L.; Schwager, S.J.; González, R.N.; Quimby, F.W.; Anderson, K.L. Multifactorial relationships between intramammary invasion by *Staphylococcus aureus* and bovine leukocyte markers. *Can. J. Vet. Res.* **2007**, *71*, 135–144.
105. Eder, J.M.; Gorden, P.J.; Lippolis, J.D.; Reinhardt, T.A.; Sacco, R.E. Lactation stage impacts the glycolytic function of bovine CD4+ T cells during ex vivo activation. *Sci. Rep.* **2020**, *10*. [CrossRef]
106. Wei, G.; Wei, L.; Zhu, J.; Zang, C.; Hu-Li, J.; Yao, Z.; Cui, K.; Kanno, Y.; Roh, T.Y.; Watford, W.T.; et al. Global Mapping of H3K4me3 and H3K27me3 Reveals Specificity and Plasticity in Lineage Fate Determination of Differentiating CD4+ T Cells. *Immunity* **2009**, *30*, 155–167. [CrossRef]
107. Bochniarz, M.; Zdzisińska, B.; Wawron, W.; Szczubiał, M.; Dąbrowski, R. Milk and serum IL-4, IL-6, IL-10, and amyloid A concentrations in cows with subclinical mastitis caused by coagulase-negative *staphylococci*. *J. Dairy Sci.* **2017**, *100*, 9674–9680. [CrossRef]
108. Kiyici, M.J.; Bilal, A.; Mahmut, K.; Korhan, A.; Esma, G.A.; Mehmet, U.C. Association of *GH, STAT5A, MYF5* gene polymorphisms with milk somatic cell count, EC and pH levels of Holstein dairy cattle. *Ani. Biotechnol.* **2020**. [CrossRef]
109. Cai, Z.; Guldbrandtsen, B.; Lund, M.S.; Sahana, G. Prioritizing candidate genes for fertility in dairy cows using gene-based analysis, functional annotation and differential gene expression. *BMC Genom.* **2019**, *20*, 255. [CrossRef]
110. Shuai, K. Regulation of cytokine signaling pathways by PIAS proteins. *Cell Res.* **2006**, *16*, 196–202. [CrossRef]
111. Henenstreit, D.; Horeks-Hoeck, J.; Duschl, A. JAK/STAT-dependent gene regulation by cytokines. *Drug News Perspect.* **2005**, *18*, 243. [CrossRef]
112. Krebs, D.L.; Hilton, D.J. SOCS proteins: Negative regulators of cytokine signaling. *Stem Cells* **2001**, *19*, 378–387. [CrossRef] [PubMed]

113. Niu, G.J.; Xu, J.D.; Yuan, W.J.; Sun, J.J.; Yang, M.C.; He, Z.H.; Zhao, X.F.; Wang, J.X. Protein Inhibitor of Activated STAT (PIAS) Negatively Regulates the JAK/STAT Pathway by Inhibiting STAT Phosphorylation and Translocation. *Front. Immunol.* **2018**, *9*, 2392. [CrossRef]
114. Sharrocks, A.D. PIAS proteins and transcriptional regulation—More than just SUMO E3 ligases? *Genes Dev.* **2006**, *20*, 754–758. [CrossRef]
115. Shuai, K.; Liu, B.; Zhang, D.; Cui, Y.; Zhou, J.; Sheng, C. Regulation of gene-activation pathways by PIAS proteins in the immune system. *Nat. Rev. Immunol.* **2005**, *5*, 593–605. [CrossRef]
116. Ungureanu, D.; Vanhatupa, S.; Grönholm, J.; Palvimo, J.; Silvennoinen, O. SUMO-1 conjugation selectively modulates STAT1-mediated gene responses. *Blood* **2005**, *106*, 224–226. [CrossRef]
117. Chung, C.D.; Liao, J.; Liu, B.; Rao, X.; Jay, P.; Berta, P.; Shuai, K. Specific inhibition of Stat3 signal transduction by PIAS3. *Science* **1997**, *278*, 1803–1805. [CrossRef]
118. Tolkunova, E.; Malashicheva, A.; Parfenov, V.N.; Sustmann, C.; Grosschedl, R.; Tomilin, A. PIAS proteins as repressors of Oct4 function. *J. Mol. Biol.* **2007**, *374*, 1200–1212. [CrossRef]
119. Xu, D.; Qu, C. Protein tyrosine phosphatases in the JAK/STAT pathway. *Front. Biosci.* **2008**, *13*, 4925–4932. [CrossRef] [PubMed]
120. Latanya, S.M.; Harshani, L.R.; Said, S.M.J.; Nicholas, L.J.; Wu, J. Targeting Protein Tyrosine Phosphatases for Anticancer Drug Discovery. *Curr. Pharm. Des.* **2010**, *16*, 1843–1862.
121. Heather, B.; Dechert, U.; Jirik, F.; Schrader, J.W.; Welham, M.J. SHP1 and SHP2 Protein-tyrosine Phosphatases Associate with βc after Interleukin-3-induced Receptor Tyrosine Phosphorylation. *J. Biol. Chem.* **1997**, *272*, 14470–14476.
122. Böhmer, F.; Friedrich, K. Protein tyrosine phosphatases as wardens of STAT signaling. *JAKSTAT* **2014**, *3*, e28087. [CrossRef]
123. Yoshimura, A. Negative regulation of cytokine signaling. *Clin. Rev. Allergy Immunol.* **2005**, *28*, 205–220. [CrossRef]
124. Collins, A.S.; McCoy, C.E.; Lloyd, A.T.; O'Farrelly, C.; Stevenson, N.J. miR-19a: An Effective Regulator of *SOCS3* and Enhancer of JAK-STAT Signalling. *PLoS ONE* **2013**, *8*, e69090. [CrossRef]
125. Kubo, M.; Hanada, T.; Yoshimura, A. Suppressors of cytokine signaling and immunity. *Nat. Immunol.* **2003**, *4*, 1169–1176. [CrossRef]
126. Flowers, L.O.; Johnson, H.M.; Mujtaba, M.G.; Ellis, M.R.; Haider, S.M.I.; Subramaniam, P.S. Characterization of a Peptide Inhibitor of Janus Kinase 2 That Mimics Suppressor of Cytokine Signaling 1 Function. *J. Immunol.* **2004**, *172*, 7510–7518. [CrossRef]
127. Waiboci, L.W.; Ahmed, C.M.; Mujtaba, M.G.; Flowers, L.O.; Martin, J.P.; Haider, M.I.; Johnson, H.M. Both the Suppressor of Cytokine Signaling 1 (SOCS-1) Kinase Inhibitory Region and SOCS-1 Mimetic Bind to JAK2 Autophosphorylation Site: Implications for the Development of a SOCS-1 Antagonist. *J. Immunol.* **2007**, *178*, 5058–5068. [CrossRef]
128. Kershaw, N.J.; Murphy, J.M.; Lucet, I.S.; Nicola, N.A.; Babon, J.J. Regulation of Janus kinases by SOCS proteins. *Biochem. Soc. Trans.* **2013**, *41*, 1042–1047. [CrossRef]
129. Kimura, A.; Tetsuji, N.; Tatsushi, M.; Osamu, T.; Shizuo, A.; Ichiro, K.; Tadamitsu, K. Suppressor of cytokine signaling-1 selectively inhibits LPS-induced IL-6 production by regulating JAK-STAT. *Blood* **2004**, *102*, 17089–17094. [CrossRef]
130. Khan, M.Z.; Zhang, Z.; Liu, L.; Wang, D.; Mi, S.; Liu, X.; Liu, G.; Guo, G.; Li, X.; Wang, Y.; et al. Folic acid supplementation regulates key immunity-associated genes and pathways during the periparturient period in dairy cows. *Asian Australas. J. Anim. Sci.* **2019**, *33*, 1507–1519. [CrossRef]
131. Yasukawa, H.; Ohishi, M.; Mori, H.; Murakami, M.; Chinen, T.; Aki, D.; Hanada, T.; Takeda, K.; Akira, S.; Hoshijima, M.; et al. IL-6 induces an anti-inflammatory response in the absence of *SOCS3* in macrophages. *Nat. Immunol.* **2003**, *4*, 551–556. [CrossRef]
132. Fang, L.; Hou, Y.; An, J.; Li, B.; Song, M.; Wang, X.; Sørensen, P.; Dong, Y.; Liu, C.; Wang, Y.; et al. Genome-wide transcriptional and post-transcriptional regulation of innate immune and defense responses of bovine mammary gland to Staphylococcus aureus. *Front. Cell. Infect. Microbiol.* **2016**, *6*. [CrossRef]
133. Huang, Y.; Zhao, F.; Luo, C.; Zhang, X.; Yu, S.; Sun, Z.; Li, Z.; Li, Q.; Gao, X. SOCS3-Mediated Blockade Reveals Major Contribution of *JAK2*/STAT5 Signaling Pathway to Lactation and Proliferation of Dairy Cow Mammary Epithelial Cells in Vitro. *Molecules* **2013**, *18*, 12987–13002. [CrossRef]

134. Dif, F.; Saunier, E.; Demeneix, B.; Kelly, P.A.; Edery, M. Cytokine-inducible SH2-containing protein suppresses PRL signaling by binding the PRL receptor. *Endocrinology* **2001**, *142*, 5286–5293. [CrossRef]
135. Rupp, R.; Senin, P.; Sarry, J.; Allain, C.; Tasca, C.; Ligat, L. A Point Mutation in Suppressor of Cytokine Signalling 2 (Socs2) Increases the Susceptibility to Inflammation of the Mammary Gland while Associated with Higher Body Weight and Size and Higher Milk Production in a Sheep Model. *PLoS Genet.* **2015**, *11*, e1005629. [CrossRef]

12

Heritability of Teat Condition in Italian Holstein Friesian and its Relationship with Milk Production and Somatic Cell Score

Francesco Tiezzi [1], Antonio Marco Maisano [2], Stefania Chessa [3], Mario Luini [2,4] and Stefano Biffani [4,*]

1 Department of Animal Science, North Carolina State University, Raleigh, NC 27695, USA; f_tiezzi@ncsu.edu
2 Istituto Zooprofilattico Sperimentale Lombardia Emilia Romagna "Bruno Ubertini"—I.Z.S.L.E.R. Territorial Section of Lodi and Brescia Sector Diagnostic, Animal Health and Welfare, 26900 Lodi, Italy; antoniomarco.maisano@izsler.it (A.M.M.); mariovittorio.luini@ibba.cnr.it (M.L.)
3 Dipartimento di Scienze Veterinarie, Università degli Studi di Torino, 10095 Grugliasco, Italy; stefania.chessa@unito.it
4 Consiglio Nazionale delle Ricerche (CNR), Istituto di biologia e biotecnologia agraria (IBBA), Via Edoardo Bassini, 20133 Milano, Italy
* Correspondence: biffani@ibba.cnr.it

Simple Summary: Mammary infections in dairy cattle are still a major problem which impair animal health and jeopardize breeders' efforts to attain sustainable production. The first natural protection against pathogens' access to udder tissue is the teat canal. Teat canal morphology can be influenced by several environmental factors but the present study confirmed the existence of a genetic component. Moreover it was observed that the teat canal morphology is related to milk production and somatic cell count, the latter being an indirect indicator of mammary infections. Considering that the current selection objectives implemented in dairy cattle worldwide have shifted toward a more balanced breeding goal, with a larger emphasis on health traits, a further genetic deterioration in teat condition is not expected.

Abstract: In spite of the impressive advancements observed on both management and genetic factors, udder health still represents one of most demanding objectives to be attained in the dairy cattle industry. Udder morphology and especially teat condition might represent the first physical barrier to pathogens' access. The objectives of this study were to investigate the genetic component of teat condition and to elucidate its relationship with both milk yield and somatic cell scores in dairy cattle. Moreover, the effect of selection for both milk yield and somatic cell scores on teat condition was also investigated. A multivariate analysis was conducted on 10,776 teat score records and 30,160 production records from 2469 Italian Holstein cows. Three teat scoring traits were defined and included in the analysis. Heritability estimates for the teat score traits were moderate to low, ranging from 0.084 to 0.238. When teat score was based on a four-classes ordinal scoring, its genetic correlation with milk yields and somatic cell score were 0.862 and 0.439, respectively. The scale used to classify teat-end score has an impact on the magnitude of the estimates. Genetic correlations suggest that selection for milk yield could deteriorate teat health, unless more emphasis is given to somatic cell scores. Considering that both at national and international level, the current selection objectives are giving more emphasis to health traits, a further genetic deterioration in teat condition is not expected.

Keywords: dairy cattle; teat-end hyperkeratosis; udder health; somatic cell; genetic correlation; selection response

---

1. Introduction

Udder health still represents one of the most demanding objectives to be attained in the dairy cattle sector. In spite of the impressive advancements observed on both management and genetic factors, the diseases of the mammary gland in response to an infection, i.e., a clinical (CM) or a subclinical mastitis (SCM), is one of the most common and expensive diseases faced [1–6]. In 2015 the estimated overall cost per case of clinical mastitis in the first 30 days of lactation was $444 [7]. Moreover, 71% of the costs of a case of clinical mastitis were indirect costs. Among the several factors which can mitigate or increase the occurrence of intramammary infections, udder and teat morphology play a substantial role [8–11]. Indeed, the most relevant pathogens affecting dairy cattle, e.g., *Staphylococcus aureus (S. aureus)* [12] gain access to udder tissues primarily via the teat canal. Teat-end hyperkeratosis (THK), i.e., the hyperplasia of the teat orifice's keratin layer [13], is considered one of the most common teat condition changes observed in dairy cattle [14]. THK is commonly evaluated using an ordinal scale ranging from 1 (no THK) to 4 (severe THK) [15]. Results presented in a recent review show that a condition of severe THK is an important risk factor for both CM and SCM, while a mild THK can mitigate possible SCM [11]. Alterations in teat condition across lactation and parities are expected as a consequence of machine milking [14] but the existence of a genetic component has also been investigated [16,17]. In a first study enrolling 1740 US Holstein cows from nine herds, Chrystal and colleagues [16] found that heritability estimates of teat end shape for first, second, and all lactations combined were 0.53, 0.44, and 0.56, respectively. Teat diameter heritability estimates were 0.23, 0.27, and 0.35, respectively across the three lactations. Teat-end shape and diameter repeatability estimates were 0.75 and 0.36, respectively. In a subsequent study with 1259 cows from a single herd, Chrystal et al [17] found heritability estimates of teat-end shape for first, second, and third and later lactations of 0.34, 0.21, and 0.13, respectively. Repeatability ranged from 0.34 to 0.46.

An additional and widely used phenotypic indicator of udder health is somatic cell count (SCC). After being transformed to somatic cell score (SCS) using a logarithmic transformation [18], it is used as a predictor in the selection for mastitis resistance [3,19]. Some studies [20–27] have investigated the relationship between THK and SCC and most of them reported positive associations, especially when THK is scored as severe. However THK scoring can be confounded with other factors, e.g., parity, and its relationship with SCC might not be clearly identified. Chrystal and colleagues investigated the relationship between teat end shape and SCS in two subsequent studies [16,17]. They used SCS as a dependent variable in a mixed model and included teat end shape as a covariate. In both cases, the effect of teat end shape was not significant. Among the possible explanations the authors hypothesized some genetic factors that would control SCS and prevail over the effect of teat end shape.

The main objectives of this work were to further investigate the genetic component of THK and to elucidate its relationship with both milk yield (MY) and SCS. Moreover, the genetic change in THK when selecting for both MY and SCS was also investigated.

2. Materials and Methods

2.1. Dataset

Animal welfare and use committee approval was not needed for this study as datasets were obtained from pre-existing databases based on routine animal recording procedures. Data used in the present study were collected between September 2011 and August 2012 and between March 2016 and January 2017 in 48 Italian Holstein dairy farms located in the Lombardy region (Northern Italy, 45.4791° N, 9.8452° E). The average herd size was 106 milking cows, ranging from 38 to 285 cows. The original data set included 3087 cows [28].

Teat condition score (TCS) was evaluated visually for each cow during milk sampling and assigned a score using the methodology proposed by Neijenhuis et al. [15]: an absent callosity was evaluated as TCS = 1, a smooth callous ring around the orifice was evaluated as TCS = 2; a rough and very rough callous rings were evaluated as TCS = 3 and 4, respectively. Scores were applied on each single teat, generating four records for each cow scored, each one was assigned to the respective teat position (FL: front left; FR: front right; RL: rear left; RR: rear right). In addition to scoring values, date of scoring and hygiene scoring were obtained. Hygiene of udder, flanks and legs was scored based on a 4-point scale system [29], from very clean (score 1) to very dirty skin (score 4). Both TCS and hygiene score were collected by a group composed of four technicians who were previously trained to harmonize the scoring procedure.

Production records for daily milk yield (MY) and SCC per ml were obtained by the Regional Breeders' Association (ARAL, Crema, Italy). The variable SCC was log-transformed into SCS by using the formula SCS = $\log_2$(SCC/100,000) + 3 [18]. Together with production records, calving dates, herd number and pedigree information were obtained. Using calving date, it was possible to extract the parity order and days in milk at teat scoring and production recording.

Teat scoring was organized in a dataset where the four quarters appeared as repeated information of the same phenotype. Each herd was visited and scored only once although the scoring was conducted over two consecutive days in two of the herds. Teat position information was assigned to each record, so that each cow showed four records with the respective position indicator. Only cows showing all four records were included in the analysis.

Production records from the same cows were retained and were organized as repeated measures on the same individuals. For each cow, only production records from the same lactation number of the scoring were retained. The median number of records per cow was 10, each record reported MY and SCS for that cow in that test-day.

The final dataset was built stacking the teat score and production datasets. Records that showed teat scoring did not show production records, and vice versa.

The final dataset included 10,776 scoring records and 30,160 production records, for a total of 40,936 records available for analyses. All records came from 2649 cows, daughters of 869 sires and 2408 dams, while 275 cows appeared also as dams. All animals were raised in a total of 48 herds.

The choice of building a dataset where test scores and production records were not aligned was dictated by practical modeling decisions. The alignment of the teat score records with the closest production record could have been done. However, the repeated nature of the teat score record would have forced the production record to be repeated four times, which was not appropriate. At the same time, repeated records for both teat scores and production records allowed us to disentangle the additive genetic and permanent environmental effects. By not aligning records, the residual covariance between the teat scores and the production records could not be estimated. Nevertheless, such covariance should be forced to zero, because the phenotypes came from different data capture and recording systems. The cow permanent environmental effect allowed us to estimate a non-genetic covariance between the two sets of traits.

2.2. Statistical Analysis

Three teat scoring traits were defined and included in the analysis. A four-classes ordinal scoring (1, 2, 3, 4) was maintained for the trait hereinafter called TS. In addition, two binary traits were created. Classes 2, 3 and 4 were combined into a single class creating the trait hereinafter called TS_a; classes 1 and 2 vs. 3 and 4 were combined to create trait TS_b. Relative frequencies for all trait classes are reported in Table 1.

A tri-variate threshold-linear model was used for analyzing traits combination such as TS-MY-SCS, TS_a-MY-SCS, TS_b-MY-SCS. Model specifications were:

$$y(\lambda) = \boldsymbol{X}b + \boldsymbol{Z}_h h + \boldsymbol{Z}_p p + \boldsymbol{Z}_s s + e$$

where y is the phenotype vector for MY and SCS, λ is the underlying liability for TS, TS_a or TS_b, $\boldsymbol{X}$ and b are the incidence matrix and vector of solutions for fixed effects, $\boldsymbol{Z}_h$ and h are the incidence matrix and vector of solutions for the herd environmental random effect, $\boldsymbol{Z}_p$ and p are the incidence matrix and vector of solutions for the cow permanent environmental random effect, $\mathbf{Z}_s$ and s are the incidence matrix and vector of solutions for the sire additive genetic random effect, e is the vector of residuals. Fixed effects common to all traits were parity by stage of lactation class (36 classes), defined by pasting the parity class (first, second and later lactations) with the stage of lactation month (last class including records until the 15th month of lactation). Additional fixed effects for TS, TS_a and TS_b were hygiene (4 classes) and teat position (4 classes). The vector of solutions for random effects were assumed to be normally and independently distributed. Specifically for the herd random effect:

$$\begin{bmatrix} h_1 \\ h_2 \\ h_3 \end{bmatrix} \sim N(0, \mathbf{I} \otimes \mathbf{H})$$

where **I** is an identity matrix and **H** is the following variance-covariance matrix:

$$\begin{bmatrix} \sigma^2_{h11} & \sigma_{h12} & \sigma_{h13} \\ \sigma_{h12} & \sigma^2_{h22} & \sigma_{h23} \\ \sigma_{h13} & \sigma_{h23} & \sigma^2_{h33} \end{bmatrix}$$

Similarly, for the cow permanent environmental effect:

$$\begin{bmatrix} p_1 \\ p_2 \\ p_3 \end{bmatrix} \sim N(0, \mathbf{I} \otimes \mathbf{P})$$

where **I** is an identity matrix and **P** is the following variance-covariance matrix:

$$\begin{bmatrix} \sigma^2_{p11} & \sigma_{p12} & \sigma_{p13} \\ \sigma_{p12} & \sigma^2_{p22} & \sigma_{p23} \\ \sigma_{p13} & \sigma_{p23} & \sigma^2_{p33} \end{bmatrix}$$

For the sire additive genetic effect:

$$\begin{bmatrix} s_1 \\ s_2 \\ s_3 \end{bmatrix} \sim N(0, \mathbf{A} \otimes \mathbf{S})$$

where **A** is the numerator relationship matrix constructed on the pedigree and **S** is the following variance-covariance matrix:

$$\begin{bmatrix} \sigma^2_{s11} & \sigma_{s12} & \sigma_{s13} \\ \sigma_{s12} & \sigma^2_{s22} & \sigma_{s23} \\ \sigma_{s13} & \sigma_{s23} & \sigma^2_{s33} \end{bmatrix}$$

and for the residual effect:

$$\begin{bmatrix} e_1 \\ e_2 \\ e_3 \end{bmatrix} \sim N(0, \mathbf{I} \otimes \mathbf{R})$$

where **I** is an identity matrix and **R** is the following variance-covariance matrix:

$$\begin{bmatrix} 1 & 0 & 0 \\ 0 & \sigma^2_{e22} & \sigma_{e23} \\ 0 & \sigma_{e23} & \sigma^2_{e33} \end{bmatrix}$$

Therefore, residual variance for any teat scoring trait was fixed to 1 for identifiability in the threshold liability model and the covariance between the teat scoring and production traits was fixed to 0, due to lack of records showing both traits.

Variance components estimates were obtained using software THRGIBBS1F90 version 3.1 [30]. Solutions for TS_a and TS_b were then obtained using the package 'MCMCglmm' implemented in R version 3.6.1 [31] by fixing the variance components to the estimated values. This package was chosen for easier manipulation of solutions in the R environment. In both cases, a total of 300,000 iterations were run, removing the first 50,000 as burn-in and thinning every 50 iterations. Convergence was assessed by visual inspection of trace plots and Geweke's test conducted using the 'coda' package in R [32].

Table 1. Frequency of observations for each teat score in the dataset (n = 10,776).

Score	Number of Records	Relative Frequency		
		TS [1]	TS_a [1]	TS_b [1]
1	7078	65.7	65.7	90.6
2	2687	24.9		
3	838	7.78	34.3	9.4
4	173	1.61		

[1] TS = teat scoring trait based on a four-classes ordinal scoring (1 = absent callosity, 2 = smooth callous ring, 3 = rough callous ring, 4 = very rough callous ring). TS_a: binary teat scoring trait where classes 2, 3 and 4 were combined into a single class. TS_b: binary teat scoring trait where classes 1 and 2 vs. 3 and 4 were combined.

2.3. Genetic Parameters

Heritability was calculated as:

$$h^2 = \frac{4\sigma_s^2}{\sigma_s^2 + \sigma_p^2 + \sigma_h^2 + \sigma_e^2}$$

Intra-herd heritability was calculated as:

$$h_{IH}^2 = \frac{4\sigma_s^2}{\sigma_s^2 + \sigma_p^2 + \sigma_e^2}$$

Cow repeatability was calculated not considering the genetic effect as a source of cow repeatability, therefore:

$$r^2 = \frac{\sigma_p^2}{\sigma_s^2 + \sigma_p^2 + \sigma_h^2 + \sigma_e^2}$$

Herd repeatability was calculated as:

$$he^2 = \frac{\sigma_h^2}{\sigma_s^2 + \sigma_p^2 + \sigma_h^2 + \sigma_e^2}$$

In all formulas, σ_e^2 was '1' for the teat score traits. Genetics, cow and herd correlations were calculated by dividing the covariance by the product of the standard deviations. Parameters were calculated at every iteration and posterior mean and 95% empirical confidence intervals were used as estimates of their standard error.

Least square means for all effects were calculated on the liability scale at every iteration and transformed to the phenotypic (probability) scale. Posterior mean and 95% empirical confidence intervals were used as estimates and their error. Plots were created using package 'ggplot2' implemented in R [33].

2.4. Genetic Change in Teat Score Traits

Expected selection response on the teat score traits was calculated for economic indices that combined MY and SCS with different values of relative emphasis. One economic index for each of the three teat score traits was built, including three traits (the teat score traits, MY and SCS). Relative emphasis was applied on MY and SCS, starting with 100% emphasis on MY and 0% emphasis on SCS and ending with 0% emphasis on MY and 100% on SCS, with step increases of 1% unit. While MY was given positive emphasis, SCS was given negative emphasis. Following [34–36] the genetic response on the teat score trait was calculated as:

$$r = \frac{\mathrm{w}'\mathrm{g}_{\circ 1}}{\sqrt{\mathrm{w}'\mathbf{G}\mathrm{w}}}$$

where r is the genetic response for the teat score trait (TS, TS_a or TS_b); w is the vector of index weight; **G** is the variance-covariance between the teat score trait, MY and SCS; $g_{\circ 1}$ is the first column of **G**. The genetic response was then expressed in genetic standard deviation units for the respective teat score trait.

3. Results

3.1. Data

Descriptive statistics for the teat score traits are in Table 1. Mean values and SD for daily milk production (MY) and daily linear score (SCS) were 29.73 ± 9.05 for and 3.97 ± 1.99 (not reported in table). The observed phenotypic trend for MY and SCS by parity and month of lactation are in Figures 1 and 2, respectively.

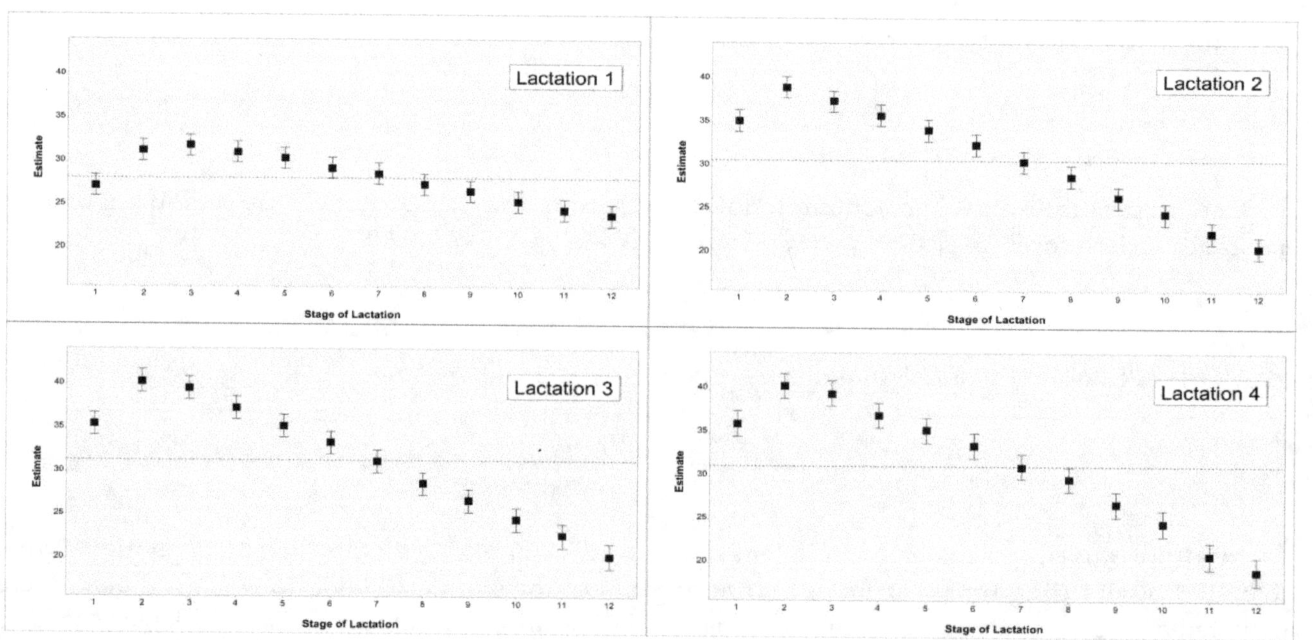

Figure 1. Milk yield across parity and stage of lactation for cows with a teat-score evaluation.

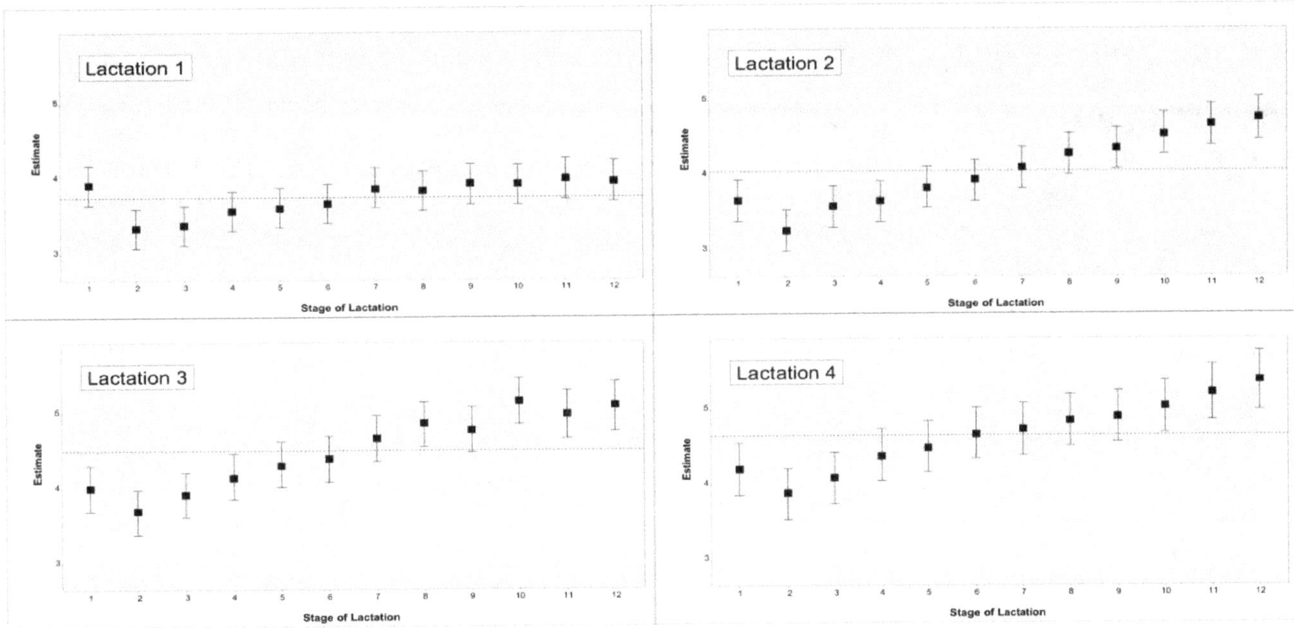

Figure 2. Somatic cell score across parity and stage of lactation for cows with a teat-score evaluation.

3.2. Heritability and Environmental Effects Estimates

Estimates of variance components, heritability, intra-herd heritability, cow repeatability and herd repeatability for all traits are reported in Table 2. Estimates for MY and SCS came from the model where TS was the correlated trait, though posterior distribution estimates for production traits in the other models largely overlapped the values shown.

Table 2. Estimates (posterior mean and 95% highest probability density intervals) of variance components and genetic parameter estimates for the traits considered in this study.

Parameter	Trait				
	TS	TS_a [1]	TS_b [1]	MY [1]	SCS [1]
Sire genetic variance	0.438 (0.233; 0.702)	0.128 (0.072; 0.188)	0.036 (0.010; 0.066)	0.958 (0.450; 1.608)	0.148 (0.084; 0.214)
Cow permanent environmental variance	3.998 (3.465; 4.532)	1.449 (1.324; 1.577)	0.430 (0.371; 0.488)	15.12 (14.05; 16.15)	1.488 (1.398; 1.591)
Herd-test day variance	1.648 (0.902; 2.548)	0.506 (0.288; 0.768)	0.160 (0.078; 0.249)	15.04 (7.85; 23.06)	0.624 (0.292; 0.925)
Residual variance	1.281 (1.217; 1.343)	1.073 (1.051; 1.095)	1.085 (1.060; 1.105)	28.01 (27.57; 28.51)	1.788 (1.758; 1.817)
Heritability (h^2)	0.238 (0.116; 0.364)	0.162 (0.090; 0.235)	0.084 (0.025; 0.155)	0.065 (0.030; 0.109)	0.146 (0.080; 0.210)
Intra-Herd heritability (h^2-IH)	0.289 (0.153; 0.45)	0.248 (0.061; 0.434)	0.250 (0.135; 0.363)	0.126 (0.025; 0.217)	0.234 (0.114; 0.343)
Cow repeatability	0.544 (0.469; 0.603)	0.460 (0.417; 0.503)	0.251 (0.222; 0.282)	0.257 (0.220; 0.290)	0.368 (0.333; 0.401)
Herd-test-day repeatability	0.221 (0.141; 0.313)	0.159 (0.096; 0.224)	0.093 (0.051; 0.141)	0.251 (0.164; 0.353)	0.153 (0.093; 0.224)

[1] TS = teat scoring trait based on a four-classes ordinal scoring (1 = absent callosity, 2 = smooth callous ring, 3 = rough callous ring, 4 = very rough callous ring). TS_a: binary teat scoring trait where classes 2, 3 and 4 were combined into a single class. TS_b: binary teat scoring trait where classes 1 and 2 vs. 3 and 4 were combined. MY = daily milk yield. SCS = daily somatic cell score.

Heritability estimates for the teat score traits were moderate to low, with TS showing the largest value (0.238) followed by TS_a with 0.162 and TS_b with 0.084. A similar but weaker trend was found for the intra-herd heritability, TS showed an estimate of 0.289, TS_a showed 0.248 and TS_b showed 0.250. The weaker trend was due to the herd effect also decreasing from 0.221 for TS to 0.159 for TS_a to 0.093 for TS_b. Cow repeatability (free of genetic variance) was 0.554 for TS, 0.46 for TS_a and 0.251 for TS_b.

Heritability and intra-herd heritability estimates were larger for SCS than MY (0.146 vs. 0.065 and 0.234 vs. 0.126, respectively). Also cow repeatability was stronger for SCS than MY (0.368 vs. 0.257) while herd effect was weaker for SCS than MY (0.153 vs. 0.251, respectively).

3.3. Genetic and Environmental Correlations

Correlations between teat scoring and production traits for all random effects are reported in Table 3. Correlations were considered significant when the 95% empirical confidence intervals did not include the '0' value.

Table 3. Estimates (posterior mean and 95% highest probability density intervals) of genetic correlations between teat score and production traits.

Item	MY [1]			SCS [1]		
	TS [1]	TS_a [1]	TS_b [1]	TS [1]	TS_a [1]	TS_b [1]
Genetic correlation	0.86 (0.71; 0.98)	0.89 (0.61; 0.99)	0.54 (−0.11; 0.96)	0.44 (0.10; 0.80)	0.36 (−0.02; 0.70)	0.38 (−0.09; 0.90)
Cow permanent environmental correlation	0.01 (−0.04; 0.06)	0.02 (−0.03; 0.07)	−0.003 (−0.08; 0.06)	0.14 (0.09; 0.19)	0.12 (0.07; 0.18)	0.15 (0.08; 0.22)
Herd-test day Correlation	0.30 (−0.06; 0.64)	0.30 (−0.03; 0.62)	0.46 (0.13; 0.72)	−0.25 (−0.57; 0.10)	−0.25 (−0.58; 0.08)	−0.47 (−0.76; −0.17)

[1] TS = teat scoring trait based on a four-classes ordinal scoring (1 = absent callosity, 2 = smooth callous ring, 3 rough callous ring, 4 = very rough callous ring). TS_a: binary teat scoring trait where classes 2, 3 and 4 were combined into a single class. TS_b: binary teat scoring trait where classes 1 and 2 vs. 3 and 4 were combined. MY = daily milk yield. SCS = daily somatic cell score.

Genetic correlations for TS and TS_a with MY were positive and significant, showing values of 0.862 and 0.893, respectively. The correlation between MY and TS_b was not significant. Only the genetic correlation between TS and SCS was significant showing a value of 0.439.

None of the cow permanent environmental correlations of teat scoring traits with MY were significant. All correlations with SCS were significant and positive but weak, showing values of 0.141, 0.125 and 0.152 for TS, TS_a and TS_b.

For the herd environmental correlations, the only significant estimate was found between TS_b and MY with a value of 0.463. However, for all estimates the tendency was for a positive relationship between teat scoring traits and MY and a negative relationship with SCS.

3.4. Influence of Fixed Effects on Teat Scores

Least square mean estimates for the hygiene score are reported in Table 4 while estimates for the teat position effect are reported in Table 5. Estimates are expressed on the phenotypic scale (probability of a TS greater than 1 for TS_a or TS greater than 2 for TS_b).

The hygiene effect did not appear to be relevant for any traits, since the posterior distributions of the estimates overlapped.

A relationship was observed among teat positions and TS_a. Indeed front quarters showed a higher probability of a TS greater than 1 or TS greater than 2. The same pattern was found for TS_b, with probabilities for front left and front right quarters at 0.095 and probabilities for rear left and rear right quarters at 0.094. While the front-back contrast could not be declared significant at the chosen α threshold of 0.05, the trend appeared evident.

Table 4. Least square mean estimates (posterior mean and 95% highest probability density intervals) for the influence of Hygiene score on TS_a and TS_b traits. Estimates are expressed on the phenotypic scale (probability of a TS greater than 1 for TS_a or TS greater than 2 for TS_b).

Trait	Hygiene Score [2]			
	1	2	3	4
TS_a [1]	0.326 (0.285; 0.375)	0.364 (0.314; 0.423)	0.382 (0.309; 0.451)	0.317 (0.248; 0.397)
TS_b [1]	0.093 (0.092; 0.094)	0.094 (0.094; 0.094)	0.094 (0.094; 0.096)	0.095 (0.094; 0.097)

[1] TS_a: binary teat scoring trait where TS classes 2, 3 and 4 were combined into a single class. TS_b: binary teat scoring trait where TS classes 1 and 2 vs. 3 and 4 were combined. [2] Hygiene of udder, flanks and legs was scored based on a 4-point scale system, from very clean (score 1) to very dirty skin (score 4).

Table 5. Least square mean estimates (posterior mean and 95% highest probability density intervals) for the influence of udder quarter on on TS_a and TS_b traits. Estimates are expressed on the phenotypic scale (probability of a TS greater than 1 for TS_a or TS greater than 2 for TS_b).

Trait	Udder Quarters			
	Front Left	Front Right	Rear Left	Rear Right
TS_a [1]	0.393 (0.327; 0.462)	0.388 (0.323; 0.455)	0.302 (0.265; 0.34)	0.312 (0.271; 0.356)
TS_b [1]	0.095 (0.093; 0.097)	0.095 (0.093; 0.097)	0.094 (0.092; 0.096)	0.094 (0.092; 0.096)

[1] TS_a: binary teat scoring trait where TS classes 2, 3 and 4 were combined into a single class. TS_b: binary teat scoring trait where TS classes 1 and 2 vs. 3 and 4 were combined.

Least square mean estimates expressed on the phenotypic scale (i.e., probability) for each parity by month of lactation effect are in Figure 3. Results for TS_a are in the upper part while results for TS_b in the lower part of the figure.

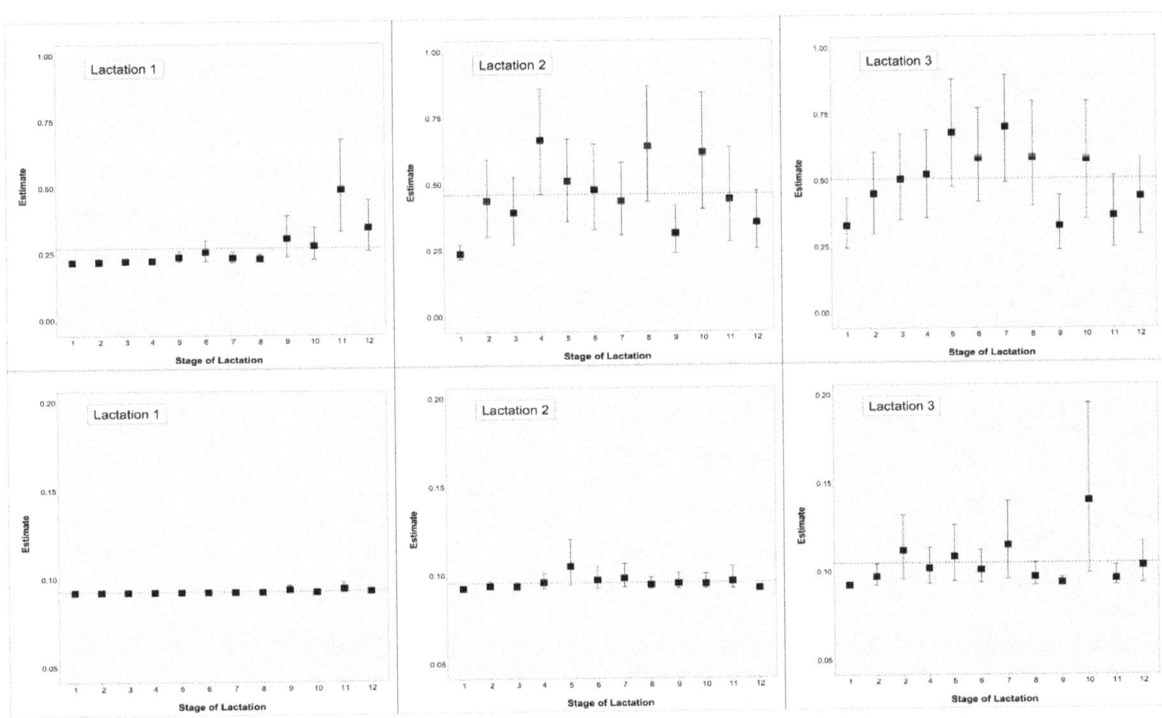

Figure 3. Least square mean estimates expressed on the phenotypic scale (posterior mean and 95% highest probability density intervals) for the lactation by stage of lactation effect on TS_a (upper figures) and TS_b (lower figures) traits. The dashed horizontal line represents the estimate for that lactation across stages.

Estimates for TS_a in lactation 1 showed an increase in the higher scores towards the end of lactation with estimates going from below 0.25 to 0.30. Values similar to the end of lactation 1 were maintained in lactation 2 and subsequently, suggesting that the deterioration of teats is carried over (it is worth considering that this is a cross-sectional study, and not a longitudinal study). Estimates within lactations 2 and subsequently did not show as clear a pattern, though a small increase was shown until the peak of lactation. Lactation estimates across stages for TS_a increased from 0.28 to 0.47 to 0.51 in lactation 1, 2 and 3, respectively. Similarly, lactation estimates across stages for TS_b increased from 0.094 to 0.097 to 0.106 for lactation 1, 2 and subsequently. Conversely, estimates within-lactation for TS_b did not show relevant differences.

3.5. Genetic Response in Teat Score Traits

The genetic response in teat score traits (TS, TS_a and TS_b) after selecting for both MY and SCS applying different relative emphasis is reported in Figure 4. The x-axis gives, from left to right, the relative emphasis as shifting from MY to SCS, the y-axis gives the genetic response in genetic standard deviation units for the respective trait given the overall relative emphasis. The values on the left side of the graph show the response when low emphasis is given to MY, which is positively (unfavorably) correlated with the three traits, and high emphasis is given to SCS, which is still positively correlated but it was given negative emphasis.

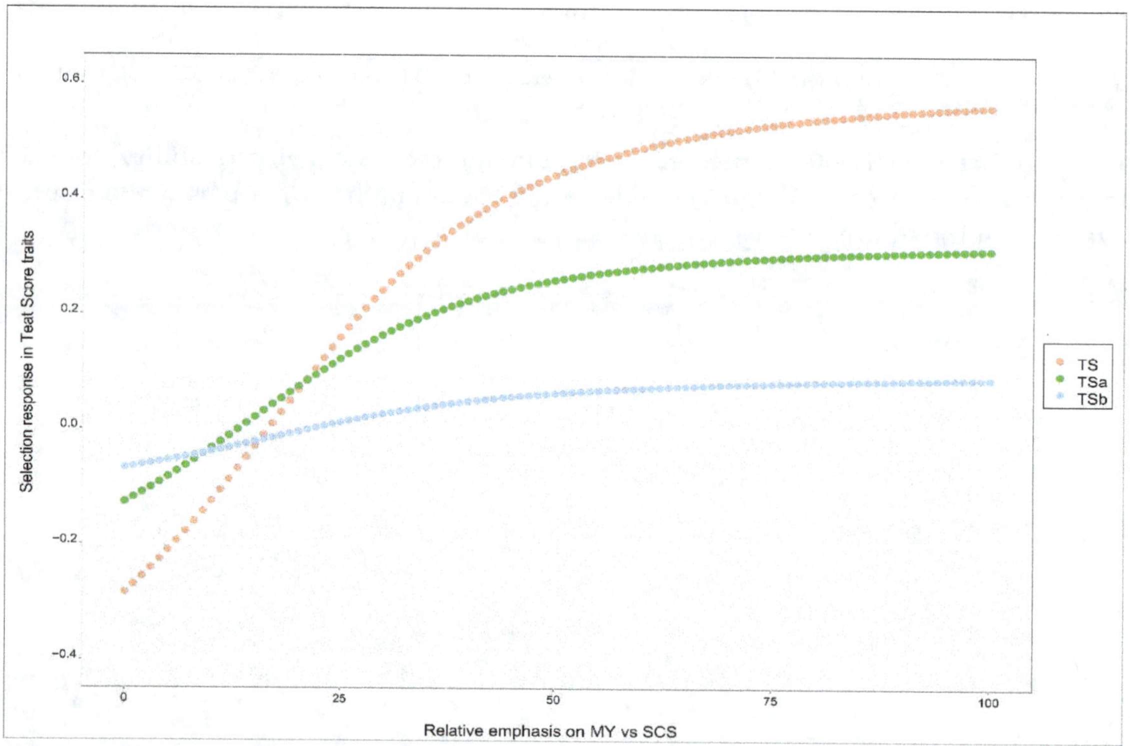

Figure 4. Expected genetic progress in Teat Score traits (y-axis) when shifting relative economic emphasis (x-axis) on milk yield (MY) vs. somatic cell score (SCS). Negative values mean an improvement in teat score (less teat-end hyperkeratosis).

When the emphasis on MY was below 12 (and subsequently the emphasis on SCS was over −88) genetic response for all three teat score traits was negative, i.e., teat score improved. The response for TS became positive at the value of MY emphasis of 17 (i.e., −83 for SCS), became positive for TS_a at the MY emphasis value of 14 (i.e., −86 for SCS) and at the value of 22 for TS_b (i.e., −78 for SCS). All the response curves reached a plateau around the value of 40 for emphasis on MY. At large values of MY emphasis, genetic response became strong and positive (unfavorable) for TS (0.56 genetic standard deviation units), moderately positive for TS_a (0.32 genetic standard deviation units) and almost null for TS_b (0.09 units). The genetic response was therefore mostly unfavorable for all traits unless most of the emphasis was given to SCS (at least 90%). While genetic correlations with other productive and reproductive traits are missing, we could infer that strong index emphasis should be given to udder health if the deterioration of teat score at the genetic level needs to be avoided. The response was stronger, in either direction, for TS than TS_a, probably due to the larger heritability since the genetic correlations with MY and SCS were about the same for both traits. The response was small to null for TS_b.

4. Discussion

The results of the present study confirm that THK has a genetic component. Indeed, heritability ranged from 0.084 for TS_b (binary trait) to 0.238 for TS (scored using a 1 to 4 scale). These results agree well with the estimates previously reported by Chrystal et al. [17] but are lower than those presented by Lojda et al. [37], Seykora and McDaniel [38], and Chrystal et al. [16]. An interesting aspect regards the scale used to score THK which might influence heritability estimates. Pantoja et al [11], in their systematic review of the association between THK and mastitis, support the idea that THK should be scored using a reduced number of categories. This approach will guarantee an adequate number of records per THK score, hence a better statistical power. However reducing the number of THK scores will partly jeopardize its actual variation and, as [17] suggested, possibly lead to lower heritability estimates. In the present study, the relative frequency of a TS = 4 (i.e., very rough callous ring) was below 2%, lower than that reported by Pantoja et al [11]. However, the 95% highest probability density intervals of the posterior mean heritability estimate for TS trait ranged from 0.116 to 0.364, suggesting that a 4-point scale is still a viable solution. A similar pattern was observed for cow repeatability, with larger estimates when THK was scored on a 4-point scale. This result is quite interesting because it suggests that reducing the scale and treating the THK as a binary trait could be a less accurate measure if recorded only once per cow.

Parity and DIM strongly affect THK [11] and the results found in the present study, even if modulated by the scoring scale, confirm this finding.

The relationship between THK and other breeding goals (e.g., milk yields and somatic cell score) has been mainly investigated considering the former as the dependent variable (Y) and the latter as possible factors affecting Y. The relationship, especially with SCS, was not always clear and significant [11,16,17]. In the present study a different approach has been applied. Indeed, previous studies, not only in dairy cattle [3] but also in other dairy species [39], have suggested a non-zero genetic correlation between udder traits and milk and/or SCS. This aspect is not negligible and should be taken into consideration when implementing a selection index. If the genetic correlation is statistically different from zero there could have been a correlated favorable or unfavorable response on THK. This is particularly true if we consider that selection on milk yield has been the primary objective in dairy cattle for many years [40]. The genetic correlation between THK and milk yield was large and positive, i.e., unfavorable, confirming previous findings [41] in dairy cattle. However, a recent and large study by Tribout [42] in dairy cattle did not confirm the existence of a single quantitative trait locus (QTL) with pleiotropic effect on both milk production and udder morphology suggesting instead the presence of neighboring QTLs that show linkage disequilibrium, eventually leading to a non-null genetic correlation. When using THK scored on 1–4 scale, the genetic correlation was positive and significant (95% empirical confidence intervals not including the '0' value). A positive genetic correlation means that an increase in SCS causes an increase in THK hence selection for lower **SCS** should have a positive impact on teat-end condition. When the relative emphasis on milk yield is below 15%, the response in teat score traits is favorable. Nowadays the focus of selection has moved away from being purely production oriented toward a more balanced breeding goal, even if milk yield has still a relative emphasis not less than 40–50% [40].

In this study we also estimated cow-level correlations as well as herd-test-day correlations. While the former expresses trait associations that are driven by any cow-related factor other than additive genetics, the latter expresses an association at the herd-level, which is likely due to management alone. In management, we include any strategic choice made by the farmer as well as the equipment used for milking, which is known to affect the insurgence of THK.

Cow correlations were not significant when MY was the correlated trait, but were positive, though weak, when SCS was the correlated trait. This suggests that, beyond genetics, there is a common factor that drives SCS to increase and THK to appear more frequently. At the herd level, correlations were not significant when TS and TS_a were the correlated traits. TS_b was positively correlated with MY and negatively correlated with SCS. This suggest that herd management (and equipment) that leads to higher MY also leads to higher THK. Also, the herd management that leads to lower SCS also leads to higher THK (moving from classes 1 and 2 to classes 3 and 4, specifically).

The different direction of the correlation between TS_b and SCS depending on the additive genetic, cow permanent or herd level suggests that there are counter-acting factors. While cows themselves could show a positive association for which higher SCS means higher THK, the herd management (and equipment) shows the opposite direction, i.e., herds with lower SCS have higher THK and vice versa. The milking practice, for example, could be a factor determining this association.

5. Conclusions

In the current study, multivariate analysis conducted on 10,776 scoring records and 30,160 production records from 2469 Italian Holstein cows enabled the estimation of the genetic parameters for teat-end score and its relationship with milk yields and SCS. Teat-end score has a genetic background and is genetically related to both production and SCS. The scale used to classify teat-end score has an impact on the magnitude of the estimates which however were always statistically different from zero. Teat-end score was also genetically related to SCS, reinforcing the idea that udder morphology is still a fundamental piece in the control of mammary infection. Finally, an unfavorable genetic correlation of teat score with milk yield was observed. However, considering that the current selection objectives implemented in dairy cattle worldwide have shifted toward a more balanced breeding goal a further genetic deterioration in teat-score is not expected. The importance of the negative effects of some environmental aspects, such as milking routine, should not be forgotten.

Author Contributions: Conceptualization, F.T. and S.B.; methodology, F.T. and S.B.; software, F.T. and S.B.; investigation, S.B. and S.C.; resources, S.B.; data curation, A.M.M. and M.L.; writing—original draft preparation, F.T. and S.B.; writing—review and editing, F.T., S.B., S.C., A.M.M. and M.L.; supervision, S.B.; funding acquisition, F.T. and S.B. All authors have read and agreed to the published version of the manuscript.

Acknowledgments: Data were provided by the Lombardy Region: Project N. 1745–MASTFIELD "Applicazione di sistemi molecolari innovativi per il controllo in campo delle mastiti bovine." The authors thank the agronomists and veterinarians involved in the project for their important contributions in sampling milk and recording management scores: Lucio Zanini, Rosangela Garlappi, Carla Cattaneo, Giorgio Oldani (ARAL, Associazione Regionale Allevatori Lombardia, Italy).

References

1. Bobbo, T.; Penasa, M.; Finocchiaro, R.; Visentin, G.; Cassandro, M. Alternative somatic cell count traits exploitable in genetic selection for mastitis resistance in Italian Holsteins. *J. Dairy Sci.* **2018**, *101*, 10001–10010. [CrossRef]
2. Santman-Berends, I.M.G.A.; Swinkels, J.M.; Lam, T.J.G.M.; Keurentjes, J.; van Schaik, G. Evaluation of udder health parameters and risk factors for clinical mastitis in Dutch dairy herds in the context of a restricted antimicrobial usage policy. *J. Dairy Sci.* **2016**, *99*, 2930–2939. [CrossRef]
3. Martin, P.; Barkema, H.W.; Brito, L.F.; Narayana, S.G.; Miglior, F. Symposium review: Novel strategies to genetically improve mastitis resistance in dairy cattle. *J. Dairy Sci.* **2018**, *101*, 2724–2736. [CrossRef]
4. Weigel, K.A.; Shook, G.E. Genetic Selection for Mastitis Resistance. *Vet. Clin. N. Am. Food Anim. Pract.* **2018**, *34*, 457–472. [CrossRef]
5. Zhao, X.; Ponchon, B.; Lanctôt, S.; Lacasse, P. Invited review: Accelerating mammary gland involution after drying-off in dairy cattle. *J. Dairy Sci.* **2019**, *102*, 6701–6717. [CrossRef]

6. Dufour, S.; Fréchette, A.; Barkema, H.W.; Mussell, A.; Scholl, D.T. Invited review: Effect of udder health management practices on herd somatic cell count. *J. Dairy Sci.* **2011**, *94*, 563–579. [CrossRef]
7. Rollin, E.; Dhuyvetter, K.C.; Overton, M.W. The cost of clinical mastitis in the first 30 days of lactation: An economic modeling tool. *Prev. Vet. Med.* **2015**, *122*, 257–264. [CrossRef]
8. Seykora, A.J.; McDaniel, B.T. Udder and teat morphology related to mastitis resistance: A review. *J. Dairy Sci.* **1985**, *68*, 2087–2093. [CrossRef]
9. Neijenhuis, F.; Barkema, H.W.; Hogeveen, H.; Noordhuizen, J.P. Relationship between teat-end callosity and occurrence of clinical mastitis. *J. Dairy Sci.* **2001**, *12*, 2664–2672. [CrossRef]
10. Mein, G.A. The role of the milking machine in mastitis control. *Vet. Clin. N. Am. Food Anim. Pract.* **2012**, *28*, 307–320. [CrossRef]
11. Pantoja, J.C.F.; Correia, L.B.N.; Rossi, R.S.; Latosinski, G.S. Association between teat-end hyperkeratosis and mastitis in dairy cows: A systematic review. *J. Dairy Sci.* **2020**, *103*, 1843–1855. [CrossRef]
12. Magro, G.; Biffani, S.; Minozzi, G.; Ehricht, R.; Monecke, S.; Luini, M.; Piccinini, R. Virulence Genes of *S. aureus* from Dairy Cow Mastitis and Contagiousness Risk. *Toxins* **2017**, *9*, 195. [CrossRef]
13. Blowey, R.W.; Weaver, A.D. Chapter 11—Udder and teat disorders. In *Color Atlas of Diseases and Disorders of Cattle*, 3nd ed.; Blowey, R.W., Weaver, A.D., Eds.; Mosby Elsevier: New York, NY, USA, 2011; Volume 3, pp. 203–219.
14. Odorčić, M.; Rasmussen, M.D.; Paulrud, C.O.; Bruckmaier, R.M. Review: Milking machine settings, teat condition and milking efficiency in dairy cows. *Animal* **2019**, *13*, 94–99. [CrossRef]
15. Neijenhuis, F.; Barkema, H.W.; Hogeveen, H.; Noordhuizen, J.P. Classification and longitudinal examination of callused teat ends in dairy cows. *J. Dairy Sci.* **2000**, *3*, 2795–2804. [CrossRef]
16. Chrystal, M.A.; Seykora, A.J.; Hansen, L.B. Heritabilities of teat end shape and teat diameter and their relationships with somatic cell score. *J. Dairy Sci.* **1999**, *82*, 2017–2022. [CrossRef]
17. Chrystal, M.A.; Seykora, A.J.; Hansen, L.B.; Freeman, A.E.; Kelley, D.H.; Healey, M.H. Heritability of teat-end shape and the relationship of teat-end shape with somatic cell score for an experimental herd of cows. *J. Dairy Sci.* **2001**, *84*, 2549–2554. [CrossRef]
18. Ali, A.K.A.; Shook, G.E. An optimum transformation for somatic cell concentration in milk. *J. Dairy Sci.* **1980**, *63*, 487–490. [CrossRef]
19. Parker Gaddis, K.L.; VanRaden, P.M.; Cole, J.B.; Norman, H.D.; Nicolazzi, E.; Dürr, J.W. Symposium review: Development, implementation, and perspectives of health evaluations in the United States. *J. Dairy Sci.* **2020**, *103*, 5354–5365. [CrossRef]
20. Gleeson, D.; Meaney, W.; O'Callaghan, E. Effect of teat hyperkeratosis on somatic cell counts of dairy cows. *Int. J. Appl. Res. Vet.* **2004**, *2*, 115–122.
21. Bhutto, A.L.; Murray, R.D.; Woldehiwet, Z. Udder shape and teat-end lesions as potential risk factors for high somatic cell counts and intra-mammary infections in dairy cows. *Vet. J.* **2010**, *183*, 63–67. [CrossRef]
22. Haghkhah, M.; Ahmadi, M.R.; Gheisari, H.R.; Kadivar, A. Preliminary bacterial study on subclinical mastitis and teat condition in dairy herds around Shiraz. *Turk. J. Vet. Anim. Sci.* **2011**, *35*, 387–394. [CrossRef]
23. de Pinho Manzi, M.; Nobrega, D.B.; Faccioli, P.Y.; Troncarelli, M.Z.; Menozzi, B.D. Langoni. Relationship between teat-end condition, udder cleanliness and bovine subclinical mastitis. *Res. Vet. Sci.* **2012**, *93*, 430–434. [CrossRef]
24. Mitev, J.E.; Gergovska, I.; Miteva, T.M. Effect of teat end hyperkeratosis on milk somatic cell counts in Bulgarian black-andwhite dairy cattle. *Bulg. J. Agric. Sci.* **2012**, *18*, 451–454.
25. Sandrucci, A.; Bava, L.; Zucali, M.; Tamburini, A. Management factors and cow traits influencing milk somatic cell counts and teat hyperkeratosis during different seasons. *Rev. Bras. Zootec.* **2014**, *43*, 505–511. [CrossRef]
26. Asadpour, R.; Bagherniaee, H.; Houshmandzad, M.; Fatehi, H.; Rafat, A.; Nofouzi, K.; Maftouni, K. Relationship between teat end hyperkeratosis with intra mammary infection and somatic cell counts in lactating dairy cattle. *Rev. Med. Vet.* **2015**, *166*, 266–270.
27. Guarin, J.F.; Paixao, M.G.; Ruegg, P.L. Association of anatomical characteristics of teats with quarter-level somatic cell count. *J. Dairy Sci.* **2017**, *100*, 643–652. [CrossRef]
28. Cremonesi, P.; Pozzi, F.; Raschetti, M.; Bignoli, G.; Capra, E.; Graber, H.U.; Vezzoli, F.; Piccinini, R.; Bertasi, B.; Biffani, S.; et al. Genomic characteristics of Staphylococcus aureus strains associated with high within-herd prevalence of intramammary infections in dairy cows. *J Dairy Sci.* **2015**, *10*, 6828–6838. [CrossRef]

29. Schreiner, D.A.; Ruegg, P.L. Relationship between udder and leg hygiene scores and subclinical mastitis. *J. Dairy Sci.* **2003**, *86*, 3460–3465. [CrossRef]
30. Tsuruta, S.; Misztal, I. THRGIBBS1F90 for estimation of variance components with threshold linear models. In Proceedings of the 8th World Congress on Genetics Applied to Livestock Production, Belo Horizonte, Minas Gerais, Brazil, 13–18 August 2006; pp. 27–31.
31. Hadfield, J.D. MCMC Methods for Multi-Response Generalized Linear Mixed Models: The MCMCglmm R Package. *J. Stat. Softw.* **2010**, *33*, 1–22. [CrossRef]
32. Plummer, M.; Best, N.; Cowles, K.; Vines, K. CODA: Convergence Diagnosis and Output Analysis for MCMC. *R News* **2006**, *6*, 7–11.
33. Wickham, H. *Ggplot2: Elegant Graphics for Data Analysis*; Springer: New York, NY, USA, 2016.
34. Cameron, N.D. *Selection Indices and Prediction of Genetic Merit in Animal Breeding*; CAB International: Wallingford, UK, 1997.
35. Schneeberger, M.; Barwick, S.A.; Crow, G.H.; Hammond, K. Economic indices using breeding values predicted by BLUP. *J. Anim. Breed. Genet.* **1992**, *109*, 180–187. [CrossRef]
36. Pretto, D.; López-Villalobos, N.; Penasa, M.; Cassandro, M. Genetic response for milk production traits, somatic cell score, acidity and coagulation properties in Italian Holstein–Friesian population under current and alternative selection indices and breeding objectives. *Livestock Sci.* **2012**, *150*, 59–66. [CrossRef]
37. Lojda, L.; Stavikova, M.; Matouskova, O. The shape of the teat and teat-end and the location of the teat canal orifice in relation to subclinical mastitis in cattle. *Acta Vet. Brno* **1976**, *45*, 181–185.
38. Seykora, A.J.; McDaniel, B.T. Heritabilities of Teat Traits and their Relationships with Milk Yield, Somatic Cell Count, and Percent Two-Minute Milk. *J. Dairy Sci.* **1985**, *68*, 2670–2683. [CrossRef]
39. Biffani, S.; Tiezzi, F.; Fresi, P.; Stella, A. Giulietta Minozzi, Genetic parameters of weeping teats in Italian Saanen and Alpine dairy goats and their relationship with milk production and somatic cell score. *J. Dairy Sci.* **2020**, *103*, 9167–9176. [CrossRef]
40. Miglior, F.; Fleming, A.; Malchiodi, F.; Brito, L.F.; Martin, P.; Baes, C.F. A 100-Year Review: Identification and genetic selection of economically important traits in dairy cattle. *J. Dairy Sci.* **2017**, *100*, 10251–10271. [CrossRef]
41. Rupp, R.; Boichard, D. Genetic parameters for clinical mastitis, somatic cell score, production, udder type traits, and milking ease in first lactation Holsteins. *J. Dairy Sci.* **1999**, *82*, 2198–2204. [CrossRef]
42. Tribout, T.; Croiseau, P.; Lefebvre, R.; Barbat, A.; Boussaha, M.; Fritz, S.; Boichard, D.; Hoze, C.; Sanchez, M.P. Confirmed effects of candidate variants for milk production, udder health, and udder morphology in dairy cattle. *Genet. Sel. Evol.* **2020**, *52*, 55–67. [CrossRef]

13

Genome-Wide DNA Methylation Changes of Perirenal Adipose Tissue in Rabbits Fed a High-Fat Diet

Jiahao Shao [1,†], Xue Bai [1,†], Ting Pan [2], Yanhong Li [1], Xianbo Jia [1], Jie Wang [1] and Songjia Lai [1,*]

1 College of Animal Science and Technology, Sichuan Agricultural University, Chengdu 611130, China; shaojh1997@163.com (J.S.); baixue333work@163.com (X.B.); lyh81236718@163.com (Y.L.); jaxb369@sicau.edu.cn (X.J.); wjie68@163.com (J.W.)
2 College of Veterinary Medicine, Sichuan Agricultural University, Chengdu 611130, China; panting555666@163.com
* Correspondence: laisj5794@163.com
† These authors contributed equally to this work.

Simple Summary: Obesity is spreading rapidly in most countries and regions, becoming a considerable public health concern because it is associated with type II diabetes mellitus, fatty liver disease, hypertension, and even certain cancers. The biological effects of caloric restriction are closely related to epigenetic mechanisms, including DNA methylation. Here, rabbits were used as a model to study the effect of a high-fat diet on the DNA methylation profile of perirenal adipose tissue. The results indicate that 2906 genes associated with differentially methylated regions were obtained and were involved in the PI3K-AKT signaling pathway (KO04151), linoleic acid metabolism (KO00591), DNA replication (KO03030), and MAPK signaling pathway (KO04010). In conclusion, high-fat diet may cause changes in the DNA methylation profile of adipose tissue and lead to obesity.

Abstract: DNA methylation is an epigenetic mechanism that plays an important role in gene regulation without an altered DNA sequence. Previous studies have demonstrated that diet affects obesity by partially mediating DNA methylation. Our study investigated the genome-wide DNA methylation of perirenal adipose tissue in rabbits to identify the epigenetic changes of high-fat diet-mediated obesity. Two libraries were constructed pooling DNA of rabbits fed a standard normal diet (SND) and DNA of rabbits fed a high-fat diet (HFD). Differentially methylated regions (DMRs) were identified using the option of the sliding window method, and online software DAVID Bioinformatics Resources 6.7 was used to perform Gene Ontology (GO) terms and KEGG (Kyoto Encyclopedia of Genes and Genomes) pathway enrichment analysis of DMRs-associated genes. A total of 12,230 DMRs were obtained, of which 2305 (1207 up-regulated, 1098 down-regulated) and 601 (368 up-regulated, 233 down-regulated) of identified DMRs were observed in the gene body and promoter regions, respectively. GO analysis revealed that the DMRs-associated genes were involved in developmental process (GO:0032502), cell differentiation (GO:0030154), and lipid binding (GO:0008289), and KEGG pathway enrichment analysis revealed the DMRs-associated genes were enriched in linoleic acid metabolism (KO00591), DNA replication (KO03030), and MAPK signaling pathway (KO04010). Our study further elucidates the possible functions of DMRs-associated genes in rabbit adipogenesis, contributing to the understanding of HFD-mediated obesity.

Keywords: DNA methylation; high-fat diet; rabbits

1. Introduction

From the last 5 decades, the incidence of obesity has sharply increased, becoming one of the most considerable threats to human health because it is associated with the risk of type II diabetes mellitus, fatty liver disease, hypertension, and even certain cancers [1]. Obesity is a multifactorial pathological process, and genetic, environmental, and behavioral factors influence the development of obesity [2]. Nowadays, an imbalance between energy intake and expenditure is a major contributor to fat deposition in individuals predisposed to obesity [3]. Fat deposition is characterized by an increase in the number and size of adipocytes, and its process is closely related to physiological homeostasis, far beyond simple fat storage [4]. HFD has been shown to induce obesity in animal models and humans, and further induce a variety of obesity-related clinical diseases, such as osteoporosis, inflammation, and even neurodegeneration [5–7]. Perirenal fat, as part of abdominal visceral fat, is often used to elucidate the molecular and pathophysiological mechanisms of metabolic disorders associated with obesity or adipose development, because it is closely related to kidney injury, metabolism of triacylglycerol, and other metabolic regulation [8]. For example, detailed studies have shown that the perirenal fat thickness in obese patients could be a valuable marker to define the risk of developing hypertension and kidney dysfunction [9,10]. The expression profile of perirenal fat microRNA was changed during different growth stages of rabbits, and the differential microRNA expression was enriched for the MAPK signaling pathway, Wnt signaling pathway, aldosterone synthesis, and secretion pathways [11].

First proposed by Waddington in 1942, epigenetics refers to heritable changes in gene expression without an altered DNA sequence [12]. Epigenetics is caused by the interaction of environmental factors and intracellular genetic material, such as dietary factors, microRNA, and genomic imprinting, etc. Noteworthily, the biological effects of caloric intake are closely related to epigenetic mechanisms, including chromatin remodeling and DNA methylation [13]. DNA methylation of leptin and adiponectin promoters in obese children is associated with BMI, dyslipidemia, and insulin resistance [14]. These observations support the hypothesis that epigenetic modifications might underpin the development of obesity and related metabolic disorders. Hypermethylation of the pro-opiomelanocortin and serotonin transporter genes has been positively associated with childhood or adult obesity [15]. HFD changes the methylation status of *Casp1* and *Ndufb9* genes in obese mice, which are related to liver lipid metabolism and liver steatosis [16]. In addition, the leptin promoter was hypermethylated and *Ppar-α* promoter was hypomethylated in oocytes of mice fed with HFD, and the same changes were also observed in the liver of female offspring [17]. However, few studies have reported the changes in perirenal adipose tissue methylation profile in HFD-induced obese rabbits.

To further understand the epigenetic mechanisms influencing fat metabolism in obese rabbits, we investigated the role of DNA methylation in perirenal adipose tissue by sequencing and analyzing DNA methylation libraries from rabbits fed a standard normal diet (SND) and a high-fat diet (HFD).

2. Materials and Methods

2.1. Animals

A total of 24 female Tianfu black rabbits from a strain breed at the Sichuan Agricultural University in China were randomly divided into two groups and fed either a standard normal diet (SND) or a high-fat diet (HFD; 10% lard was added to the standard normal diet) for four weeks. The composition and nutrient content of the standard normal diet (SND) and the high-fat diet (HFD) were described in our previous report [18]. At the beginning of the trial, all rabbits were 35 days of age and housed individually in a clean iron cage (600 × 600 × 500 mm) and kept in an environmentally controlled room. Rabbits were free to access water and fed twice a day. At the end of the trial, rabbits were screened for obesity using the body mass index (BMI; BMI = bodyweight (kg)/height^2 (m)), and three rabbits from each group meeting the experimental requirements were selected for sampling. All experimental protocols were performed under the direction of the Institutional Animal Care and

Use Committee from the College of Animal Science and Technology, Sichuan Agricultural University, China (DKY-B2019202015, 5 December 2019).

2.2. DNA Extraction

Perirenal adipose tissue samples were collected immediately after rabbits were euthanized (shock and bleed treatment). Tissue blocks were placed in 4 mL EP tubes and stored in a −80 °C freezer. Total DNA from perirenal adipose tissue was extracted using a commercial TIANamp Genomic DNA extraction kit (Tiangen, Beijing, China), following the manufacturer's instructions. Subsequently, the purity and concentration of DNA were assessed by Agilent 2100 Bioanalyzer (Agilent Technologies, Carlsbad, CA, USA), and only DNA meeting quality criteria (thresholds: $A_{260}/A_{280} \approx 1.8$; concentration ≥ 200 ng/μL) was used for the trial.

2.3. DNA Methylation Library Construction and Sequencing

To identify genome-wide DNA methylation changes in perirenal adipose tissue induced by HFD, two libraries were constructed by pooling the DNA samples from three SND rabbits and three HFD rabbits. Briefly, DNA was fragmented by sonication to 100 to 500 bp fragments. The fragments were end-repaired using T4 DNA polymerase and Klenow enzyme and adaptors were ligated after generating 3′dA overhangs. Bisulfite treatment was conducted using the ZYMO EZ DNA Methylation-Gold kit (Zymo Research, Orange, CA, USA), following the manufacturer's protocol. After desalting, fragments of sizes ranging from 220 to 320 bp were isolated using a 15% PAGE gel and amplified by adaptor-mediated PCR. Lastly, the libraries were sequenced using the Illumina HiSeq 4000 platform (Illumina, San Diego, CA, USA) by Chengdu Life Baseline Technology Corporation, China.

2.4. Processing and Comparison of Sequencing Data

By removing adapter sequences and low-quality reads containing more than 50% low-quality bases (quality score < 5), clean reads were retained. Clean reads were aligned to the rabbit reference genome (GCF_000003625.3) with software BSMAP 2.90 (http://code.google.com/p/bsmap). Two forward strands, i.e., BSW (++) and BSC (−+) were used as references. The accuracy of DNA methylation detection depends on the conversion efficiency of cytosine, and the incomplete transformation of cytosine in sequences may lead to false-positive results. Here, lambda phage DNA was used as a control group to calculate the bisulfite conversion rate.

2.5. Methylation Site Detection

The methylation C sites were determined using the method described in a previous study [19]. Briefly, a binomial distribution test was performed for methylated reads number and non-methylated reads number at C sites. C sites were identified as the methylation C sites when the number of reads was greater than or equal to the binomial distribution expected value and the total effective coverage was greater than or equal to four.

2.6. Methylation Level Analysis

The average genome-wide methylation level reflects the overall characteristics of the methylation pattern of the genome. DNA methylation occurs in three sequence contexts: CG, CHG, and CHH (H = A, C, or T). The average methylation levels of CG, CHG, and CHH were calculated based on the percentage of methylated cytosine in the entire genome, chromosome, and genomic functional elements. For each type of sequence (CG, CHG, and CHH), the average methylation level was calculated according to the following formula: the average methylation level = methylated reads / (methylated reads + non-methylated reads) × 100%. To assess the association between sequence characteristics and methylation bias, we calculated the methylation percentage of nine bases upstream and downstream of the methylation site.

2.7. *Searching for Differentially Methylated Regions (DMRs)*

DMRs were identified using the option of a sliding window method. Briefly, the sliding windows, which were used for further analysis, had to meet the following criteria: (a) the depth in each cytosine should be more than four in each sample, and each C site should cover at least four methylation reads; (b) the number of selected cytosine should be larger than five; (c) after calculating mean methylation level of each sample, the fold change of mean methylation level between the two samples should be larger than two. After repeating extension steps, the merged regions with $p < 0.05$ were defined as DMRs.

2.8. *Functional Enrichment Analysis of Differentially Methylated Genes*

To explore the role of epigenetic variation in biological processes and pathways, online software DAVID Bioinformatics Resources 6.7 (http://david.abcc.ncifcrf.gov/home.jsp) was used to perform Gene Ontology (GO) terms and KEGG (Kyoto Encyclopedia of Genes and Genomes) pathway enrichment analysis of DMRs-associated genes. GO analysis can be used to identify the performance of the gene product and contains three types of information: cellular component, molecular function, and biological processes. KEGG is the main public database that integrates the genome, chemistry, and system function information, particularly the set of genes associated with the systemic functions of cells, organisms, and ecosystems. Differences were considered to be statistically significant at $p < 0.05$.

3. Results

3.1. *Quality Assessment of Sequencing Data*

After raw reads were processed, a total of 1,221,455,488 clean reads were obtained from methylation sequencing libraries (Table S1). The clean reads were mapped to the rabbit reference genome, and the mapping rate was 84.910% in the SND group and 84.730% in the HFD group, respectively. The bisulfite conversion rate was 99.550% for SND, and 99.520% for HFD. In addition, the effective coverage rate of C base in each chromosome ranged from 89.892% to 97.577% and ranged from 91.822% to 97.804% in different functional genomic elements (Tables S2 and S3).

3.2. *Methylation Level Analysis*

Genome-wide methylation level analysis showed that the methylation level of C, CHG, and CHH in the HFD group was higher than in the SND group but the CG methylation level in the HFD group was lower than in the SND group (Table S4). Results of the methylation level C, CG, CHG, and CHH on different chromosomes are shown in Table S5. The greatest differences in C, CG, CHG, and CHH between the two groups were found on chromosome 20, chromosome X, chromosome 1, and chromosome 11, reaching 0.569%, 2.736%, 0.056%, and 0.047%, respectively. In addition, we classified the various functional genomic elements into promoter, CDS, intron, mRNA, downstream, CpGIsland, ncRNA, and transposons. Compared with the SND group, the methylation level of C, CHG, and CHH in each functional genomic element was increased in the HFD group (Table S6). However, based on comparison with the SND group, promoter, intron, mRNA, downstream, and ncRNA methylation levels were decreased in CG, and only CDS, CpGIsland, and transposons methylation levels were increased in CG.

3.3. *Genome-Wide Characteristics of Methylated C Bases*

The percentage of methylated C bases in CG were highest, reaching 94.795% (SND) and 94.843% (HFD) but rarely cytosine methylation was found in CHH and CHG. In addition, we calculated the methylation percentage of nine bases (methylated C at the fourth base) upstream and downstream of the methylated site. As shown in Figure 1, CG, CAG, and CAC were the most likely sites to be methylated in both SND and HFD groups.

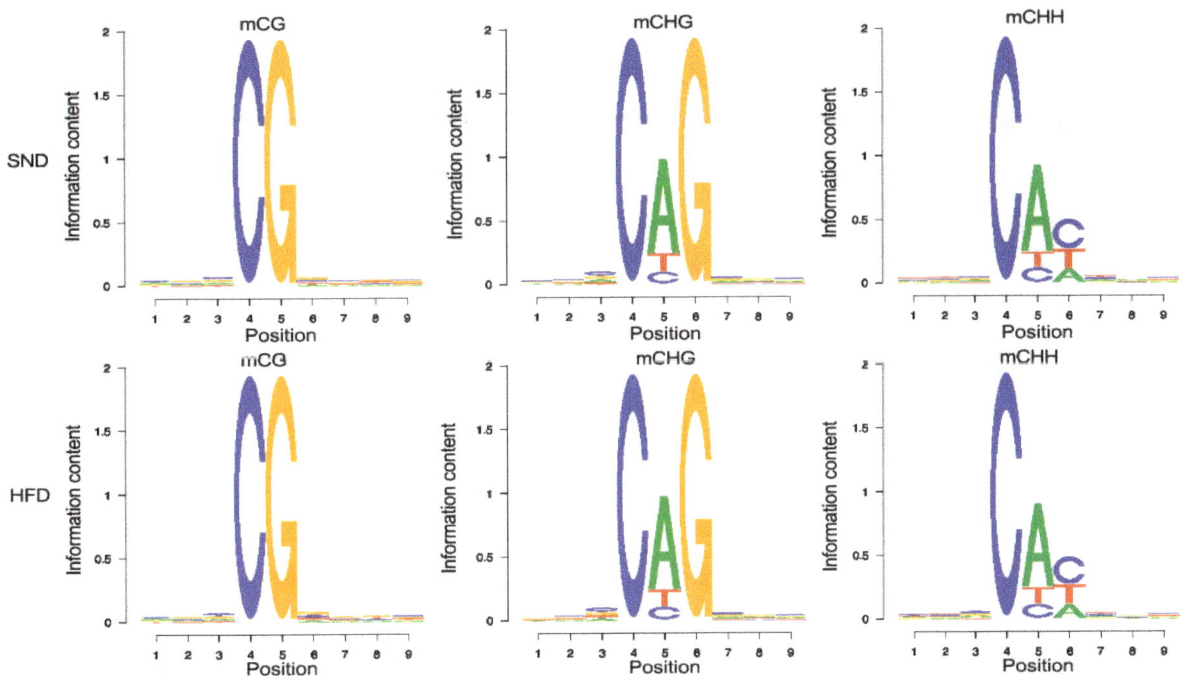

Figure 1. Genome-wide characteristics of methylated C bases. Sequence characteristics of bases near mCG, mCHG, and mCHH in the SND and HFD group.

3.4. Analysis of Differentially Methylated Regions (DMRs)

A total of 12,230 DMRs were identified in the genome of the HFD group compared to the SND group. Chromosome 21 was the chromosome with the least amount of DMRs and chromosome 13 was the chromosome with the most amount of DMRs (Figure 2a,b). The total length of DMRs in each chromosome is shown in Table S7. In addition, the DMRs were mapped to the gene body and promoter regions, and 2305 (1207 up-regulated, 1098 down-regulated) and 601 (368 up-regulated, 233 down-regulated) methylated genes were obtained, respectively. Some genes involved in adipocyte growth and development have also been identified, including *ACE2*, *AGTR1*, *IGF1R*, and *ACSL4*.

3.5. GO and KEGG Enrichment Analysis

To better study the biological functions of the DMRs-associated genes, we used online software DAVID Bioinformatics Resources 6.7 (http://david.abcc.ncifcrf.gov/home.jsp) to carry out gene ontology (GO) terms and KEGG (Kyoto Encyclopedia of Genes and Genomes) pathway enrichment analysis. GO analysis of the overlapping DMRs-associated genes in the gene body regions found a total of 6310 enriched GO terms (4796 biological processes (BP), 579 cellular components (CC), and 935 molecular functions (MF)), of which 12.570% were significantly enriched ($p < 0.05$) (Table S8). The main GO terms involved in overlapping DMRs-associated genes in the gene body regions included the developmental process (GO:0032502), cell differentiation (GO:0030154), and lipid binding (GO:0008289). The top 10 significantly enriched terms in the BP, CC, and MF categories are shown in Figure 3a. The KEGG pathway analysis showed that overlapping DMRs-associated genes in the gene body regions were enriched in 314 pathways including the PI3K-AKT signaling pathway (KO04151), linoleic acid metabolism (KO00591), and pathways for DNA replication (KO03030). Thirty-nine of these pathways (12.420%) were significantly enriched ($p < 0.05$, Table S9). In addition, a scatter analysis was carried out for the 20 most significant pathways to intuitively show the significance of these pathways (Figure 3b).

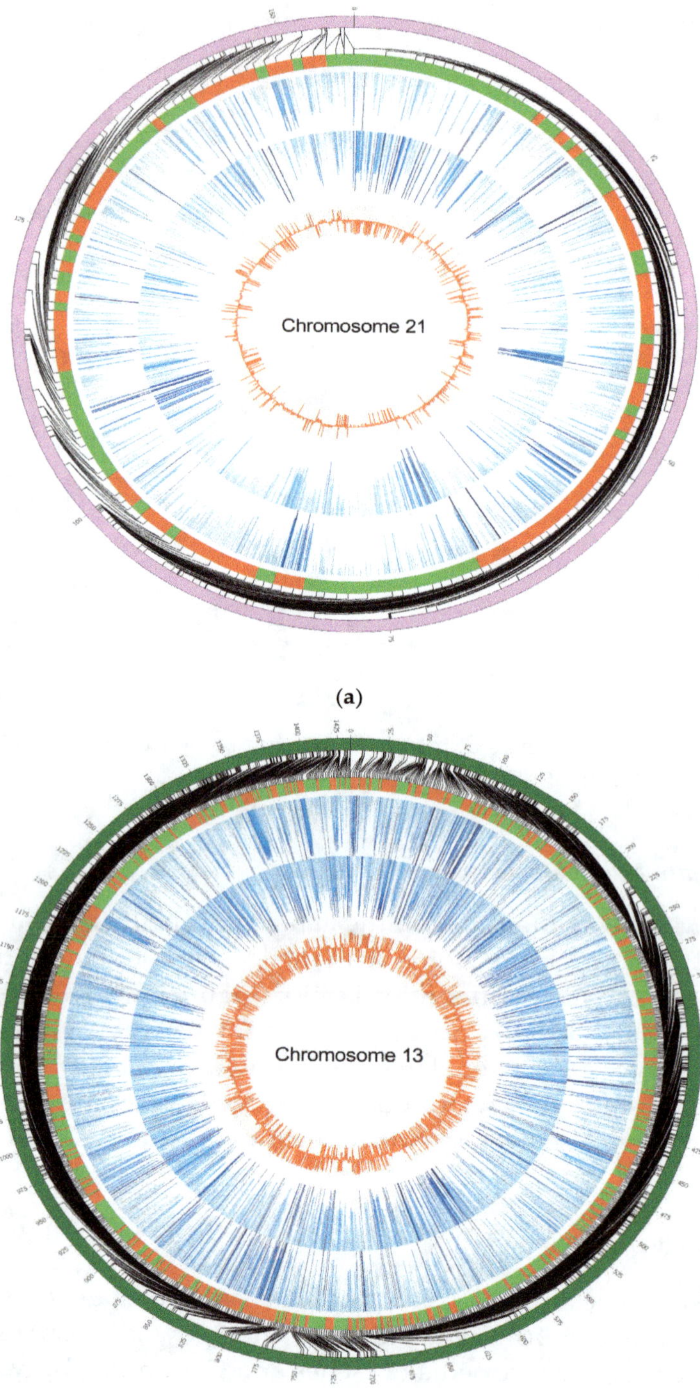

(b)

Figure 2. Analysis of differentially methylated regions (DMRs). Two chromosomes with the least (**a**) and the most (**b**) amount of DMRs. The outer ring represents the position of the genomic chromosome; the second circle is the DMRs region: the red area represents the higher methylation level of HFD compared to the SND group and the green area represents the lower methylation level of HFD compared to the SND group; the third circle represents the methylation rate of each site of sample HFD; the fourth circle represents the methylation rate of each site of sample SND; the fifth circle represents the difference of methylation rate.

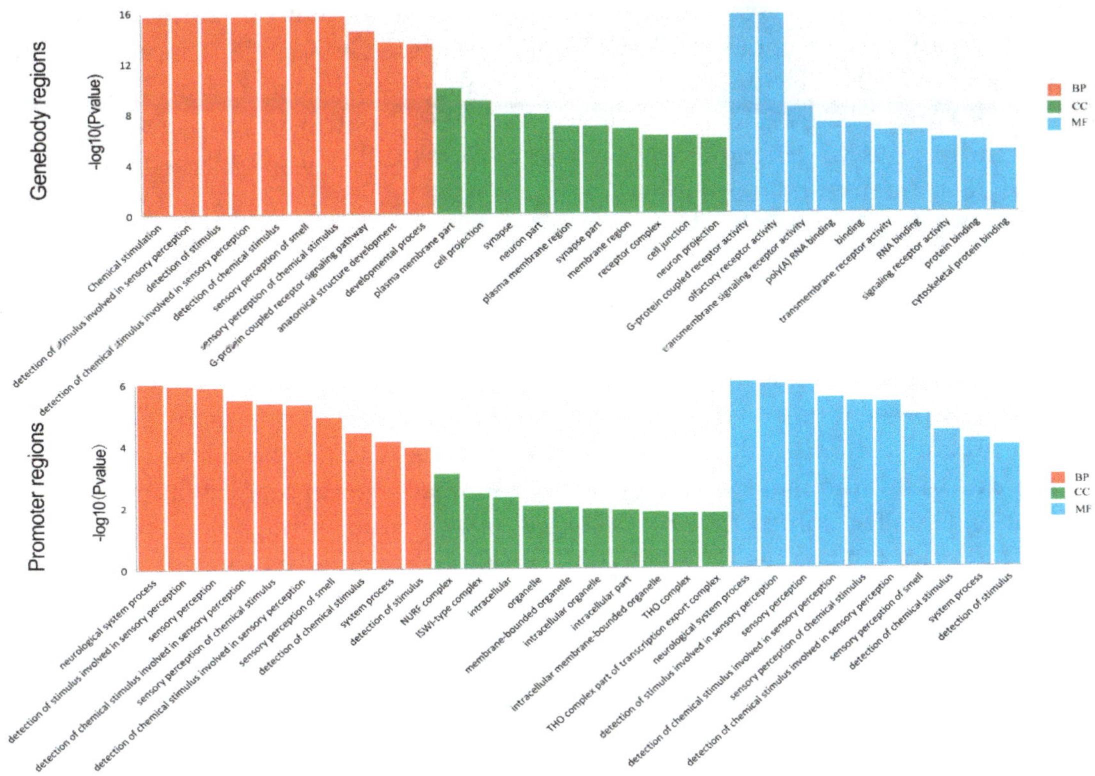

(**a**)

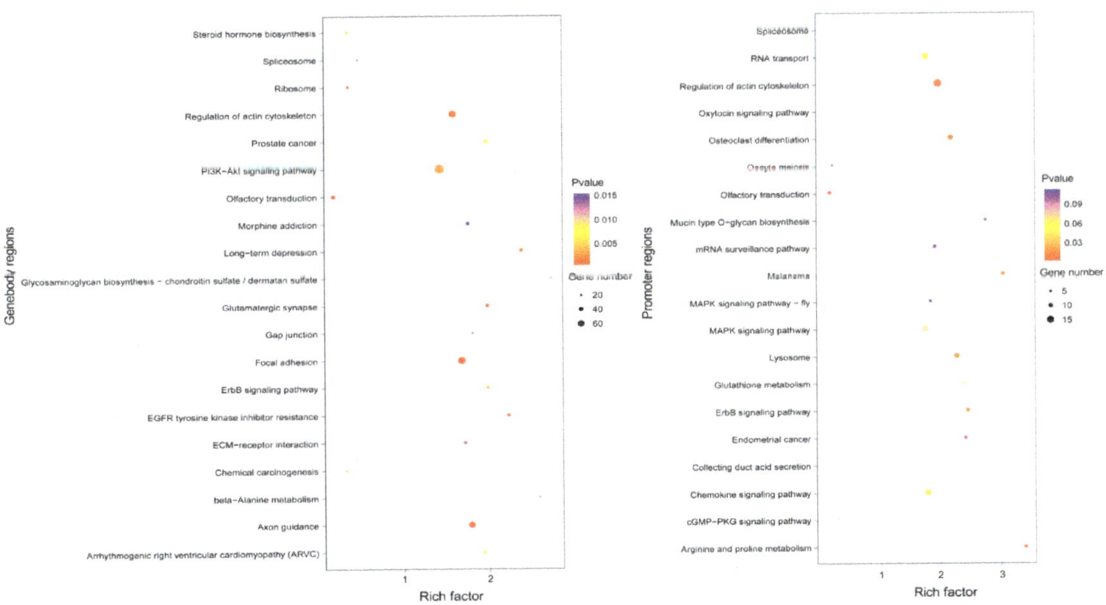

(**b**)

Figure 3. GO and KEGG enrichment analysis. (**a**) GO analysis of the overlapping DMRs-associated genes in the gene body regions and promoter regions. (**b**) KEGG pathway analysis of the overlapping DMRs-associated genes in the gene body regions and promoter regions. Rich factor = (DMRs-associated genes annotation in term/genes annotation in term)/(DMRs-associated genes with KEGG annotation / all genes with KEGG annotation).

GO analysis of the overlapping DMRs-associated genes in the promoter regions showed enrichment of 2223 biological processes (BP), 311 cellular components (CC), and 405 molecular functions (MF), of which 173 BP (7.780%), 20 CC (6.430%), and 37 MF (9.140%) were significantly enriched (Table S10).

The significantly enriched GO terms mainly include positive regulation of lipid biosynthetic process (GO:0046889), regulation of cholesterol metabolic process (GO:0090181), and regulation of lipid biosynthetic process (GO:0046890). The top 10 significantly enriched GO terms in the BP, CC, and MF categories of GO analysis are shown in Figure 3a. KEGG pathway analysis found 266 enriched pathways including the MAPK signaling pathway (KO04010) (Table S11). The top 20 significantly enriched pathways are presented in Figure 3b.

4. Discussion

DNA methylation represents an important epigenetic marker because it is associated with chromosomal structural changes, embryonic development, expression of imprinted genes, and causing corresponding diseases, including X chromosome inactivation and DNA unwinding [20–22]. Nowadays, obesity prevention and treatment strategies have been unsuccessful, and DNA methylation is one of the epigenetic modifications associated with obesity [23]. The rabbit is an ideal material to study obesity due to its lipid metabolism and obesity-related clinical manifestations similar to those of humans [24,25]. Thus far, some DNA methylation related studies have been investigated in rabbit models but studies of the changes in perirenal adipose tissue methylation profile in HFD-induced obese rabbits have not been carried out. In this study, DNA methylation patterns were investigated in rabbit models to understand obesity-related DNA methylation changes.

Here, the mapping rates were 84.910% and 84.730% in the SND group and HDF group, respectively. The bisulfite conversion rates were 99.550% (SND) and 99.520% (HFD) in the two groups, which was consistent with previous research, indicating that the libraries were high quality and reliable [26,27]. Methylation is a dynamic process in cells, which can be regulated by methylation and demethylation. The average methylation level of the whole genome reflects the overall characteristics of the genome methylation profile. The results of the genome-wide methylation level analysis in this study were similar to those in mice [28]. The methylation level of CG was higher than the methylation level in C, CHG, and CHH. However, this result is different from that of plant Arabidopsis Thaliana. The plant genome has extensive methylation at the CHG site [29]. CG methylation was maintained by Dnmt1. CHH methylation and some CHG methylation is usually maintained by the activity of the conserved Dnmt3. The high level of CHG methylation seen in Arabidopsis thaliana is maintained by plant-specific methyltransferase [30]. In addition, research on chickens suggests that promoter DNA methylation generally affects chromatin structure and is a signal to inhibit gene transcription, and promoter regions are lowly methylated [31]. Our study also found that promoter regions showed a lower methylation level than other regions. However, a study in mice fed with HFD showed that promoter regions are hypermethylated [32]. Therefore, we hypothesized that differences in methylation level may be species-specific.

The results of genome-wide characteristics of methylated C bases showed that the proportion of mCG was the highest, while the cytosine methylation was low in CHH and CHG. Some studies have shown that no enzyme can maintain mCHG during DNA replication in animals, so the sites of CHG type in animal cells generally show a very low level of methylation. CHH can only rely on the methylation mechanism, so CHH methylation is easily lost in the process of DNA replication and is generally in the state of hypomethylation [33]. The results of this study showed that the characteristics of methylation in the rabbit genome were similar to those in other animals.

DMRs refer to the regions of DNA molecules with different methylation status in two samples. The identification of DMRs is the first step towards the study of DMRs-associated genes [34]. In our study, a total of 2906 DMRs were identified, and 2305 (1207 up-regulated, 1098 down-regulated) and 601 (368 up-regulated, 233 down-regulated) methylated genes were associated with differentially methylated regions. Many genes are related to adipocyte growth and development. For example, as the members of the renin-angiotensin system (RAS), *ACE2* and *AGTR1* were reported to participate in the development and progression of obesity [35,36]. *PPARγ* and *aP2* are important transcription factors in the development and function of the adipose tissue and marker of lipogenesis [37]. Previous studies showed that inhibition of *IGF1R* decreased the expression of PPARγ, thereby inhibiting lipogenesis [38]. Moreover, *ACSL4* plays a role in the regulation of lipid metabolism. *ACSL4* was expressed throughout the entire differentiation process in pig preadipocytes and showed a similar expression trend with lipogenesis-associated genes *PPARγ* and *aP2* [39].

Gene ontology (GO) analysis is a reliable bioinformatics tool for understanding the characteristics of genes and gene products. The significantly enriched terms in the BP, CC, and MF categories indicated the possible roles of the DMRs-associated genes in regulating obesity. The significantly enriched GO terms showed correlation with adipocyte lipid metabolism and metabolisms, such as lipid binding (GO:0008289), positive regulation of lipid biosynthetic process (GO:0046889), regulation of cholesterol metabolic process (GO:0090181), developmental process (GO:0032502), and cell differentiation (GO:0030154). Some terms were related to adipocyte development, including cytoskeletal protein binding (GO:0008092), tubulin binding (GO:0015631), calcium ion binding (GO:0005509). Cytoskeletal remodeling and cell–cell interaction are a necessary step in the transformation of preadipocytes into mature adipocytes, and adipocyte development is dependent on α-tubulin [40,41]. Calcium is a complex mediator in adipogenesis because it regulates numerous cellular processes [42]. Furthermore, other GO items related to hormones and enzymes were also significantly enriched, such as regulation of glucocorticoid secretion (GO:2000849), N-acetyltransferase activity (GO:0008080), and phosphoric diester hydrolase activity (GO:0008081). Increasing evidence suggests that excess glucocorticoids leads to increased fat mass and obesity through the accumulation of adipocytes [43]. Acetyltransferase is a regulator of adipogenesis and lipid metabolism, and its regulatory mechanism is mainly transcription and post-translation modifications [44]. Phosphoric diester hydrolase is a regulator of systemic glucose and insulin homeostasis [45]. Interference of phosphoric diester hydrolase expression in 3T3-L1 adipocytes caused a dramatic decrease in adipocyte differentiation key gene (*PPARγ*, *aP2*) and lipid accumulation [46].

Adipogenesis is a complex process involving an elaborate network of transcription factors and signaling pathways. Results of KEGG analysis showed that DMRs-associated genes were mainly involved in the PI3K-AKT signaling pathway (ko04151), linoleic acid metabolism (KO00591), DNA replication (KO03030), and MAPK signaling pathway (KO04010). The PI3K-AKT signaling pathway is a key regulator in cell proliferation, differentiation, and apoptosis [47]. Activation of the PI3K-AKT signaling pathway promotes the expression of marker genes involved in adipogenesis and glucose uptake [48]. In our study, 70 DMRs-associated genes were enriched in the PI3K-AKT signaling pathway, thereby revealing that these DMRs-associated genes may be essential for adipogenesis. Linoleic acid metabolism (KO00591) is also associated with adipogenesis. Linoleic acid can be converted to the metabolically active arachidonic acid, which has roles in inducing inflammation and adipogenesis. Excessive intake of linoleic acid results in increasing magnitudes of adiposity, inflammatory cytokines, and insulin resistance [49]. In addition, it is becoming clear that DNA replication (KO03030) and the MAPK signaling pathway (KO04010) play an important role in adipocyte growth and development [50,51]. Thus, the results of our study indicate that these DMRs-associated genes might be an important regulator in adipogenesis. However, due to the limitation of experimental conditions, such as pooled samples, only one library per group, sequencing methods, etc., functional verification of these DMRs-associated genes will be important to consider in the future.

5. Conclusions

In conclusion, our study indicates that a high-fat diet may affect genes associated with adipogenesis by altering DNA methylation patterns. We identified 2906 methylated genes, of which, *ACE2*, *AGTR1*, *IGF1R*, and *ACSL4* may have a key role in adipogenesis. These genes may be involved in the regulation of adipogenesis through the PI3K-AKT signaling pathway (KO04151), linoleic acid metabolism (KO00591), DNA replication (KO03030), and MAPK signaling pathway (KO04010).

Supplementary Materials:
Table S1: Data output and comparative statistics, Table S2: The effective coverage rate of C base in each chromosome, Table S3: The effective coverage rate of C base in different functional genomic elements, Table S4: Results of genome-wide methylation level analysis, Table S5: Results of the methylation level C, CG, CHG, and CHH on different chromosomes, Table S6: Methylation level in various functional genomic elements between standard normal diet (SND) and high-fat diet (HFD) group, Table S7: DMRs number and length statistics of standard normal diet (SND) and high-fat diet (HFD) group, Table S8: GO analysis of the overlapping DMRs-associated genes in the gene body regions, Table S9: KEGG pathway analysis of the overlapping DMRs-associated genes in the gene body regions, Table S10: GO analysis of the overlapping DMRs-associated genes in the promoter regions, Table S11: KEGG pathway analysis of the overlapping DMRs-associated genes in the promoter regions.

Author Contributions: X.J., J.W., and S.L. conceived and designed the study; T.P. and Y.L. collected data and conducted the research; J.S. and X.B. wrote the paper. All authors have read and agreed to the published version of the manuscript.

References

1. Blüher, M. Obesity: Global epidemiology and pathogenesis. *Nat. Rev. Endocrinol.* **2019**, *15*, 288–298. [CrossRef] [PubMed]
2. Bray, G.A.; Heisel, W.E.; Afshin, A.; Jensen, M.D.; Dietz, W.H.; Long, M.; Kushner, R.F.; Daniels, S.R.; Wadden, T.A.; Tsai, A.G. The Science of Obesity Management: An Endocrine Society Scientific Statement. *Endocr. Rev.* **2018**, *39*, 79–132. [CrossRef] [PubMed]
3. Richard, D. Cognitive and autonomic determinants of energy homeostasis in obesity. *Nat. Rev. Endocrinol.* **2015**, *11*, 489–501. [CrossRef] [PubMed]
4. Trayhurn, P.; Beattie, J.H. Physiological role of adipose tissue: White adipose tissue as an endocrine and secretory organ. *Proc. Nutr. Soc.* **2001**, *60*, 329–339. [CrossRef] [PubMed]
5. Xie, H.; Wang, Q.; Zhang, X.; Wang, T.; Hu, W.; Manicum, T.; Chen, H.; Sun, L. Possible therapeutic potential of berberine in the treatment of STZ plus HFD-induced diabetic osteoporosis. *Biomed. Pharmacother.* **2018**, *108*, 280–287. [CrossRef]
6. Cani, P.D.; Bibiloni, R.; Knauf, C.; Waget, A.; Neyrinck, A.M.; Delzenne, N.M.; Burcelin, R. Changes in gut microbiota control metabolic endotoxemia-induced inflammation in high-fat diet-induced obesity and diabetes in mice. *Diabetes* **2008**, *57*, 1470–1481. [CrossRef]
7. Nuzzo, D.; Galizzi, G.; Amato, A.; Terzo, S.; Carlo, M.D. Regular Intake of Pistachio Mitigates the Deleterious Effects of a High Fat-Diet in the Brain of Obese Mice. *Antioxidants* **2020**, *9*, 317. [CrossRef]
8. Hou, N.; Han, F.; Wang, M.; Huang, N.; Zhao, J.; Liu, X.; Sun, X. Perirenal fat associated with microalbuminuria in obese rats. *Int. Urol. Nephrol.* **2014**, *46*, 839–845. [CrossRef]
9. Anastasia, R.M.; Matteo, S.; Stefano, M.; Stefano, D.V.; Giacomo, P.; Graziana, L. Morbid obesity and hypertension: The role of perirenal fat. *J. Clin. Hypertens.* **2018**, *20*, 1430–1437.
10. Olga, L.; Vincenzo, N.; Donatella, C.; Umberto, V.; Rosaria, G.; Loreto, G.; Mauro, C. Para- and perirenal fat thickness is an independent predictor of chronic kidney disease, increased renal resistance index and hyperuricaemia in type-2 diabetic patients. *Nephrol. Dial. Transplant. Off. Publ. Eur. Dial. Transpl. Assoc. Eur. Ren. Assoc.* **2011**, *26*, 892–898.
11. Wang, G.; Guo, G.; Tian, X.; Hu, S.; Lai, S. Screening and identification of MicroRNAs expressed in perirenal adipose tissue during rabbit growth. *Lipids Health Dis.* **2020**, *19*, 35. [CrossRef] [PubMed]
12. Waddington, C.H. Canalization of Development and the Inheritance of Acquired Characters. *Nature* **1942**, *150*, 91–97. [CrossRef]
13. Milagro, F.I.; Campion, J.; Cordero, P.; Goyenechea, E.; Gomez-Uriz, A.M.; Abete, I.; Zulet, M.A.; Martinez, J.A. A dual epigenomic approach for the search of obesity biomarkers: DNA methylation in relation to diet-induced weight loss. *FASEB J.* **2011**, *25*, 1378–1389. [CrossRef] [PubMed]
14. García-Cardona, M.C.; Huang, F.; García-Vivas, J.M.; López-Camarillo, C.; del Río Navarro, B.E.; Navarro Olivos, E.; Hong-Chong, E.; Bolanos-Jiménez, F.; Marchat, L.A. DNA methylation of leptin and adiponectin promoters in children is reduced by the combined presence of obesity and insulin resistance. *Int. J. Obes.* **2014**, *38*, 1457–1465. [CrossRef] [PubMed]

15. Zhao, J.; Goldberg, J.; Vaccarino, V. Promoter methylation of serotonin transporter gene is associated with obesity measures: A monozygotic twin study. *Int. J. Obes.* **2013**, *37*, 140–145. [CrossRef] [PubMed]
16. Ahram, Y.; Tammen, S.A.; Soyoung, P.; Han, S.N.; Sang-Woon, C. Genome-wide hepatic DNA methylation changes in high-fat diet-induced obese mice. *Nutr. Res. Pract.* **2017**, *11*, 105–113.
17. Ge, Z.; Luo, S.; Lin, F.; Liang, Q.; Sun, Q. DNA methylation in oocytes and liver of female mice and their offspring: Effects of high-fat-diet-induced obesity. *Environ. Health Perspect* **2014**, *122*, 159–164. [CrossRef]
18. Shao, J.; Wang, J.; Li, Y.; Elzo, M.A.; Tang, T.; Lai, T.; Ma, Y.; Gan, M.; Wang, L.; Jia, X.; et al. Growth, behavioural, serum biochemical and morphological changes in female rabbits fed high-fat diet. *J. Anim. Physiol. Anim. Nutr.* **2020**, 1–9. [CrossRef]
19. Lister, R.; Pelizzola, M.; Dowen, R.H.; Hawkins, R.D.; Hon, G.; Tonti-Filippini, J.; Nery, J.R.; Lee, L.; Ye, Z.; Ngo, Q.M.; et al. Human DNA methylomes at base resolution show widespread epigenomic differences. *Nature* **2009**, *462*, 315–322. [CrossRef]
20. Dvir, A.; Gidon, T.; Michael, R.; Asaf, H. Replication timing-related and gene body-specific methylation of active human genes. *Hum. Mol. Genet.* **2011**, *20*, 670–680.
21. Jjingo, D. On the presence and role of human gene-body DNA methylation. *Oncotarget* **2012**, *3*, 462–474. [CrossRef] [PubMed]
22. Reik, W. Stability and flexibility of epigenetic gene regulation in mammalian development. *Nature* **2007**, *447*, 425–432. [CrossRef]
23. Cordero, P.; Campion, J.; Milagro, F.I.; Martinez, J.A. Transcriptomic and epigenetic changes in early liver steatosis associated to obesity: Effect of dietary methyl donor supplementation. *Mol. Genet. Metab.* **2013**, *110*, 388–395. [CrossRef] [PubMed]
24. Jerez, S.; Scacchi, F.; Sierra, L.; Karbiner, S.; María, P.D.B. Vascular Hyporeactivity to Angiotensin II and Noradrenaline in a Rabbit Model of Obesity. *J. Cardiovasc. Pharmacol.* **2012**, *59*, 49. [CrossRef] [PubMed]
25. Zhang, X.; Chinkes, D.L.; Asle, A.; Herndon, D.N.; Wolfe, R.R. Lipid metabolism in diet-induced obese rabbits is similar to that of obese humans. *J. Nutr.* **2008**, *138*, 515–518. [CrossRef]
26. An, X.; Ma, H.; Han, P.; Zhu, C.; Cao, B.; Bai, Y. Genome-wide differences in DNA methylation changes in caprine ovaries between oestrous and dioestrous phases. *J. Anim. Sci. Biotechnol.* **2019**, *10*, 29–36. [CrossRef]
27. Jin, L.; Jiang, Z.; Xia, Y.; Lou, P.; Chen, L.; Wang, H. Genome-wide DNA methylation changes in skeletal muscle between young and middle-aged pigs. *BMC Genom.* **2014**, *15*, 1–12. [CrossRef]
28. Feng, S.; Cokus, S.J.; Zhang, X. Conservation and divergence of methylation patterning in plants and animals. *Proc. Natl. Acad. Sci. USA* **2010**, *107*, 8689–8694. [CrossRef]
29. Chan, W.L.; Henderson, I.R.; Jacobsen, S.E. Gardening the genome: DNA methylation in Arabidopsis thaliana. *Nat. Rev. Genet.* **2005**, *6*, 351–360. [CrossRef]
30. Klose, R.J.; Bird, A.P.; Klose, R.J.; Bird, A.P. Genomic DNA methylation: The mark and its mediators. *Trends Biochem. Sci.* **2006**, *31*, 89–97. [CrossRef]
31. Li, Q.; Li, N.; Hu, X.; Li, J.; Du, Z.; Chen, L.; Yin, G.; Duan, J.; Zhang, H.; Zhao, Y. Genome-Wide Mapping of DNA Methylation in Chicken. *PLoS ONE* **2011**, *6*, e19428. [CrossRef] [PubMed]
32. Milagro, F.I.; Campión, J.; García-Díaz, D.F.; Goyenechea, E.; Paternain, L.; Martínez, J.A. High fat diet-induced obesity modifies the methylation pattern of leptin promoter in rats. *J. Physiol. Biochem.* **2009**, *65*, 1–9. [CrossRef] [PubMed]
33. Fouse, S.D.; Nagarajan, R.P.; Costello, J.F. Genome-scale DNA methylation analysis. *Epigenomics* **2010**, *2*, 105–117. [CrossRef] [PubMed]
34. Condon, D.E.; Tran, P.V.; Lien, Y.C.; Schug, J.; Georgieff, M.K.; Simmons, R.A.; Won, K.J. Defiant: (DMRs: Easy, fast, identification and ANnoTation) identifies differentially Methylated regions from iron-deficient rat hippocampus. *BMC Bioinform.* **2018**, *19*, 31. [CrossRef] [PubMed]
35. Riedel, J.; Badewien-Rentzsch, B.; Kohn, B.; Hoeke, L.; Einspanier, R. Characterization of key genes of the renin–angiotensin system in mature feline adipocytes and during invitro adipogenesis. *J. Anim. Physiol. Anim. Nutr.* **2016**, *100*, 1139–1148. [CrossRef]
36. Pahlavani, M.; Kalupahana, N.S.; Ramalingam, L.; Moustai-Moussa, N. Regulation and Functions of the Renin-Angiotensin System in White and Brown Adipose Tissue. *Compr. Physiol.* **2017**, *7*, 1137–1150.
37. Siersbæk, R.; Nielsen, R.; Mandrup, S. PPARγ in adipocyte differentiation and metabolism—Novel insights from genome-wide studies. *FEBS Lett.* **2010**, *584*, 3242–3249. [CrossRef]

38. Wang, F.; Yin, H.; Lou, J.; Xie, D.; Cao, X. Insulinlike growth factor I promotes adipogenesis in hemangioma stem cells from infantile hemangiomas. *Mol. Med. Rep.* **2019**, *19*, 2825–2830.
39. Peng, Y.; Xiang, H.; Chen, C.; Zheng, R.; Jiang, S. MiR-224 impairs adipocyte early differentiation and regulates fatty acid metabolism. *Int. J. Biochem. Cell Biol.* **2013**, *45*, 1585–1593. [CrossRef]
40. Yang, W.; Guo, X.; Thein, S.; Xu, F.; Sugii, S.; Baas, P.W.; Radda, G.K.; Han, W. Regulation of adipogenesis by cytoskeleton remodelling is facilitated by acetyltransferase MEC-17-dependent acetylation of α-tubulin. *Biochem. J.* **2013**, *449*, 605–612. [CrossRef]
41. Massimo, B.; Elisa, M.; Wheeler, M.B.; Li, W.J. Transcription Adaptation during In Vitro Adipogenesis and Osteogenesis of Porcine Mesenchymal Stem Cells: Dynamics of Pathways, Biological Processes, Up-Stream Regulators, and Gene Networks. *PLoS ONE* **2015**, *10*, e0137644.
42. Goudarzi, F.; Mohammadalipour, A.; Khodadadi, I.; Karimi, S.; Mostoli, R.; Bahabadi, M.; Goodarzi, M.T. The Role of Calcium in Differentiation of Human Adipose-Derived Stem Cells to Adipocytes. *Mol. Biotechnol.* **2018**, *60*, 279–289. [CrossRef] [PubMed]
43. Barclay, J.L.; Agada, H.; Jang, C.; Ward, M.; Wetzig, N.; Ho, K.K.Y. Effects of glucocorticoids on human brown adipocytes. *J. Endocrinol.* **2015**, *224*, 139–147. [CrossRef]
44. Zhou, Y.; Peng, J.; Jiang, S. Role of histone acetyltransferases and histone deacetylases in adipocyte differentiation and adipogenesis. *Eur. J. Cell Biol.* **2014**, *93*, 170–177. [CrossRef] [PubMed]
45. Song, D.; Chen, Y.; Li, Z.; Guan, Y.; Zou, D.; Miao, C. Protein tyrosine phosphatase 1B inhibits adipocyte differentiation and mediates TNFα action in obesity. *Biochim. Biophys. Acta-Mol. Cell Biol. Lipids* **2013**, *1831*, 1368–1376. [CrossRef] [PubMed]
46. Glondu-Lassis, M.; Dromard, M.; Chavey, C.; Puech, C.; Fajas, L.; Hendriks, W.; Freiss, G. Downregulation of protein tyrosine phosphatase PTP-BL represses adipogenesis. *Int. J. Biochem. Cell Biol.* **2009**, *41*, 2173–2180. [CrossRef]
47. Zhong, X.; Shen, X.; Wen, J.; Kong, Y.; Chu, J.; Yan, G.; Li, T.; Liu, D.; Wu, M.; Zeng, G. Osteopontin-induced brown adipogenesis from white preadipocytes through a PI3K-AKT dependent signaling. *Biochem. Biophys. Res. Commun.* **2015**, *459*, 553–559. [CrossRef]
48. Wang, J.; Hu, X.; Ai, W.; Zhang, F.; Yang, K.; Wang, L.; Zhu, X.; Gao, P.; Shu, G.; Jiang, Q. Phytol increases adipocyte number and glucose tolerance through activation of PI3K/Akt signaling pathway in mice fed high-fat and high-fructose diet. *Biochem. Biophys. Res. Commun.* **2017**, *489*, 432–438. [CrossRef]
49. Naughton, S.S.; Mathai, M.L.; Hryciw, D.H.; McAinch, A.J. Linoleic acid and the pathogenesis of obesity. *Prostaglandins Other Lipid Mediat.* **2016**, *125*, 90–99. [CrossRef]
50. Johmura, Y.; Osada, S.; Nishizuka, M.; Imagawa, M. FAD24 Acts in Concert with Histone Acetyltransferase HBO1 to Promote Adipogenesis by Controlling DNA Replication. *J. Biol. Chem.* **2008**, *283*, 2265–2274. [CrossRef]
51. Lee, H.W.; Rhee, D.K.; Kim, B.O.; Pyo, S. Inhibitory effect of sinigrin on adipocyte differentiation in 3T3-L1 cells: Involvement of AMPK and MAPK pathways. *Biomed. Pharmacother.* **2018**, *102*, 670–680. [CrossRef] [PubMed]

14

Overview of Research Development on the Role of NF-κB Signaling in Mastitis

Muhammad Zahoor Khan [1], Adnan Khan [2], Jianxin Xiao [1], Jiaying Ma [1], Yulin Ma [1], Tianyu Chen [1], Dafu Shao [3] and Zhijun Cao [1,*]

1 State Key Laboratory of Animal Nutrition, Beijing Engineering Technology Research Center of Raw Milk Quality and Safety Control, College of Animal Science and Technology, China Agricultural University, Beijing 100193, China; zahoorkhattak91@163.com (M.Z.K.); dairyxiao@gmail.com (J.X.); majiaying@cau.edu.cn (J.M.); ma18810318038@163.com (Y.M.); 18355593440@163.com (T.C.)

2 Key Laboratory of Animal Genetics, Breeding, and Reproduction, Ministry of Agriculture & National Engineering Laboratory for Animal Breeding, College of Animal Science and Technology, China Agricultural University, Beijing 100193, China; dr.adnan93@cau.edu.cn

3 Institute of Agricultural Information of CAAS, Beijing 100081, China; shaodafu@caas.cn

* Correspondence: caozhijun@cau.edu.cn;

Simple Summary: NF-κB signaling has been widely studied for its role in inflammatory and immunity-related diseases. Mastitis is considered one of the inflammatory and immunity associated diseases which are a serious threat to the global dairy industry. Having such a critical role in immunity and inflammation, NF-κB signaling is currently under target for therapeutic purposes in mastitis control research. The virulent factor, lipopolysaccharides (LPS), of bacteria after attachment with relevant Toll-like receptors (TLRs) on mammary epithelial cells starts its pathogenesis by using NF-κB signaling to cause mastitis. Several studies have proved that the blocking of NF-κB signaling could be a useful strategy for mastitis control.

Abstract: Mastitis is the inflammation of the mammary gland. *Escherichia coli* and *Staphylococcus aureus* are the most common bacteria responsible for mastitis. When mammary epithelial cells are infected by microorganisms, this activates an inflammatory response. The bacterial infection is recognized by innate pattern recognition receptors (PRRs) in the mammary epithelial cells, with the help of Toll-like receptors (TLRs). Upon activation by lipopolysaccharides, a virulent agent of bacteria, the TLRs further trigger nuclear factor-κB (NF-κB) signaling to accelerate its pathogenesis. The NF-κB has an essential role in many biological processes, such as cell survival, immune response, inflammation and development. Therefore, the NF-κB signaling triggered by the TLRs then regulates the transcriptional expression of specific inflammatory mediators to initiate inflammation of the mammary epithelial cells. Thus, any aberrant regulation of NF-κB signaling may lead to many inflammatory diseases, including mastitis. Hence, the inhibiting of NF-κB signaling has potential therapeutic applications in mastitis control strategies. In this review, we highlighted the regulation and function of NF-κB signaling in mastitis. Furthermore, the role of NF-κB signaling for therapeutic purposes in mastitis control has been explored in the current review.

Keywords: mastitis; bovine mammary epithelial cells; inflammatory cytokines; NF-κB signaling; PRRs; TLRs

1. Introduction

Mastitis is the inflammation of the mammary gland, which is associated with pathological changes in udder tissue and decreases in the quantity and quality of milk [1,2]. Based on its duration and symptoms, mastitis might be acute or chronic [3,4]. Udder swelling, reduced milk yield, clots and increase somatic cell counts in milk are the most common clinical signs of mastitis [5]. All these factors are associated with pathogenic invasion, which is followed by the involvement of neutrophils under a specific stimulus. The inflammatory conditions may lead to chronic inflammation if not properly controlled and treated [6,7]. Different types of etiological invading bacterial pathogens are involved in bovine mastitis, of which *Coliforms, Escherichia coli, Streptococci* and *Staphylococcus aureus* are the most common bacteria [8–11]. Gram-negative bacteria, such as *E. coli*, can often cause clinical mastitis, and Gram-positive bacteria, such as *S. aureus*, are involved in subclinical mastitis infection [12–14].

Previous reports have documented that mammary epithelial cells work as the first line of defense of the mammary gland by generating multiple inflammatory cytokines against bacteria invading the epithelial cells [15,16]. Toll-like receptors (TLRs) are pattern recognition receptors (PRRs) expressed by many cell types, including mammary epithelial and immune cells [17]. In addition, it has been reported that innate immune systems recognize pathogens through TLRs [18–20].

The TLRs are distributed on the host cell surface that regulates the initial sensation of infection [21,22]. Every pathogen uses specific receptors on host cells—for example, *S. aureus* uses TLR2 and TLR6 [23], while *E. coli* utilizes TLR2 and TLR4—to transmit their signals inside the cell [21]. This specificity to TLRs depends on the virulent factor of pathogens. The cell wall of *S. aureus* is composed of lipoteichoic acid and peptidoglycan [24], while Gram-negative bacteria, such as *E. coli*, have lipopolysaccharides (LPS) in their cell wall [25]. The binding of pathogenic virulent factors to TLRs leads to the activation of several signaling components, including nuclear factor kappa-light-chain-enhancer of activated B (NF-κB) [26], which is considered one of the key players associated with inflammatory action. Besides, NF-κB signaling has been widely studied for its role in regulation of immunity and inflammation. Keeping in view the versatile functions of NF-κB signaling, the current review has specifically concentrated on summarizing possible research development on the role of NF-κB signaling activation and regulation of immunity and inflammation in bovine mastitis.

2. Materials and Methods

All studies which have discussed the role of NF-κB signaling in mammary gland infection, mainly bovine mastitis, were screened through authentic sources, such as PubMed, ScienceDirect, Web of Science, SpringerLink, Scopus and Google Scholar. The major keywords used for the search of literature were milk production, mastitis, NF-κB signaling, TLRs, MYD88, PPRs, cytokines, *E. coli*- and *S. aureus*-mastitis. The related data published in the English language in well-reputed peer-reviewed journals have been included for discussion in the current review. Furthermore, we excluded all content available in the form of conference abstracts, books, book chapters and unpublished findings.

3. General Regulatory Pattern of NF-κB Signaling

NF-κB is a common term used for inducible dimeric transcription factors. It is composed of a Rel family DNA binding protein which distinguishes common sequence motifs. Mammals express 5 Rel (NF-κB) proteins which are composed of two classes including Rel A (p65), c-Rel and Rel-B proteins which do not need proteolytic processing as the class is composed of NF-κB1 and NF-κB2 genes, encoded for p105 and p100, respectively, which do not require proteolytic processing to synthesize mature p50 and p52 NF-κB proteins [27]. The NF-κB protein was first found in murine B-lymphocytes, but currently, it has been identified in many cell types, including mammary epithelial cells [28]. Different external stimuli, such as tumor necrosis factor Alpha (TNF-α) [29], interleukin 1-beta (IL-1β) [30], LPS and reactive oxygen species (ROS) [31] after attachment with TLRs, activate NF-κB [32]. NF-κB signaling has an essential role in the regulation of immunity and inflammation [33], cell apoptosis, cell survival and proliferation (Figure 1) [34,35].

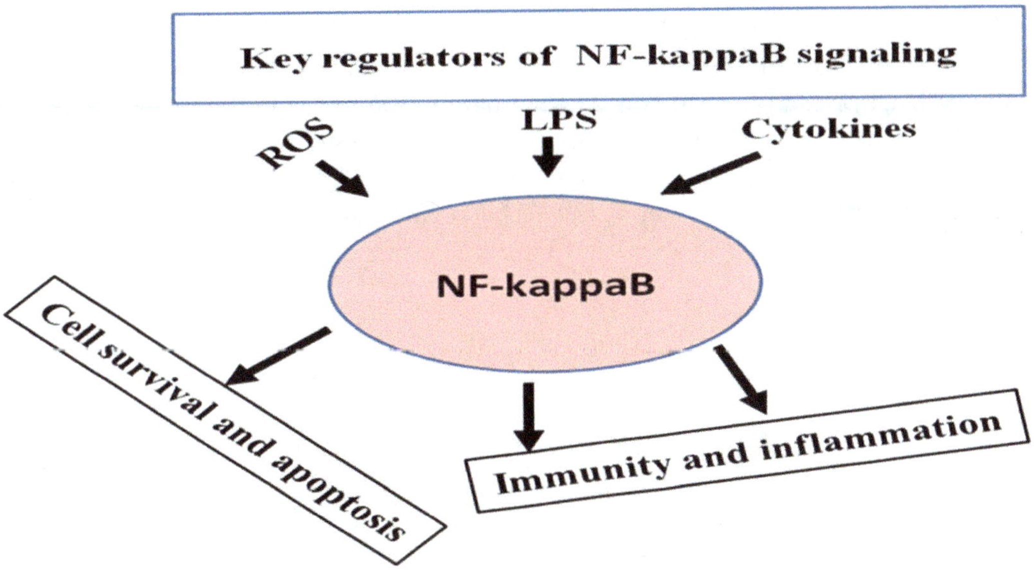

Figure 1. The key inducers of the NF-κB pathway and regulation of immunity, inflammation, cell survival and apoptosis by NF-κB signaling.

In addition, NF-κB signaling plays a vital role in the regulation of inflammatory cytokines, adhesion molecules, chemokines and growth factors involved in mammary gland inflammation [36]. Adhesion molecules are important proteins of tight junctions [37], which are closely related to the link between cell membranes and are required for normal lactation in mammals [38]. Song et al. has shown that LPS disrupt the permeability of the blood–milk barrier by activating the NF-κB signaling pathway. The pro-inflammatory cytokines regulated by the NF-κB signaling pathway promote the process of inflammation and interrupt the integrity of tight junction structures in the mammary epithelial cells [39]. The disruption in the blood–milk barrier has been reported during mastitis, which might be due to damage of the tight junctions responsible for normal lactation [40]. The disruption of tight junctions also may lead to loss of milk which is one of the common signs of mastitis in dairy cattle. Having such a critical role in inflammation and immunity, the NF-κB pathway has been widely targeted in mastitis research [41–46].

4. Role of NF-κB Signaling in Normal Physiology of Mammary Gland Development

A regulated pattern of activation of NF-κB during the various stages of the development of mammary glands has been demonstrated [46]. NF-κB activation rises during pregnancy and decreases during lactation, followed by elevation during the mammary gland involution, again [47,48]. This change in pattern suggests that NF-κB plays a significant role during pregnancy and involution. Mammary gland involution is associated with apoptosis of the secretory alveolar epithelium [49], and NF-κB has been explored to mediate the anti-apoptotic proteins [50]. These findings revealed the role of NF-κB in promoting the survival of epithelial cells [51]. It has been demonstrated that NF-κB activates the two essential lactogenic hormones, namely prolactin and oxytocin [52,53]. In addition to playing a role in the developmental process of normal mammary glands, NF-κB activation was found to be associated with mammary gland infections.

5. Role of NF-κB Signaling in Mastitis

The murine model and bovine reports have shown the link of NF-κB regulation with mastitis [43]. Most of the studies investigated the role of NF-κB in mastitis as a regulator of inflammatory cytokines [54,55]. Considerable losses of milk have been observed during mastitis and mammary gland involution which showed the link of both with the up-regulation of NF-κB during a time of milk loss and mammary gland remodeling.

5.1. *Mechanism of NF-κB Signaling Activation by Bacteria during Mastitis*

LPS, a bacterial virulence factor, interacts with TLRs which are residing on surface mammary epithelial cells [56]. Upon activation, the TLRs further engage myeloid differentiation factor 88 (MyD88) [57] and c-Jun N-terminal kinase (JNK) [58], which triggers NF-κB [32] and mitogen-activated protein kinase (MAPK) signaling. The translocation of NF-κB and MAPK signaling further regulates the production of target inflammatory genes [59–62]. The mechanism of NF-κB signaling activated by *S. aureus* and *E. coli* during mastitis is shown in Figure 2.

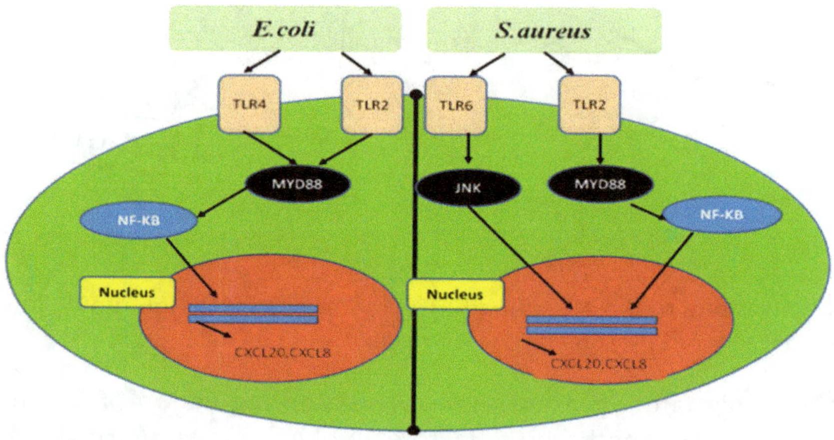

Figure 2. The interactive mechanism of *E. coli* and *S. aureus* with TLR2, TLR4 and TLR6, and the regulation of NF-κB signaling to activate the inflammatory genes.

5.2. *Mechanism of NF-κB Signaling Activation by Inflammatory Cytokines*

Besides *S. aureus* and *E. coli*, various inflammatory cytokines activate NF-κB signaling regulation in mammary epithelial cells. The NF-κB and MAPK pathways activate pro-inflammatory cytokines interleukin 6 (IL-6), IL-1β and TNF-α [63]. Nuclear factor-κB is a nuclear transcription factor that exists in an inactive form in the cytoplasm and is bound to its inhibitor IκB [64,65]. Once activated, the NF-κB unit p65 separates from IκB and translocates from the cytoplasm to the nucleus, where it regulates inflammatory gene expression [66]. The pathogenic message usually causes the liberation of NF-κB from IκB [65]. The regulation of the inflammation through NF-κB by pro-inflammatory cytokines is shown in Figure 3. The promoter of the inflammatory genes contains binding sites for NF-κB, and thus mostly depends on NF-κB for its regulation [67]. It has been reported that active NF-κB complexes cannot be detected in healthy cow milk cells, while the NF-κB elevated level was noticed in the milk cells of cows with acute mastitis. In addition, the activity of NF-κB in milk cells varies from low to high in chronic mastitis [67]. Stimulation of LPS causes mammary epithelial cells to produce cytokines TNF-α, IL-6 and IL-1β [68]. The increased levels of TNF-α, IL-6 and IL-1β have been observed in LPS-infused mammary glands [69]. Furthermore, Blum et al. reported the high level of cytokines (TNF-α, IL-6 and IL-17), somatic cell count (SCC), and up-regulation of TLR4 expression in leukocytes of the milk of an *E. coli*-induced mastitic cow [70]. In the mammary glands, inflammation is associated with an increased level of neutrophil chemo-attractants and the cytokines IL-1ß, IL-6, IL8 and TNF-α [71,72]. The expression level reported for IL8 and TNF-α in *E. coli* induced-mastitis in bovine mammary epithelial cells (BMECs) was much higher than for *S. aureus*, which is due to the weak Lipoteichoic acid (LTA) induction of TNF-α, or inactivation of NF-κB signaling [73]. Boulanger et al. observed that NF-κB was highly associated with the level of the expression of interleukin-8 and granulocyte/macrophage colony-stimulating factors, two NF-κB-dependent cytokines critically linked to the regulation and continuation of neutrophilic inflammation. Altogether, these findings suggested the crucial role of NF-κB in the pathogenesis of mastitis.

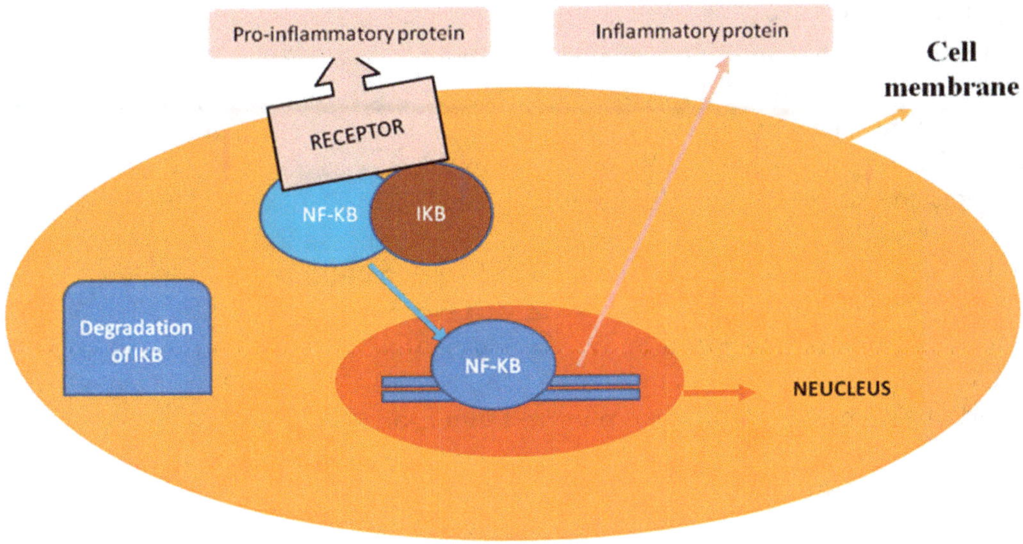

Figure 3. The regulation of the inflammation process by pro-inflammatory cytokines through NF-κB signaling; the cytokines, after attachment with receptors, cause the degradation of IKB from NF-κB. Upon activation, NF-κB directly binds to the promoters of target genes on DNA in the nucleus and regulates the specific inflammatory proteins.

5.3. Bovine Myeloid Differentiation Primary Response 88 (MYD88), NFKBIA and TRAPPC9 Role as a Regulator of Lipopolysaccharide (LPS)-Induced NF-κB Signaling Pathways

MYD88 is the main adopter molecule for TLR2, 4, 5, 7, 8 and 9 signaling [74]. The TLRs, when activated by mastitis-induced bacteria, pass the signal to MYD88, which is considered the critical immune regulator adapter molecule against various pathogens [75,76]. MYD88 acts as the key regulator of NF-κB by causing the degradation of IKB. Wang and his co-authors compared the expression level of MYD88 in healthy and mastitic cows. It was observed that MYD88 expression, which works as a bridge between TLRs and NF-κB, was elevated in mastitic cows compared to healthy ones [69,77,78]. It was noticed in a study that inhibition of MYD88, along with its inhibitor, Pepinh-MYD, significantly reduced the level of NF-κB [63].

Another essential protein is the nuclear factor of kappa light polypeptide gene enhancer in B-cells inhibitor, alpha (NFKBIA), which encodes IκB and is responsible for the negative activation of NF-κB transcription factors. It has been shown in a report that LPS cause the degradation of IκBα; they facilitate the translocation of NF-κB in the nucleus, which in response accelerates the re-synthesis of IκBα [79]. Fang et al. noticed the up-regulation of NFKBIA in *S. aureus*-induced mastitis [80]. The trafficking protein particle complex 9 (TRAPPC9), also called NIK-and-IKK2-binding protein (NIBP), is a key regulator of NF-κB signaling [72,81,82]. An in-vitro study revealed NIBP low expression results in the down-regulation of TNF-α-induced NF-κB [83]. Wang et al. noticed through a genome-wide association study (GWAS) that the mutation in TRAPPC9 is associated with milk SCS [84]. The high expression level of the TRAPPC9 gene was reported in mammary epithelial cells infected with *S. aureus*. Furthermore, it was revealed that the TRAPPC9 gene might be considered a potential marker against mastitis [85]. The above-published studies showed that MYD88, NFKBIA and TRAPPC9 might work as a bridge between cell surface receptors and NF-κB. Thus, any change in these genes may disturb NF-κB signaling, which facilitates the pathogenesis of mastitis.

5.4. NF-κB Regulates the Immunity and Inflammatory Linked Genes during Mastitis

When NF-κB signaling is activated by external stimuli, such as bacteria or cytokines, it starts to regulate the production of inflammatory chemokines (IL-8, CXCL1, CXCL10, etc.), cytokines (IL-6, TNF-α, IFN-gamma and IL-1β), adhesion molecules (ICAM-1 and MMPs), growth factors (CSF) and apoptotic associated genes [76,86,87]. For the site of infection, many proteins are required; these proteins are: adhesion factors, such as ICAM-1 and VCAM-1, which facilitate neutrophil margination, diapedesis and transepithelial migration; chemokines, such as interleukin (IL)-8, which are responsible for chemotactic of neutrophils; IL-1β and TNF-α, which regulate neutrophils [67]. When bacteria enter the teat, the mammary epithelial cells secrete chemokines (CXCL8 and CXCL20) and cytokines (TNF-α and IL-1β). Production of cytokines and chemokines in the milk of the mastitic mammary gland is considered the key player of inflammation [72,88]. The TNF-α and fatty acid synthetase (FAS) mRNA expression was significantly up-regulated in LPS-challenged quarters [89]. A study reported the up-regulation of CXCL8 and TNF-α in *E. coli* induced mastitis in mammary epithelial cells [88]. In addition, the high expression of CXCL10, CCL2, CCL5 *and* CCL20 was noticed in bovine mammary epithelial cells in *E. coli* induced mastitis, which is essential for the recruitment of leucocytes [90]. The expression levels of IL-6, complement factor 3 (C3), NFKBIA and MMP9 were also elevated during mammary gland infection [90]. It has been reported that monocytes, natural killer cells and activated lymphocytes are majorly regulated by the chemokines CXCL10 and CCL5 [91]. Apart from the above functions, CXCL10 directs the recruitment and activation of neutrophils towards LPS-infection spots in mice and humans [83,92,93]. In addition, CXCL10 was reported as a highly expressed gene in response to *E. coli* infection in mammary glands [94]. The levels of CXCL10 and ICAM1 were noticed to be significantly elevated in the *S. aureus*-mastitic mammary glands of cows [95]. Similarly, the high expression of CCl5 has also reported in *E. coli*-induced mastitis in BMECs [96]. The expression levels of CXCL8, IL6 and CSF3 were higher in *S. aureus* challenged BMECs [80]. Additionally, many other immunity and inflammatory associated genes, such as SAA3, CCL5, C3 and CSF3, were also documented in mastitis-infected mammary glands [69]. Furthermore, the high expressions of CXCL10, IL6, CXCL8, IFN-gamma and IL-1β induced by LPS in BMECs are able to regulate inflammation [97]. It has been demonstrated in previous reports that inflammatory cytokines and chemokines create protection against foreign invading pathogens in bovine mammary glands, by increasing the movement of leucocytes from the blood into the mammary tissue [98]. Similarly, a study reported the protecting role of IL-1β by recruiting neutrophils into the mammary gland [99].

5.5. *Research Progress on Target of NF-κB Signaling as a Therapeutic in Mastitis Control*

It is well known that TLRs, upon recognition of external stimuli, activate NF-κB regulation to produce inflammatory linked genes to eliminate the cause of infection in mammary epithelial cells. TLR4, a pro-inflammatory cytokine, and LPS, a component of the cell wall of bacteria, are common inducers of NF-κB signaling. The LPS-induced inflammation in mammary epithelial cells causes the up-regulation of TLR4 [100,101]. Recently, NF-κB signaling is being widely targeted as a therapeutic choice against mastitis resistance. A study proved, experimentally, that selenium restricts *S. aureus*-induced mastitis through inhibition of the MAPK and NF-κB pathways and TLR2 [102]. Cytokines, an important group of inflammatory mediators, play a major role in the process of inflammation [103]. Stimulation by LPS causes mammary epithelial cells to produce the cytokines TNF-α, IL-6 and IL-1β [60]. Increased levels of TNF-α, IL-6 and IL-1β have been observed in LPS-infused mammary glands. Similarly, Akhter et al. [104] noticed the up-regulation of pro-inflammatory cytokines in *S. aureus*-induced mammary epithelial cells. Further, they proved that the expression levels of genes associated with TLR2/TLR4-mediated NF-κB/MAPKs pathways were higher in *S. aureus*-infected mammary epithelial cells. The excessive expression of pro-inflammatory IL1β may lead to pathological conditions [105]. Dai et al. noticed that methionine and arginine attenuated the proinflammatory action by preventing the regulation of NF-κB. Furthermore, methionine and arginine down-regulated the levels of TLR4 and IL1β in LPS-induced mastitis, which caused the excessive regulation of inflammatory changes, and thus damaged the cells [106]. Taken together, it has been concluded here that methionine and arginine, being blockers of NF-κB, can be considered as prophylactic agents of mastitis.

Exogenous hydrogen sulfide has the ability to suppress inflammatory cytokine production, ROS [107–109], and promotes anti-inflammatory proteins [110]. The high level of ROS is associated with the imbalance between cellular redox states and oxidative stress, which has a significant role in the promotion of inflammation [111]. It was noticed that LPS alone diminished cell viability and caused inflammatory changes in mammary epithelial cells. However, it was found that the hydrogen sulfide (H2S) combined with LPS restored the viability of the cells [112]. Sun et al. revealed that H2S, after entry into the cells, first blocked the TLR4 and ROS, and thereby no signal was given for NF-κB to produce a high level of inflammatory proteins in mammary epithelial cells [113]. In addition, the mRNA expression of TNF-α, IL-1β, IL-8 and IL-6 was also very low in H2S-treated mammary epithelial cells.

Morin has anti-inflammatory properties [114] and inhibits the release of the inflammatory cytokines IL-6 and IL-8 and tumor necrosis factor (TNF) from mast cells [115]. It was experimentally proved that morin is associated with inhibition of TNF-α, IL-6 and IL-1β in LPS-induced bovine mammary epithelial cells (bMECs). To suppress the level of cytokines, morin down-regulates the levels of MAPK and NF-κB pathways in LPS-induced mammary epithelial cells [78]. NLRP3 inflammasome is the key regulator of IL-1β, while a recent study noticed that morin significantly down-regulated the level of IL-1β [116] in LPS-induced bovine mammary epithelial cells by suppression of NF-κB and nucleotide-binding domain, leucine-rich repeat-containing family, pyrin domain containing 3 (NLRP3) inflammasome [117]. Furthermore, it has been noticed that morin also maintained the integrity of the tight junction from the action of the inflammatory cytokines regulated by NF-κB [63]. Likewise, polydatin has anti-inflammatory efficiency and can be used to control *S. aureus*-induced mastitis. The most in-depth mechanism showed that polydatin decreased the expression of TLR2 and MyD88, which further suppressed the level of NF-κB in mammary epithelial cells of *S. aureus*- induced mastitis [60].

Tea tree oil (TTO) is an essential oil which has antibacterial and anti-inflammatory properties and promotes the movement of polymorphonuclear leukocytes towards the infection. TTO also inhibits NFKBIA and TNF-α [118]. In addition, TTO act as an inhibitor of the NF-κB pathway, which is essential for the regulation of immunity and inflammatory responses in mammary glands. Nucleotide-binding oligomerization domain (NOD) is a type of PRR that plays an important role in the regulation of innate immunity [119]. Recently, it was documented that by blocking NOD1/NF-κB signaling, LPS stimulation reduced neutrophil migration and phagocytic killing ability. Further, it was proved that the activation of NOD1/NF-κB in vitro restricted the action of LPS by promoting the functional capacity of neutrophil [60]. Chlorogenic acid has anti-inflammatory and antibacterial effects [120,121]. A study reported that chlorogenic acid inhibits cytokine production in LPS-stimulated RAW264.7 cells by suppressing the phosphorylation of NF-κB [122]. Similarly, chlorogenic acid was noticed to reduce the level of cytokines followed by inhibition of TLR4 and phosphorylation of NF-κB in LPS-induced mastitic mammary epithelial cells [123]. Thymol was found to be very effective in mastitis treatment. The mechanism for the association of thymol was tested in BMECs. The western blot result showed that thymol treatment significantly inhibited the production of IL-6 and TNF-α, followed by suppression of the NF-κB pathway [124]. In Table 1, we summarized those studies which targeted the NF-κB signaling to control mastitis.

Table 1. Chemicals and their anti-inflammatory effect in mastitis by suppression NF-κB signaling.

Authors	Agent	Function	Targets
Sun et al. [113]	H2S		Block TLR4, ROS, NF-κB
Garcia et al. [125]	Citrus oils	Antibacterial	Down-regulate TLR2, NFKBIA, IL8, TNF-α
Wang et al. [78]	Morin	Anti-inflammatory	Inhibit IL-6, TNF-α, IL-1β, suppress NF-κB phosphorylation
Li et al. [126]	8-Methoxypsoralen	Anti-inflammatory	Inhibit IL-6, TNF-α, IL-8, IL-1β, suppress NF-κB phosphorylation
Chen et al. [36]	Nuciferine	Anti-inflammatory	Inhibit TLR4, TNF-α, IL-1β, suppress NF-κB phosphorylation
Yang et al. [127]	Oxymatrine	Anti-inflammatory	Suppress NF-κB phosphorylation
Ershun et al. [128]	Cepharanthine	Anti-inflammatory	Inhibit IL6, TNF-α, IL-1β, suppress NF-κB phosphorylation
Su et al. [129]	Rutin		Decrease level of IL-1β, IL-6, and TNF-α, suppress NF-κB phosphorylation
Liu et al. [112]	Sodium houttuyfonate	Antinflammatory	Inhibit NF-κB phosphorylation
Li et al. [130]	Emodin ameliorates	Anti-inflammatory, antibacterial	Decrease level of IL-1β, IL-6, and TNF-α, suppress NF-κB phosphorylation
Hu et al. [42]	Cynatratoside-C from Cynanchum atratum	Anti-inflammatory	Suppress TLR4, inhibit NF-κB phosphorylation
He et al. [131]	Docosahexaenoic acid	Anti-inflammatory	Decrease level of IL-1β, IL-6, and TNF-α, suppress NF-κB phosphorylation
He et al. [132]	Baicalein	Anti-inflammatory	Suppress TLR4, inhibit NF-κB phosphorylation

From the above discussion, it has been cleared that NF-κB signaling plays a role of backbone in the pathogenesis of mastitis by promoting cytokine production. Thus, by targeting NF-κB, mastitis can be effectively controlled [124].

6. Conclusions

Overall, the current review, based on published studies, revealed that activation of NF-κB resulted in decreased of milk and apoptotic signaling, which could be minimized through selective modulation of NF-κB signals. Furthermore, the review suggested that NF-κB is a vital regulator of milk loss during mammary gland involution and infection, and recognized the NF-κB signaling pathway as a possible target for preventing mastitis induced milk loss in dairy cattle. In addition, based on published literature, we concluded that TLR4, IL-1β, IL-6, TNF-α and MYD88 are key players in NF-κB signaling and also have an essential role in mastitis development. From the literature studies, it was revealed that *S. aureus* and *E. coli*, after attachment with TLRs, used NF-κB pathway for pathogenesis. Thus, the utilization of NF-κB as a therapeutic target in mastitis control showed successful outcomes. In addition, TLR4, IL-1β, IL-6, TNF-α, MYD88 and NF-κB might be a useful addition as markers in mastitis control strategies.

Author Contributions: Conceptualization, M.Z.K. and Z.C.; writing—original draft preparation, M.Z.K. and Z.C.; editing and technical review, A.K., J.M., Y.M., T.C., D.S., J.X. and Z.C.; visualization, Z.C.; supervision, Z.C. All authors have read and agreed to the published version of the manuscript.

Acknowledgments: We acknowledge the financial support of the National Key Research and Development Program of China (2018YFD0501600). We also acknowledge the China Agricultural University, Beijing, China, for providing us with an environment of learning. Without this platform, the completion of this work would not have been an easy task.

References

1. Gomes, F.; Henriques, M. Control of Bovine Mastitis: Old and Recent Therapeutic Approaches. *Curr. Microbiol.* **2016**, *72*, 377–382. [CrossRef] [PubMed]
2. Zhao, X.; Lacasse, P. Mammary tissue damage during bovine mastitis: Causes and control. *J. Anim. Sci.* **2008**, *86*, 57–65. [CrossRef] [PubMed]
3. Abebe, R.; Hatiya, H.; Abera, M.; Megersa, B.; Asmare, K. Bovine mastitis: Prevalence, risk factors and isolation of Staphylococcus aureus in dairy herds at Hawassa milk shed, South Ethiopia. *BMC Vet. Res.* **2016**, *12*, 270. [CrossRef] [PubMed]
4. Heikkilä, A.M.; Liski, E.; Pyörälä, S.; Taponen, S. Pathogen-specific production losses in bovine mastitis. *J. Dairy Sci.* **2018**, *101*, 9493–9504. [CrossRef] [PubMed]
5. Skarbye, A.P.; Krogh, M.A.; Sørensen, J.T. The effect of individual quarter dry-off in management of subclinical mastitis on udder condition and milk production in organic dairy herds: A randomized field trial. *J. Dairy Sci.* **2018**, *101*, 11186–11198. [CrossRef] [PubMed]
6. Havixbeck, J.J.; Rieger, A.M.; Wong, M.E.; Hodgkinson, J.W.; Barreda, D.R. Neutrophil contributions to the induction and regulation of the acute inflammatory response in teleost fish. *J. Leukoc. Biol.* **2016**, *99*, 241–252. [CrossRef] [PubMed]
7. Pisanu, S.; Cubeddu, T.; Pagnozzi, D.; Rocca, S.; Cacciotto, C.; Alberti, A.; Marogna, G.; Uzzau, S.; Addis, M.F. Neutrophil extracellular traps in sheep mastitis. *Vet. Res.* **2015**, *46*, 59. [CrossRef]
8. Lavon, Y.; Leitner, G.; Kressel, Y.; Ezra, E.; Wolfenson, D. Comparing effects of bovine Streptococcus and Escherichia coli mastitis on impaired reproductive performance. *J. Dairy Sci.* **2019**, *102*, 10587–10598. [CrossRef]
9. Poutrel, B.; Bareille, S.; Lequeux, G.; Leboeuf, F. Prevalence of Mastitis Pathogens in France: Antimicrobial Susceptibility of Staphylococcus aureus, Streptococcus uberis and Escherichia coli. *J. Vet. Sci. Technol.* **2018**, *9*, 2. [CrossRef]
10. Biswas, S.; Chakravarti, S.; Barui, A. Emergence of coagulase positive methicillin resistant Staphylococcus Aureus isolated from buffalo mastitis milk samples. *Explor. Anim. Med. Res.* **2018**, *8*, 190–196.

11. Li, T.; Lu, H.; Wang, X.; Gao, Q.; Dai, Y.; Shang, J.; Li, M. Molecular characteristics of Staphylococcus aureus causing bovine mastitis between 2014 and 2015. *Front. Cell. Infect. Microbiol.* **2017**, *7*, 127. [CrossRef] [PubMed]
12. Jensen, K.; Günther, J.; Talbot, R.; Petzl, W.; Zerbe, H.; Schuberth, H.J.; Seyfert, H.M.; Glass, E.J. Escherichia coli- and Staphylococcus aureus-induced mastitis differentially modulate transcriptional responses in neighbouring uninfected bovine mammary gland quarters. *BMC Genom.* **2013**, *14*, 36. [CrossRef] [PubMed]
13. Jing, X.Q.; Zhao, Y.Q.; Shang, C.C.; Yao, Y.L.; Tian, T.T.; Li, J.; Chen, D.K. Dynamics of cytokines associated with IL-17 producing cells in serum and milk in mastitis of experimental challenging with Staphylococcus aureus and Escherichia coli in dairy goats. *J. Anim. Vet. Adv.* **2012**, *11*, 475–479.
14. Pumipuntu, N.; Kulpeanprasit, S.; Santajit, S.; Tunyong, W.; Kong-ngoen, T.; Hinthong, W.; Indrawattana, N. Screening method for Staphylococcus aureus identification in subclinical bovine mastitis from dairy farms. *Vet. World* **2017**, *10*, 721–726. [CrossRef]
15. Wellnitz, O.; Bruckmaier, R.M. The innate immune response of the bovine mammary gland to bacterial infection. *Vet. J.* **2012**, *192*, 148–152. [CrossRef]
16. Brenaut, P.; Lefèvre, L.; Rau, A.; Laloë, D.; Pisoni, G.; Moroni, P.; Bevilacqua, C.; Martin, P. Contribution of mammary epithelial cells to the immune response during early stages of a bacterial infection to Staphylococcus aureus. *Vet. Res.* **2014**, *45*, 16. [CrossRef]
17. Kumar, H.; Kawai, T.; Akira, S. Pathogen recognition by the innate immune system. *Int. Rev. Immunol.* **2011**, *30*, 16–34. [CrossRef]
18. Albiger, B.; Dahlberg, S.; Henriques-Normark, B.; Normark, S. Role of the innate immune system in host defence against bacterial infections: Focus on the Toll-like receptors. *J. Intern. Med.* **2007**, *261*, 511–528. [CrossRef]
19. Akira, S.; Uematsu, S.; Takeuchi, O. Pathogen recognition and innate immunity. *Cell* **2006**, *124*, 783–801. [CrossRef]
20. Kawai, T.; Akira, S. The roles of TLRs, RLRs and NLRs in pathogen recognition. *Int. Immunol.* **2009**, *21*, 317–337. [CrossRef]
21. Bhattarai, D.; Worku, T.; Dad, R.; Rehman, Z.U.; Gong, X.; Zhang, S. Mechanism of pattern recognition receptors (PRRs) and host pathogen interplay in bovine mastitis. *Microb. Pathog.* **2018**, *120*, 64–70. [CrossRef] [PubMed]
22. Takeuchi, O.; Akira, S. Pattern Recognition Receptors and Inflammation. *Cell* **2010**, *140*, 805–820. [CrossRef] [PubMed]
23. Ren, C.; Zhang, Q.; Haan, B.J.; De Zhang, H.; Faas, M.M. Identification of TLR2 / TLR6 signalling lactic acid bacteria for supporting immune regulation. *Sci. Rep.* **2016**, *6*, 1–12. [CrossRef] [PubMed]
24. Guo, W.; Liu, B.; Hu, G.; Kan, X.; Li, Y.; Gong, Q.; Xu, D.; Ma, H.; Cao, Y.; Huang, B.; et al. Vanillin protects the blood–milk barrier and inhibits the inflammatory response in LPS-induced mastitis in mice. *Toxicol. Appl. Pharmacol.* **2019**, *365*, 9–18. [CrossRef]
25. Doyle, S.L.; O'Neill, L.A.J. Toll-like receptors: From the discovery of NF-κB to new insights into transcriptional regulations in innate immunity. *Biochem. Pharmacol.* **2006**, *72*, 1102–1113. [CrossRef]
26. Liu, C.Y.; Gao, X.X.; Chen, L.; You, Q.X. Rapamycin suppresses Abeta25–35- or LPSinduced neuronal inflammation via modulation of NF-kappaB signaling. *Neuroscience* **2017**, *355*, 188–199. [CrossRef]
27. Ghosh, S.; May, M.J.; Kopp, E.B. NF-kB and Rel proteins: Evolutionary conserved mediators of the immune response. *Annu. Rev. Immunol.* **1998**, *16*, 225–260. [CrossRef]
28. Tripathi, P.; Aggarwal, A. NF-kB transcription factor: A key player in the generation of immune response. *Curr. Sci.* **2006**, *90*, 25.
29. Fitzgerald, D.C.; Meade, K.G.; McEvoy, A.N.; Lillis, L.; Murphy, E.P.; MacHugh, D.E.; Baird, A.W. Tumour necrosis factor-α (TNF-α) increases nuclear factor κB (NFκB) activity in and interleukin-8 (IL-8) release from bovine mammary epithelial cells. *Vet. Immunol. Immunopathol.* **2007**, *116*, 59–68. [CrossRef]
30. Renard, P.; Zachary, M.D.; Bougelet, C.; Mirault, M.E.; Haegeman, G.; Remacle, J.; Raes, M. Effects of antioxidant enzyme modulations on interleukin-1-induced nuclear factor kappa B activation. *Biochem. Pharmacol.* **1997**, *53*, 149–160. [CrossRef]
31. Chandel, N.S.; Trzyna, W.C.; McClintock, D.S.; Schumacker, P.T. Role of Oxidants in NF-κB Activation and TNF-α Gene Transcription Induced by Hypoxia and Endotoxin. *J. Immunol.* **2000**, *165*, 1013–1021. [CrossRef] [PubMed]

32. Oliveira-Nascimento, L.; Massari, P.; Wetzler, L.M. The Role of TLR2 in Infection and Immunity. *Front. Immunol.* **2012**, *18*, 3–79. [CrossRef] [PubMed]
33. Ghosh, S.; Hayden, M.S. New regulators of NF-κB in inflammation. *Nat. Rev. Immunol.* **2008**, *8*, 837–848. [CrossRef] [PubMed]
34. Oeckinghaus, A.; Ghosh, S. The NF-kappaB family of transcription factors and its regulation. *Cold Spring Harb. Perspect. Biol.* **2009**, *1*, a000034. [CrossRef]
35. Fu, Z.H.; Liu, S.Q.; Qin, M.B.; Huang, J.A.; Xu, C.Y.; Wu, W.H.; Zhu, L.Y.; Qin, N.; Lai, M.Y. NIK- and IKKβ-binding protein contributes to gastric cancer chemoresistance by promoting epithelial-mesenchymal transition through the NF-κB signaling pathway. *Oncol. Rep.* **2018**, *39*, 2721–2730. [CrossRef]
36. Chen, X.; Zheng, X.; Zhang, M.; Yin, H.; Jiang, K.; Wu, H.; Dai, A.; Yang, S. Nuciferine alleviates LPS-induced mastitis in mice via suppressing the TLR4-NF-κB signaling pathway. *Inflamm. Res.* **2018**, *67*, 903–911. [CrossRef]
37. Stelwagen, K.; Singh, K. The role of tight junctions in mammary gland function. *J. Mammary Gland Biol. Neoplasia* **2014**, *19*, 131–138. [CrossRef]
38. Quesnell, R.R.; Erickson, J.; Schultz, D.B. Apical electrolyte concentration modulates barrier function and tight junction protein localization in bovine mammary epithelium. *Am. J. Physiol. Cell. Physiol.* **2007**, *292*, C305–C318. [CrossRef]
39. Song, X.; Zhang, W.; Wang, T.; Jiang, H.; Zhang, Z.; Fu, Y.; Yang, Z.Y.; Cao, Y.; Zhang, N. Geniposide plays an anti-inflammatory role via regulating TLR4 and downstream signaling pathways in lipopolysaccharide-induced mastitis in mice. *Inflammation* **2014**, *37*, 1588–1598. [CrossRef]
40. Guo, W.; Liu, B.; Yin, Y.; Kan, X.; Gong, Q.; Li, Y.; Cao, Y.; Wang, J.; Xu, D.; Ma, H.; et al. Licochalcone A protects the blood-milk barrier integrity and relieves the inflammatory response in LPS-induced mastitis. *Front. Immunol.* **2019**, *10*, 287. [CrossRef]
41. Glynn, D.J.; Hutchinson, M.R.; Ingman, W.V. Toll-Like Receptor 4 Regulates Lipopolysaccharide-Induced Inflammation and Lactation Insufficiency in a Mouse Model of Mastitis1. *Biol. Reprod.* **2014**, *90*, 1–11. [CrossRef] [PubMed]
42. Hu, G.; Hong, D.; Zhang, T.; Duan, H.; Wei, P.; Guo, X.; Mu, X. Cynatratoside-C from Cynanchum atratum displays anti-inflammatory effect via suppressing TLR4 mediated NF-κB and MAPK signaling pathways in LPS-induced mastitis in mice. *Chem. Biol. Interact.* **2018**, *279*, 187–195. [CrossRef]
43. Notebaert, S.; Carlsen, H.; Janssen, D.; Vandenabeele, P.; Blomhoff, R.; Meyer, E. In vivo imaging of NF-κB activity during Escherichia coli-induced mammary gland infection. *Cell. Microbiol.* **2008**, *10*, 1249–1258. [CrossRef] [PubMed]
44. Wu, J.; Li, L.; Sun, Y.; Huang, S.; Tang, J.; Yu, P.; Wang, G. Altered Molecular Expression of the TLR4 / NF- κ B Signaling Pathway in Mammary Tissue of Chinese Holstein Cattle with Mastitis. *PLoS ONE* **2015**, *10*, 1–15. [CrossRef] [PubMed]
45. Xiao, H.B.; Wang, C.R.; Liu, Z.K.; Wang, J.Y. LPS induces pro-inflammatory response in mastitis mice and mammary epithelial cells: Possible involvement of NF-κB signaling and OPN. *Pathol. Biol.* **2015**, *63*, 11–16. [CrossRef]
46. Connelly, L.; Barham, W.; Pigg, R.; Saint-Jean, L.; Sherrill, T.; Cheng, D.S.; Chodosh, L.A.; Blackwell, T.S.; Yull, F.E. Activation of nuclear factor kappa B in mammary epithelium promotes milk loss during mammary development and infection. *J. Cell. Physiol.* **2010**, *222*, 73–81. [CrossRef] [PubMed]
47. Brantley, D.M.; Chen, C.L.; Muraoka, R.S.; Bushdid, P.B.; Bradberry, J.L.; Kittrell, F.; Medina, D.; Matrisian, L.M.; Kerr, L.D.; Yull, F.E. Nuclear factor-kappaB (NF-kappaB) regulates proliferation and branching in mouse mammary epithelium. *Mol. Biol. Cell.* **2001**, *12*, 1445–1455. [CrossRef]
48. Brantley, D.M.; Yull, F.E.; Muraoka, R.S.; Hicks, D.J.; Cook, C.M.; Kerr, L.D. Dynamic expression and activity of NF-kappaB during post-natal mammary gland morphogenesis. *Mech. Dev.* **2000**, *97*, 149–155. [CrossRef]
49. Baxter, F.O.; Neoh, K.; Tevendale, M.C. The beginning of the end: Death signaling in early involution. *J. Mammary. Gland Biol. Neoplasia.* **2007**, *12*, 3–13. [CrossRef]
50. Karin, M.; Ben-Neriah, Y. Phosphorylation meets ubiquitination: The control of NF-[kappa]B activity. *Annu. Rev. Immunol.* **2000**, *18*, 621–663. [CrossRef]
51. Clarkson, R.W.; Heeley, J.L.; Chapman, R.; Aillet, F.; Hay, R.T.; Wyllie, A.; Watson, C.J. NF-kappaB inhibits apoptosis in murine mammary epithelia. *J. Biol. Chem.* **2000**, *275*, 12737–12742. [CrossRef] [PubMed]

52. Friedrichsen, S.; Harper, C.V.; Semprini, S.; Wilding, M.; Adamson, A.; Spiller, D.G.; Nelson, G.; Mullins, J.J.; White, M.R.H.; Davis, J.R.E. Tumor Necrosis Factor-α Activates the Human Prolactin Gene Promoter via Nuclear Factor-κB Signaling. *Endocrinology* **2006**, *147*, 773–781. [CrossRef] [PubMed]
53. Terzidou, V.; Lee, Y.; Lindstrom, T.; Johnson, M.; Thornton, S.; Phillip, R.B. Regulation of the human oxytocin receptor by nuclear factor-kB and CCAAT/enhancer-binding protein-b. *J. Clin. Endocrinol. Metab.* **2006**, *91*, 2317–2326. [CrossRef] [PubMed]
54. Boutet, P.; Sulon, J.; Closset, R.; Detilleux, J.; Beckers, J.F.; Bureau, F.; Lekeux, P. Prolactin-induced activation of nuclear factor kappaB in bovine mammary epithelial cells: Role in chronic mastitis. *J. Dairy Sci.* **2007**, *90*, 155–164. [CrossRef]
55. Notebaert, S.; Demon, D.; Vanden Berghe, T.; Vandenabeele, P.; Meyer, E. Inflammatory mediators in Escherichia coli-induced mastitis in mice. *Comp. Immunol. Microbiol. Infect. Dis.* **2008**, *31*, 551–565. [CrossRef]
56. Atabai, K.; Matthay, M.A. The pulmonary physician in critical care 5: Acute lung injury and the acute respiratory distress syndrome: Definitions and epidemiology. *Thorax* **2002**, *57*, 452–458. [CrossRef]
57. Barbalat, R.; Lau, L.; Locksley, R.M.; Barton, G.M. Toll-like receptor 2 on inflammatory monocytes induces type i interferon in response to viral but not bacterial ligands. *Nat. Immunol.* **2009**, *10*, 1200–1209. [CrossRef]
58. Fu, Y.; Gao, R.; Cao, Y.; Guo, M.; Wei, Z.; Zhou, E.; Li, Y.; Yao, M.; Yang, Z.; Zhang, N. Curcumin attenuates inflammatory responses by suppressing TLR4-mediated NF-κB signaling pathway in lipopolysaccharide-induced mastitis in mice. *Int. Immunopharmacol.* **2014**, *20*, 54–58. [CrossRef]
59. Guo, Y.F.; Xu, N.N.; Sun, W.; Zhao, Y.; Li, C.Y.; Guo, M.Y. Luteolin reduces inflammation in Staphylococcus aureus-induced mastitis by inhibiting NF-kB activation and MMPs expression. *Oncotarget* **2017**, *8*, 28481–28493. [CrossRef]
60. Jiang, K.F.; Zhao, G.; Deng, G.Z.; Wu, H.C.; Yin, N.N.; Chen, X.Y.; Qiu, C.W.; Peng, X.L. Polydatin ameliorates Staphylococcus aureus-induced mastitis in mice via inhibiting TLR2-mediated activation of the p38 MAPK/NF-κB pathway. *Acta Pharmacol. Sin.* **2017**, *38*, 211–222. [CrossRef]
61. Li, D.; Fu, Y.; Zhang, W.; Su, G.; Liu, B.; Guo, M.; Li, F.; Liang, D.; Liu, Z.; Zhang, X.; et al. Salidroside attenuates inflammatory responses by suppressing nuclear factor-kappaB and mitogen activated protein kinases activation in lipopolysaccharide-induced mastitis in mice. *Inflamm. Res.* **2013**, *62*, 9–15. [CrossRef] [PubMed]
62. Watters, T.M.; Kenny, E.F.; O'Neill, L.A. Structure, function and regulation of the Toll/IL-1 receptor adaptor proteins. *Immunol. Cell Biol.* **2007**, *85*, 411–41910. [CrossRef] [PubMed]
63. Jiang, A.; Zhang, Y.; Zhang, X.; Wu, D.; Liu, Z.; Li, S.; Yang, Z. Morin alleviates LPS-induced mastitis by inhibiting the PI3K/AKT, MAPK, NF-κB and NLRP3 signaling pathway and protecting the integrity of blood-milk barrier. *Int. Immunopharmacol.* **2020**, *78*, 105972. [CrossRef] [PubMed]
64. Baeuerle, P.A.; Baichwal, V.R. NF-κB as a frequent target for immunosuppressive and anti-inflammatory molecules. *Adv. Immunol.* **1997**, *65*, 111–137.
65. Scheidereit, C. IkappaB kinase complexes: Gateways to NF-kappaB activation and transcription. *Oncogene* **2006**, *25*, 6685–6705. [CrossRef]
66. Hoshino, K.; Takeuchi, O.; Kawai, T.; Sanjo, H.; Ogawa, T.; Takeda, Y.; Takeda, K.; Akira, S. Cutting edge: Toll-like receptor 4 (TLR4)-deficient mice are hyporesponsive to lipopolysaccharide: Evidence for TLR4 as the Lps gene product. *J. Immunol.* **1999**, *162*, 3749–3752.
67. Boulanger, D.; Bureau, F.; Mélotte, D.; Mainil, J.; Lekeux, P. Increased nuclear factor κB activity in milk cells of mastitis-affected cows. *J. Dairy Sci.* **2003**, *86*, 1259–1267. [CrossRef]
68. Wellnitz, O.; Kerr, D.E. Cryopreserved bovine mammary cells to model epithelial response to infection. *Vet. Immunol. Immunopathol.* **2004**, *101*, 191–202. [CrossRef]
69. Wang, X.G.; Ju, Z.H.; Hou, M.H.; Jiang, Q.; Yang, C.H.; Zhang, Y.; Sun, Y.; Li, R.L.; Wang, C.F.; Zhong, J.F.; et al. Correction: Deciphering Transcriptome and Complex Alternative Splicing Transcripts in Mammary Gland Tissues from Cows Naturally Infected with Staphylococcus aureus Mastitis. *PLoS ONE* **2016**, *11*, e0167666. [CrossRef]
70. Blum, S.E.; Heller, E.D.; Jacoby, S.; Krifucks, O.; Leitner, G. Comparison of the immune responses associated with experimental bovine mastitis caused by different strains of Escherichia coli. *J. Dairy Res.* **2017**, *84*, 190–197. [CrossRef]

71. Porcherie, A.; Cunha, P.; Trotereau, A.; Roussel, P.; Gilbert, F.B.; Rainard, P.; Germon, P. Repertoire of Escherichia coli agonists sensed by innate immunity receptors of the bovine udder and mammary epithelial cells. *Vet. Res.* **2012**, *43*, 14. [CrossRef] [PubMed]
72. Riollet, C.; Rainard, P.; Poutrel, B. Differential induction of complement fragment C5a and inflammatory cytokines during intramammary infections with Escherichia coli and Staphylococcus aureus. *Clin. Diagn. Lab. Immunol.* **2000**, *7*, 161–167. [CrossRef] [PubMed]
73. Yang, W.; Zerbe, H.; Petzl, W.; Brunner, R.M.; Günther, J.; Draing, C.; von Aulock, S.; Schuberth, H.J.; Seyfert, H.M. Bovine TLR2 and TLR4 properly transduce signals from Staphylococcus aureus and E. coli, but S. aureus fails to both activate NF-κB in mammary epithelial cells and to quickly induce TNFα and interleukin-8 (CXCL8) expression in the udder. *Mol. Immunol.* **2008**, *45*, 1385–1397. [CrossRef]
74. Takeda, K.; Akira, S. TLR signaling pathways. *Semin. Immunol.* **2004**, *16*, 3–9. [CrossRef]
75. O'Neill, L.A.; Bowie, A.G. The family of five: TIR-domain-containing adaptors in Toll-like receptor signalling. *Nat. Rev. Immunol.* **2007**, *7*, 353–364. [CrossRef] [PubMed]
76. Takeuchi, O.; Akira, S. Toll-like receptors; their physiological role and signal transduction system. *Int. Immunopharmacol.* **2001**, *1*, 625–635. [CrossRef]
77. Cates, E.A.; Connor, E.E.; Mosser, D.M.; Bannerman, D.D. Functional characterization of bovine TIRAP and MyD88 in mediating bacterial lipopolysaccharide-induced endothelial NF-κB activation and apoptosis. *Comp. Immunol. Microbiol. Infect. Dis.* **2009**, *32*, 477–490. [CrossRef]
78. Wang, J.; Guo, C.; Wei, Z.; He, X.; Kou, J.; Zhou, E.; Yang, Z.; Fu, Y. Morin suppresses inflammatory cytokine expression by downregulation of nuclear factorkappaB and mitogen-activated protein kinase (MAPK) signaling pathways in lipopolysaccharide-stimulated primary bovine mammary epithelial cells. *J. Dairy. Sci.* **2016**, *99*, 3016–3022. [CrossRef]
79. Vallabhapurapu, S.; Karin, M. Regulation and Function of NF-κB Transcription Factors in the Immune System. *Annu. Rev. Immunol.* **2009**, *27*, 693–733. [CrossRef]
80. Fang, L.; Hou, Y.; An, J.; Li, B.; Song, M.; Wang, X.; Sørensen, P.; Dong, Y.; Liu, C.; Wang, Y.; et al. Genome-wide transcriptional and post-transcriptional regulation of innate immune and defense responses of bovine mammary gland to Staphylococcus aureus. *Front. Cell. Infect. Microbiol.* **2016**, *6*, 193. [CrossRef]
81. Bodnar, B.; DeGruttola, A.; Zhu, Y.; Lin, Y.; Zhang, Y.; Mo, X.; Hu, W. Emerging role of NIK/IKK2-binding protein (NIBP)/trafficking protein particle complex 9 (TRAPPC9) in nervous system diseases. *Transl. Res.* **2020**, *224*, 55–70. [CrossRef]
82. Mir, A.; Kaufman, L.; Noor, A.; Motazacker, M.M.; Jamil, T.; Azam, M.; Kahrizi, K.; Rafiq, M.A.; Weksberg, R.; Nasr, T.; et al. Identification of Mutations in TRAPPC9, which Encodes the NIK- and IKK-β-Binding Protein, in Nonsyndromic Autosomal-Recessive Mental Retardation. *Am. J. Hum. Genet.* **2009**, *85*, 909–915. [CrossRef] [PubMed]
83. Qin, M.; Zhang, J.; Xu, C.; Peng, P.; Tan, L.; Liu, S.; Huang, J. Knockdown of NIK and IKKβ-binding protein (NIBP) reduces colorectal cancer metastasis through down-regulation of the canonical NF-κB signaling pathway and suppression of MAPK signaling mediated through ERK and JNK. *PLoS ONE* **2017**, *12*, e0170595. [CrossRef] [PubMed]
84. Wang, X.; Ma, P.; Liu, J.; Zhang, Q.; Zhang, Y.; Ding, X.; Jiang, L.; Wang, Y.; Zhang, Y.; Sun, D. Genome-wide association study in Chinese Holstein cows reveal two candidate genes for somatic cell score as an indicator for mastitis susceptibility. *BMC Genetics* **2015**, *16*, 111. [CrossRef] [PubMed]
85. Song, M.; Wei, Y.; Khan, Z.M.; Wang, X.; Yu, Y. Molecular marker study of inflammatory reaction in Bovine mammary epithelium cell line induced by methicillin-resistant staphylococcus areus (MRSA). *Acta Veterin Zootecn Sina* **2016**, *47*, 1995–2010.
86. Wu, D.; Zhang, X.; Liu, L.; Guo, Y. Key CMM Combinations in Prescriptions for Treating Mastitis and Working Mechanism Analysis Based on Network Pharmacology. *Evid. Based Complement. Altern. Med.* **2019**, *2019*. [CrossRef]
87. Liu, T.; Zhang, L.; Joo, D.; Sun, S.C. NF-κB signaling in inflammation. *Signal. Transduct. Target. Ther.* **2017**, *2*, 1–9. [CrossRef]
88. Bannerman, D.D.; Paape, M.J.; Lee, J.W.; Zhao, X.; Hope, J.C.; Rainard, P. Escherichia coli and Staphylococcus aureus elicit differential innate immune responses following intramammary infection. *Clin. Diagn. Lab. Immunol.* **2004**, *11*, 463–472. [CrossRef]

89. Bruckmaier, R.M. Gene expression of factors related to the immune reaction in response to intramammary Escherichia coli lipopolysaccharide challenge. *J. Dairy Res.* **2005**, *72*, 120–124. [CrossRef]
90. Gilbert, F.B.; Cunha, P.; Jensen, K.; Glass, E.J.; Foucras, G.; Robert-Granié, C.; Rupp, R.; Rainard, P. Differential response of bovine mammary epithelial cells to Staphylococcus aureus or Escherichia coli agonists of the innate immune system. *Vet. Res.* **2013**, *44*, 40. [CrossRef]
91. Jia, T.; Leiner, I.; Dorothee, G.; Brandl, K.; Pamer, E.G. MyD88 and Type I Interferon Receptor-Mediated Chemokine Induction and Monocyte Recruitment during Listeria monocytogenes Infection. *J. Immunol.* **2009**, *183*, 1271–1278. [CrossRef] [PubMed]
92. Kelly-Scumpia, K.M.; Scumpia, P.O.; Delano, M.J.; Weinstein, J.S.; Cuenca, A.G.; Wynn, J.L.; Moldawer, L.L. Type I interferon signaling in hematopoietic cells is required for survival in mouse polymicrobial sepsis by regulating CXCL10. *J. Exp. Med.* **2010**, *207*, 319–326. [CrossRef] [PubMed]
93. Zeng, X.; Moore, T.A.; Newstead, M.W.; Deng, J.C.; Lukacs, N.W.; Standiford, T.J. IP-10 mediates selective mononuclear cell accumulation and activation in response to intrapulmonary transgenic expression and during adenovirus-induced pulmonary inflammation. *J. Interf. Cytokine Res.* **2005**, *25*, 103–112. [CrossRef] [PubMed]
94. Zheng, J.; Watson, A.D.; Kerr, D.E. Genome-wide expression analysis of lipopolysaccharide-induced mastitis in a mouse model. *Infect. Immun.* **2006**, *74*, 1907–1915. [CrossRef]
95. Kosciuczuk, E.M.; Lisowski, P.; Jarczak, J.; Majewska, A.; Rzewuska, M.; Zwierzchowski, L.; Bagnicka, E. Transcriptome profiling of Staphylococci-infected cow mammary gland parenchyma. *BMC Vet. Res.* **2017**, *13*, 1–12. [CrossRef]
96. Griesbeck-Zilch, B.; Osman, M.; Kühn, C.; Schwerin, M.; Bruckmaier, R.H.; Pfaffl, M.W.; Hammerle-Fickinger, A.; Meyer, H.H.D.; Wellnitz, O. Analysis of key molecules of the innate immune system in mammary epithelial cells isolated from marker-assisted and conventionally selected cattle. *J. Dairy Sci.* **2009**, *92*, 4621–4633. [CrossRef]
97. Islam, M.A.; Takagi, M.; Fukuyama, K.; Komatsu, R.; Albarracin, L.; Nochi, T.; Suda, Y.; Ikeda-Ohtsubo, W.; Rutten, V.; van Eden, W.; et al. Transcriptome analysis of the inflammatory responses of bovine mammary epithelial cells: Exploring immunomodulatory target genes for bovine mastitis. *Pathogens* **2020**, *9*, 200. [CrossRef]
98. Rainard, P.; Riollet, C. Innate immunity of the bovine mammary gland. *Vet. Res.* **2006**, *37*, 369–400. [CrossRef]
99. Waller, K.P. Modulation of endotoxin-induced inflammation in the bovine teat using antagonists inhibitors to leukotrienes, platelet activating factor and interleukin 1beta. *Vet. Immunol. Immunopathol.* **1997**, *57*, 239–251. [CrossRef]
100. Bulgari, O.; Dong, X.; Roca, A.L.; Caroli, A.M.; Loor, J.J. Innate immune responses induced by lipopolysaccharide and lipoteichoic acid in primary goat mammary epithelial cells. *J. Anim. Sci. Biotechnol.* **2017**, *8*, 29. [CrossRef]
101. Wang, W.; Hu, X.; Shen, P.; Zhang, N.; Fu, Y. Sodium houttuyfonate inhibits LPS-induced inflammatory response via suppressing TLR4/NF-kB signaling pathway in bovine mammary epithelial cells. *Microb. Pathog.* **2017**, *107*, 12–16. [CrossRef] [PubMed]
102. Wang, H.; Bi, C.; Wang, Y.; Sun, J.; Meng, X.; Li, J. Selenium ameliorates Staphylococcus aureus-induced inflammation in bovine mammary epithelial cells by inhibiting activation of TLR2, NF-KB and MAPK signaling pathways. *BMC Vet. Res.* **2018**, *14*, 197. [CrossRef] [PubMed]
103. Sordillo, L.M.; Streicher, K.L. Mammary gland immunity and mastitis susceptibility. *J. Mammary Gland Biol. Neoplasia* **2002**, *7*, 135–146. [CrossRef]
104. Akhtar, M.; Guo, S.; Guo, Y.; Zahoor, A.; Shaukat, A.; Chen, Y.; Guo, M. Upregulated-gene expression of Pro-inflammatory cytokines (TNF-α, IL-1β and IL-6) via TLRs following NF-κB and MAPKs in bovine mastitis. *Acta Tropica* **2020**, *207*, 105458. [CrossRef] [PubMed]
105. Ren, K.; Torres, R. Role of interleukin-1β during pain and inflammation. *Brain Res. Rev.* **2009**, *60*, 57. [CrossRef]
106. Dai, H.; Coleman, D.N.; Hu, L.; Martinez-Cortés, I.; Wang, M.; Parys, C.; Shen, X.; Loor, J.J. Methionine and arginine supplementation alter inflammatory and oxidative stress responses during lipopolysaccharide challenge in bovine mammary epithelial cells in vitro. *J. Dairy Sci.* **2020**, *103*, 676–689. [CrossRef]

107. Zimmermann, K.K.; Spassov, S.G.; Strosing, K.M.; Ihle, P.M.; Engelstaedter, H.; Hoetzel, A.; Faller, S. Hydrogen Sulfide Exerts Anti-oxidative and Anti-inflammatory Effects in Acute Lung Injury. *Inflammation* **2018**, *41*, 249–259. [CrossRef]
108. Benedetti, F.; Curreli, S.; Krishnan, S.; Davinelli, S.; Cocchi, F.; Scapagnini, G.; Gallo, R.C.; Zella, D. Anti-inflammatory effects of H2S during acute bacterial infection: A review. *J. Transl. Med.* **2017**, *15*, 100. [CrossRef]
109. Zhi-Zhong, X.; Yang, L.; Jin-Song, B. Hydrogen sulfide and cellular redox homeostasis. *Oxidative Med. Cell. Longev.* **2016**, 1–12. [CrossRef]
110. Liu, W.; Xu, C.; You, X.; Olson, D.M.; Chemtob, S.; Gao, L.; Ni, X. Hydrogen sulfide delays LPS-Induced preterm birth in mice via anti-inflammatory pathways. *PLoS ONE* **2016**, *11*, e0152838. [CrossRef]
111. Ahire, J.J.; Mokashe, N.U.; Patil, H.J.; Chaudhari, B.L. Antioxidative potential of folate producing probiotic Lactobacillus helveticus CD6. *J. Food Sci. Technol.* **2013**, *50*, 26–34. [CrossRef] [PubMed]
112. Liu, P.; Yang, C.; Lin, S.; Zhao, G.; Zhang, T.; Guo, S.; Jiang, K.; Wu, H.; Qiu, C.; Guo, M.; et al. Sodium houttuyfonate inhibits LPS-induced mastitis in mice via the NF-κB signalling pathway. *Mol. Med. Rep.* **2019**, *19*, 2279–2286. [CrossRef] [PubMed]
113. Sun, L.; Chen, L.; Wang, F.; Zheng, X.; Yuan, C.; Niu, Q.; Li, Z.; Deng, L.; Zheng, B.; Li, C.; et al. Exogenous hydrogen sulfide prevents lipopolysaccharide-induced inflammation by blocking the TLR4/NF-κB pathway in MAC-T cells. *Gene* **2019**, *710*, 114–121. [CrossRef] [PubMed]
114. Gálvez, J.; Coelho, G.; Crespo, M.E.; Cruz, T.; Rodríguez-Cabezas, M.E.; Concha, A.; Gonzalez, M.; Zarzuelo, A. Intestinal anti-inflammatory activity of morin on chronic experimental colitis in the rat. *Aliment. Pharmacol. Ther.* **2001**, *15*, 2027–2039. [CrossRef] [PubMed]
115. Kempuraj, D.; Madhappan, B.; Christodoulou, S.; Boucher, W.; Cao, J.; Papadopoulou, N.; Cetrulo, C.L.; Theoharides, T.C. Flavonols inhibit pro-inflammatory mediator release, intracellular calcium ion levels and protein kinase C theta phosphorylation in human mast cells. *Br. J. Pharmacol.* **2005**, *145*, 934–944. [CrossRef]
116. van de Veerdonk, F.L.; Netea, M.G.; Dinarello, C.A.; Joosten, L.A.B. Inflammasome activation and IL-1β and IL-18 processing during infection. *Trends Immunol.* **2011**, *32*, 110–116. [CrossRef]
117. Yu, S.; Liu, X.; Yu, D.; Changyong, E.; Yang, J. Morin Protects LPS-Induced Mastitis via Inhibiting NLRP3 Inflammasome and NF-κB Signaling Pathways. *Inflammation* **2020**, *43*, 1293–1303. [CrossRef]
118. Zhan, K.; Yang, T.; Feng, B.; Zhu, X.; Chen, Y.; Huo, Y.; Zhao, G. The protective roles of tea tree oil extracts in bovine mammary epithelial cells and polymorphonuclear leukocytes. *J. Anim. Sci. Biotechnol.* **2020**, *11*, 62. [CrossRef]
119. Mahla, R.S.; Reddy, M.C.; Vijaya Raghava Prasad, D.; Kumar, H. Sweeten PAMPs: Role of sugar complexed PAMPs in innate immunity and vaccine biology. *Front. Immunol.* **2013**, *4*, 248. [CrossRef]
120. Zhao, M.; Wang, H.; Yang, B.; Tao, H. Identification of cyclodextrin inclusion complex of chlorogenic acid and its antimicrobial activity. *Food Chem.* **2010**, *120*, 1138–1142. [CrossRef]
121. Sato, Y.; Itagaki, S.; Kurokawa, T.; Ogura, J.; Kobayashi, M.; Hirano, T.; Sugawara, M.; Iseki, K. In vitro and in vivo antioxidant properties of chlorogenic acid and caffeic acid. *Int. J. Pharm.* **2011**, *403*, 136–138. [CrossRef] [PubMed]
122. Shan, J.; Fu, J.; Zhao, Z.; Kong, X.; Huang, H.; Luo, L.; Yin, Z. Chlorogenic acid inhibits lipopolysaccharide-induced cyclooxygenase-2 expression in RAW264.7 cells through suppressing NF-κB and JNK/AP-1 activation. *Int. Immunopharmacol.* **2009**, *9*, 1042–1048. [CrossRef] [PubMed]
123. Ruifeng, G.; Yunhe, F.; Zhengkai, W.; Ershun, Z.; Yimeng, L.; Minjun, Y.; Xiaojing, S.; Zhengtao, Y.; Naisheng, Z. Chlorogenic acid attenuates lipopolysaccharide-induced mice mastitis by suppressing TLR4-mediated NF-κB signaling pathway. *Eur. J. Pharmacol.* **2014**, *729*, 54–58. [CrossRef] [PubMed]
124. Liang, D.; Li, F.; Fu, Y.; Cao, Y.; Song, X.; Wang, T.; Wang, W.; Guo, M.; Zhou, E.; Li, D.; et al. Thymol inhibits LPS-stimulated inflammatory response via down-regulation of NF-κB and MAPK signaling pathways in mouse mammary epithelial cells. *Inflammation* **2014**, *37*, 214–222. [CrossRef] [PubMed]
125. Garcia, M.T.H.; Elsasser, H.T.; Biswas, D.; Moyes, M.K. The effect of citrus-derived oil on bovine blood neutrophil function and gene expression in vitro. *J. Dairy Sci.* **2014**, *98*, 1–99127. [CrossRef] [PubMed]
126. Li, J.; Yin, P.; Gong, P.; Lv, A.; Zhang, Z.; Liu, F. 8-Methoxypsoralen protects bovine mammary epithelial cells against lipopolysaccharide-induced inflammatory injury via suppressing JAK/STAT and NF-κB pathway. *Microbiol.Immunol.* **2019**, *63*, 427–437. [CrossRef]

127. Yang, Z.; Yin, R.; Cong, Y.; Yang, Z.; Zhou, E.; Wei, Z.; Zhang, N. Oxymatrine Lightened the Inflammatory Response of LPS-Induced Mastitis in Mice through Affecting NF-κB and MAPKs Signaling Pathways. *Inflammation* **2014**, *37*, 2047–2055. [CrossRef]
128. Ershun, Z.; Yunhe, F.; Zhengkai, W.; Yongguo, C.; Naisheng, Z.; Zhengtao, Y. Cepharanthine Attenuates Lipopolysaccharide-Induced Mice Mastitis by Suppressing the NF-κB Signaling Pathway. *Inflammation* **2014**, *32*, 331–337. [CrossRef]
129. Su, S.; Xiaoyu, L.; Siting, L.; Pengfei, M.; Yingying, H.; Yanli, D.; Hongyan, D.; Shibin, F.; Jinchun, L.; Xichun, W.; et al. Rutin protects against lipopolysaccharide-induced mastitis by inhibiting the activation of the NF-κB signaling pathway and attenuating endoplasmic reticulum stress. *Inflammopharmacology* **2018**, *27*, 77–88. [CrossRef]
130. Li, D.; Zhang, N.; Cao, Y.; Zhang, W.; Su, G.; Sun, Y.; Yang, Z. Emodin ameliorates lipopolysaccharide-induced mastitis in mice by inhibiting activation of NF-κB and MAPKs signal pathways. *Eur. J. Pharmacol.* **2013**, *705*, 79–85. [CrossRef]
131. He, X.; Liu, W.; Shi, M.; Yang, Z.; Zhang, X.; Gong, P. Docosahexaenoic acid attenuates LPS-stimulated inflammatory response by regulating the PPARγ/NF-κB pathways in primary bovine mammary epithelial cells. *Res. Vet. Sci.* **2017**, *112*, 7–12. [CrossRef] [PubMed]
132. He, X.; Wei, Z.; Zhou, E.; Chen, L.; Kou, J.; Wang, J.; Yang, Z. Baicalein attenuates inflammatory responses by suppressing TLR4 mediated NF-κB and MAPK signaling pathways in LPS-induced mastitis in mice. *Internat. Immunopharmacol.* **2015**, *28*, 470–476. [CrossRef] [PubMed]

15

Insight into the Possible Formation Mechanism of the Intersex Phenotype of Lanzhou Fat-Tailed Sheep using Whole-Genome Resequencing

Jie Li [1,†], Han Xu [1,2,†], Xinfeng Liu [1], Hongwei Xu [3,4,*], Yong Cai [5,6] and Xianyong Lan [1,*]

1 Animal Genome and Gene Function Laboratory, College of Animal Science and Technology, Northwest A&F University, Yangling 712100, China; lijie95@nwafu.edu.cn (J.L.); xuhan23@mail2.sysu.edu.cn (H.X.); liuxinfen227@nwafu.edu.cn (X.L.)
2 School of Medicine, Sun Yat-sen University, Guangzhou 510275, China
3 College of Life Science and Engineering, Northwest Minzu University, Lanzhou 730030, China
4 Gansu Tech Innovation Center of Animal Cell, Biomedical Research Center, Northwest Minzu University, Lanzhou 730030, China
5 Science Experimental Center, Northwest Minzu University, Lanzhou 730030, China; caiyong@xbmu.edu.cn
6 Key Laboratory of Biotechnology and Bioengineering of State Ethnic Affairs Commission, Biomedical Research Center, Northwest Minzu University, Lanzhou 730030, China
* Correspondence: xuhongwei@xbmu.edu.cn (H.X.); lanxianyong79@nwsuaf.edu.cn (X.L.)
† These authors equally contributed to this work.

Simple Summary: Individuals with hermaphroditism are a serious hazard to animal husbandry and production due to their abnormal fertility. The molecular mechanism of sheep intersex formation was unclear. This study was the first to locate the homologous sequence of the goat polled intersex syndrome (PIS) region in sheep and found that the intersex traits of Lanzhou fat-tailed sheep were not caused by the lack of this region. By detecting the selective sweep regions, vital genes associated with androgen biosynthesis and the follicle stimulating hormone response entry were found, including *steroid 5 alpha-reductase 2* (*SRD5A2*), and *pro-apoptotic WT1 regulator* (*PAWR*). Additionally, the copy number variations of the four regions on chr9, chr1, chr4, and chr16 may affect the expression of the gonadal development genes, *zinc finger protein, FOG family member 2* (*ZFPM2*), *LIM homeobox 8* (*LHX8*), *inner mitochondrial membrane peptidase subunit 2* (*IMMP2L*) and *slit guidance ligand 3* (*SLIT3*), respectively, and further affect the formation of intersex traits.

Abstract: Intersex, also known as hermaphroditism, is a serious hazard to animal husbandry and production. The mechanism of ovine intersex formation is not clear. Therefore, genome-wide resequencing on the only two intersex and two normal Lanzhou fat-tailed (LFT) sheep, an excellent but endangered Chinese indigenous sheep breed, was performed. Herein, the deletion of homologous sequences of the goat polled intersex syndrome (PIS) region (8787 bp, 247747059–247755846) on chromosome 1 of the LFT sheep was not the cause of the ovine intersex trait. By detecting the selective sweep regions, we found that the genes related to androgen biosynthesis and follicle stimulating hormone response items, such as *steroid 5 alpha-reductase 2* (*SRD5A2*), *steroid 5 alpha-reductase 3* (*SRD5A3*), and *pro-apoptotic WT1 regulator* (*PAWR*), may be involved in the formation of intersex traits. Furthermore, the copy number variations of the four regions, chr9: 71660801–71662800, chr1: 50776001–50778000, chr4: 58119201–58121600, and chr16: 778801–780800, may affect the expression of the *zinc finger protein, FOG family member 2* (*ZFPM2*), *LIM homeobox 8* (*LHX8*), *inner mitochondrial membrane peptidase subunit 2* (*IMMP2L*) and *slit guidance ligand 3* (*SLIT3*) genes, respectively, which contribute to the appearance of intersex traits. These results may supply a theoretical basis for the timely detection and elimination of intersex individuals in sheep, which could accelerate the healthy development of animal husbandry.

Keywords: sheep; intersex; whole-genome resequencing; copy number variation; forming mechanism

1. Introduction

Intersexuality, also known as hermaphroditism, refers to the phenomenon that a dioecious animal is characterized by female-to-male sex reversal or abnormal gonad development. Intersex individuals are unable to reproduce, which poses certain obstacles to the protection and breeding of endangered species, and causes production loss to animal husbandry. In vertebrates, the mechanisms of sex determination are mainly divided into two types, genetic sex determination and environmental sex determination [1]. Intersex mostly occurs in the goat population, with high occurrence frequencies (about 3%–10%) [2], while related reports on horses, donkeys, pigs, and sheep are few. In goats, it is also named polled intersex syndrome (PIS) for the phenomenon of intersex individuals often found in hornless goat populations [2]. In the previous study, a 11.7 kb deletion fragment containing a repeat sequence (AF404302) was cloned by PCR, and the complete absence of this fragment resulted in goat polled syndrome [3,4]. A recent study about long-read whole-genome sequencing of a PIS-affected goat and a horned control goat revealed the presence of a more complex structural variant consisting of a 10,159 bp deletion and an inversely inserted 480 kb duplicated segment containing two genes, *potassium inwardly rectifying channel subfamily J member 15* (*KCNJ15*) and *ETS transcription factor ERG* (*ERG*) [5]. The deletion of the PIS region was identified affecting the development of germ cell support cells, and it can also affect the expression of genes, including *Forkhead box L2* (*FOXL2*), *PIS-regulated transcript 1* (*PISRT1*), and *promoter FOXL2 inverse complementary* (*PFOXic*) [6], indicating that the lack of the PIS region is closely related to goat intersex traits.

Compared to goats, reports of intersex sheep are quite rare. Domestic sheep and domestic goats, diverging about 4 to 5 million years ago and evolving into two different branches, are relatively close in genetic distance, and they have many similar genetic targets during domestication [7]. Therefore, it was suspected that the cause of sexual traits in sheep may be similar to that of goat sex. The location of homologous sequences of goat PIS regions should be detected in sheep.

Genetic variations or regulatory regions may affect an individual's phenotypic traits by affecting the transcription or translation of key genes [8]. In bovines, a 110 kb deletion in the *MER1 repeat containing imprinted transcript 1* (*MIMT1*) gene was a prominent cause of bovine abortion and stillbirth [9]. Bovine osteosclerosis may be associated with a deletion of approximately 2.8 kb in exon 2 and part of exon 3 of the *solute carrier family 4 member 2* (*SLC4A2*) gene encoding an anion exchanger [10]. An increased copy number of the *prolactin receptor* (*PRLR*) and *sperm flagellar 2* (*SPEF2*) genes in the K locus on the Z chromosome in chickens were closely related to the slow feathering trait of the chicken [11,12]. Additionally, the copy number variation of the *sperm flagellar 2* (*ASIP*) gene in sheep was closely related to the coat color [13]. It was speculated that some mutations may lead to the abnormal expression of certain genes that affect sex formation, leading to the generation of intersex traits.

As an excellent sheep variety of meat and wool, Lanzhou fat-tailed (LFT) sheep are famous for their large and fat tail and a number of excellent characteristics, such as the crude feed tolerance, higher disease resistance, and higher resilience than other domestic sheep. In recent years, only two surviving intersexual sheep were found in the LFT sheep population. In this study, the genome-wide resequencing of two intersex LFT sheep and two normal LFT sheep was performed, and combined with the resequencing data of four normal Tan sheep to find potential genes or regions related with the formation of ovine intersex traits, and thus provide an important basis for the timely detection and elimination of intersex individuals in sheep conservation and expansion.

2. Materials and Methods

2.1. Ethics Statement

All implemented experiments were approved by the Institutional Animal Care and Use Committee and were in strict accordance with good animal practices as defined by the Northwest A&F University (protocol number NWAFAC1008).

2.2. Animal and Sequencing

In this study, the ear tissues of four sheep, including two surviving intersex (LZ1 and LZ2) and six normal (LZ3 to LZ8) Lanzhou fat-tail sheep from Lanzhou City were collected and stored in 70% alcohol at −80 °C. Genomic DNA was extracted from sheep ear tissues using the phenol-chloroform method according to a previously reported protocol [14]. The DNA samples were quantified using a Nanodrop 1000 (Thermo Scientific, Waltham, MA, USA). Four DNA libraries, two intersex (LZ1 and LZ2) and two normal LFT sheep (LZ3 and LZ4), with insert sizes of approximately 350 bp, were constructed following the manufacturer's instructions, and 150 bp paired-end reads were generated using the Illumina HiSeq X10 platform.

2.3. Sequence Quality Checking and Mapping

Considering the relatively close genetic relationship between LFT sheep and Tan sheep, the previous four resequencing data of Tan sheep were also used as a normal control group for further analysis [15,16]. Before alignment, the FastQC software was used (http://www.bioinformatics.babraham.ac.uk/projects/fastqc/) to detect the joint information, the length information, and the quality information for each base on each read of all the raw data. Based on the results of the above quality control, the adapter and low quality raw paired reads were filtered using Trimmomatic (v0.36) [17]. The high quality reads were mapped to the sheep version 4.0 reference genome (GCF_000298735.2_Oar_v4.0_genomic.fna) using the 'mem' algorithm of the Burrows–Wheeler Alignment Tool (BWA) software [18]. SAMtools (http://samtools.sourceforge.net/) was used to remove replicate sequences [19].

2.4. Calling and Validation of SNPs and CNVs

The calling of single nucleotide polymorphisms (SNPs) was performed with Genome Analysis Toolkit (GATK, version 2.4–9) UnifiedGenotyper [20], and was annotated by ANNOVAR [21]. The called SNPs with reads >4 and quality ≥20 were used for further analysis. CNVcaller software (https://github.com/JiangYuLab/CNVcaller) was used for the detection of whole-genome copy number variation (CNV) [22]. The specific steps were in accordance with a reported study [23], including segmenting the reference genome into a window of a specified size (800 bp) with a step size of 400 bp. Herein, Vst was used to measure the difference in the size of each copy number variation between different groups [24,25]. The mean log2 ratio across all probes falling within a specific CNV region was calculated. The variance of the means was for the entire set (Vt). The average variance within populations was then calculated (Vs) by taking the mean between populations (i.e., the V intersex sheep and Vnormal sheep). Vst values were finally calculated using the standard formula Vst = (Vt − Vs)/Vt.

2.5. Regional Localization and Depth Statistics for Ovine Homologous Sequences of PIS

The sequence of the PIS region was extracted from the goat reference genome (GCF_001704415.1_ASM170441v1_genomic.fna) by using SAMtools and then aligned to the sheep reference genome using BLAT v. 36 × 1 software (BLAST-Like Alignment Tool) to obtain the ovine homologous regions [26].

After that, we used the SAMtools-depth to count the reads depth for each locus in the candidate region. Furthermore, we corrected it based on the total depth of sequencing to obtain the reads depth in the homologous regions of the eight samples, including two intersex LFT sheep, two LFT sheep, and four reported Tan sheep [15,16]. If the reads depth was essentially 0, the candidate region was completely missing on the ovine genome.

2.6. PCR Amplification of PIS Candidate Region Sequences in Sheep

In order to further verify whether the PIS candidate region of the intersex individual was really missing, primers, namely PIS-1, PIS-2, PIS-3, and PIS-4, for the homologous sequence in the ovine PIS region were designed to reference the second generation genome of the sheep chr1: 247747059–247755846 sequence (Supplemental Table S1). We performed assays of amplification on two intersex and six normal LFT sheep according to previous reaction volume and amplification procedure [27]. The products were separated on 2.5% agarose gels.

2.7. Sweep Analysis of SNPs in Selected Regions

In order to identify the selection signatures in the genomes of sheep, two sequenced pools based on genetic differentiation (Fst) of each 150 KB genome window were separately performed. The specific formula of Fst was consistent with the previous studies [28,29].

After Z-transformation of Fst, the candidate selection windows were used by selecting the top 1% in Fst score intersections [30]. Finally, the geneview module of python and R were utilized for data visualization.

2.8. Gene Annotation and Functional Enrichment Analysis of Selected Signal Regions

Gene functional enrichment analysis was performed primarily on the KOBAS 3.0 website (http://kobas.cbi.pku.edu.cn/index.php) [31]. Herein, considering that the sheep database in KOBAS was not complete, a Perl script was used to compare the longest protein sequences of each gene in sheep and human by invoking Blastp, and the gene extracted in the previous step (2.4 and 2.7) was converted into a gene homologous to "human", and then human was selected as a species for annotation.

3. Results

3.1. Sequencing, Filtering, and Mapping

Whole-genome sequencing of two normal Tan sheep, as well as two intersex sheep and four normal LFT sheep, was performed on an Illumina HiSeq X10 platform using genomic DNA and 198.5 Gb of high quality paired-end reads were generated. After getting the raw data, we utilized FastQC software (http://www.bioinformatics.babraham.ac.uk/projects/fastqc/) for quality testing. According to the test results, the clean reads were obtained using trimmomatic (http://www.usadellab.org/cms/index.php/page=trimmomatic) to filter the low-quality reads (Supplemental Table S2). The clean reads of eight sheep were mapped to the sheep reference genome (GCF_000298735.2_Oar_v4.0_genomic.fna) using BWA-MEM [17,31], with an average mapping rate above 94% (Supplemental Table S3).

3.2. Single Nucleotide Polymorphisms (SNPs) Calling and Annotation

A total of 29,732,629 SNPs were obtained among eight sheep, among which, the most distributed SNPs were on chromosome 1 (n = 3,186,739), and the least distributed, lowest number of SNPs were on chromosome 24 (n = 459,707) (Supplemental Table S4). According to the results of the annotation, the proportions of transition (ts) mutations (A/G 10333679 and T/C 10308562) and transversion (tv) mutations (A/T 2050141, A/C 2457813, G/T 2450228, and G/C 2132206) were 69.4% and 30.6%, respectively, which met the 3 to 1 ratio (Figure 1).

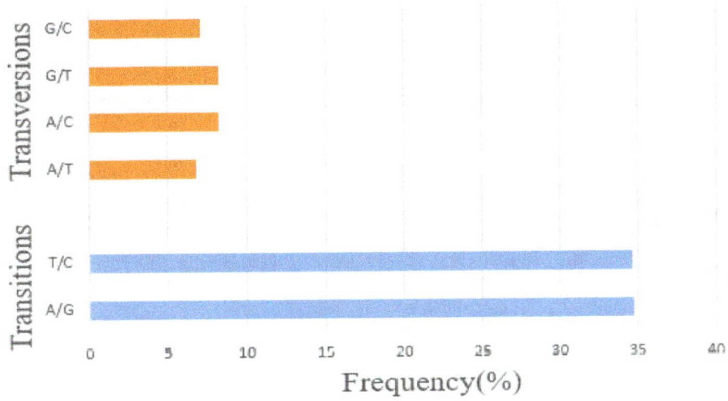

Figure 1. The statistics of mutation type of single nucleotide polymorphisms (SNPs). Note: The proportion of translation (ts) mutations and transversion (tv) mutations meet the 3 to 1 ratio.

3.3. The Localization Results of Homologous Sequences of Goat PIS Region in Sheep

According to the specific information of the goat PIS region (AF404302.1: 27015–38775) in the NCBI, the obtained sequence of this 11.76 kb segment [2] was aligned to the sheep genome using BLAT, and then the score was calculated using the pslScore.pl script provided by the BLAT software to evaluate the results of the comparison.

The BLAT results show that there were 79 alignment regions, and the alignment region with the highest score was located in the region of the ovine chromosome1 (start to end position: 247747059–250146105, 2399.046 kb) (Supplemental Table S5). Then, the detailed analysis of the 79 region revealed that the first 58 of them were a closely connected 8787 bp region (chr1: 247747059–247755846), corresponding to a segment of the 11.7 kb region of the goat (AF404302.1:30003–38775) with 100% coverage (Figure 2a). Further localization revealed that this region was located approximately 340 kb upstream of the *FOXL2* gene (chr1: 248088730–248095868) in the sheep genome, which was consistent with the position of the goat *FOXL2* gene. Therefore, the 8787 bp sequence (chr1: 247747059–247755846) was served as a candidate region for ovine intersex traits.

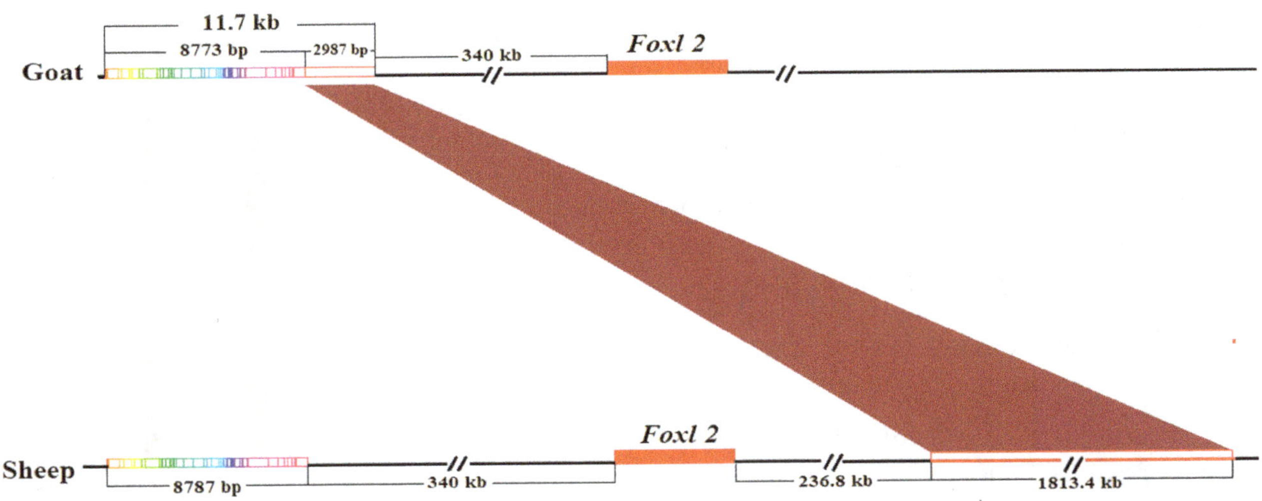

(a)

Figure 2. *Cont.*

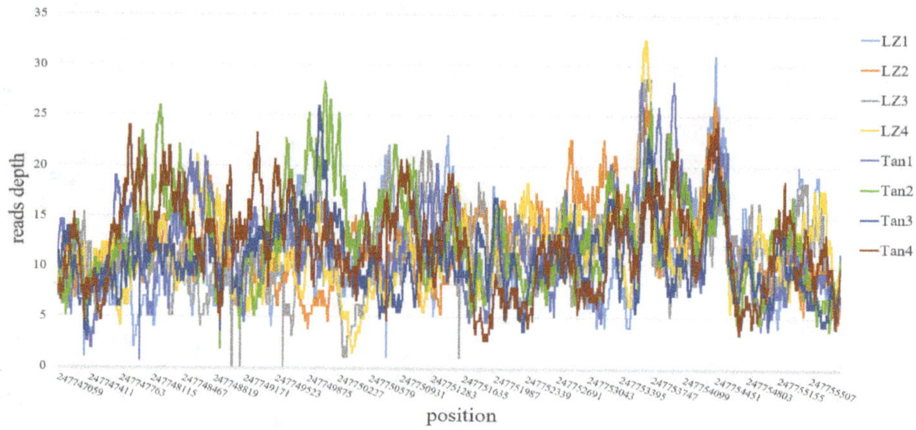

(**b**)

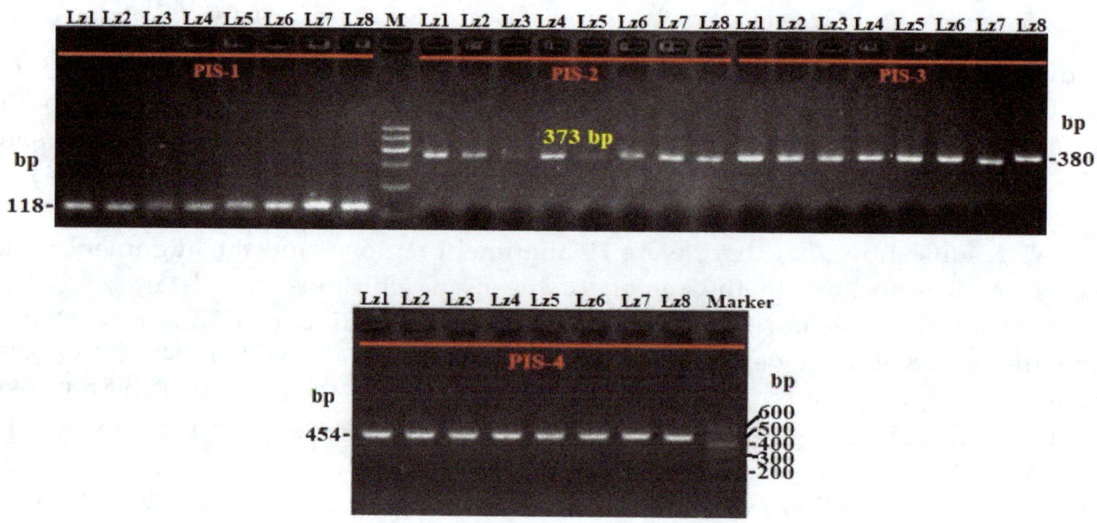

(**c**)

Figure 2. Study on the homologous sequences of the polled intersex syndrome (PIS) regions in sheep and goats. (**a**) The comparison results between the sheep chromosome 1: 247747059–250146105 and goat PIS area (the color line represents the matching relationship: goat 8773 bp matched sheep 8787 bp, and goat 2987 kb matched sheep 1813.4 kb). (**b**) The statistics of the read depth in the sheep 8787 bp candidate area. (**c**) Electrophoresis results of the four pairs of primer amplification products, indicating that the four regions of intersex sheep were not missing.

3.4. Statistics of Reads Depth and PCR Amplification of Sheep 8787 bp Candidate Sequences

In the two intersex sheep and normal individuals, the read depth was between 5 and 20, and there was no significant difference between them (Figure 2b).

According to the results of agarose gel electrophoresis, in two intersex LFT sheep (LZ1 and LZ2) and six normal LFT sheep (LZ3, LZ4, LZ5, LZ6, LZ7, and LZ8), four pairs of primers (PIS-1, PIS-2, PIS-3, and PIS-4) were able to amplify the target band in the candidate region, and the product lengths were 118, 376, 380, and 454 bp (Figure 2c), respectively, indicating that the candidate region of intersex sheep was not missing. It is further explained that the intersex traits of LFT sheep was not caused by the lack of the region.

3.5. Genome-Wide Selection Sweeping Analysis in Intersex and Normal Populations

ZFst score were calculated for the only two intersex LFT sheep and six normal sheep populations (including two LFT sheep and four Tan sheep). The top 1% percent of the windows with the highest *ZFst* score were defined as candidate selective sweep regions. The results show that most chromosomes contained windows with a higher differentiation coefficient, and chromosomes 2, 6, 7, 10, and 11 were strongly selected (Figure 3a). The region with the largest *ZFst* value was located on the X chromosome (chrX: 99675001–99825000, *ZFst* = 10.69), and the second one was located on chromosome 3 (chr3: 105000001–105150000, *ZFst* = 10.38) (Figure 3a; Supplemental Table S6).

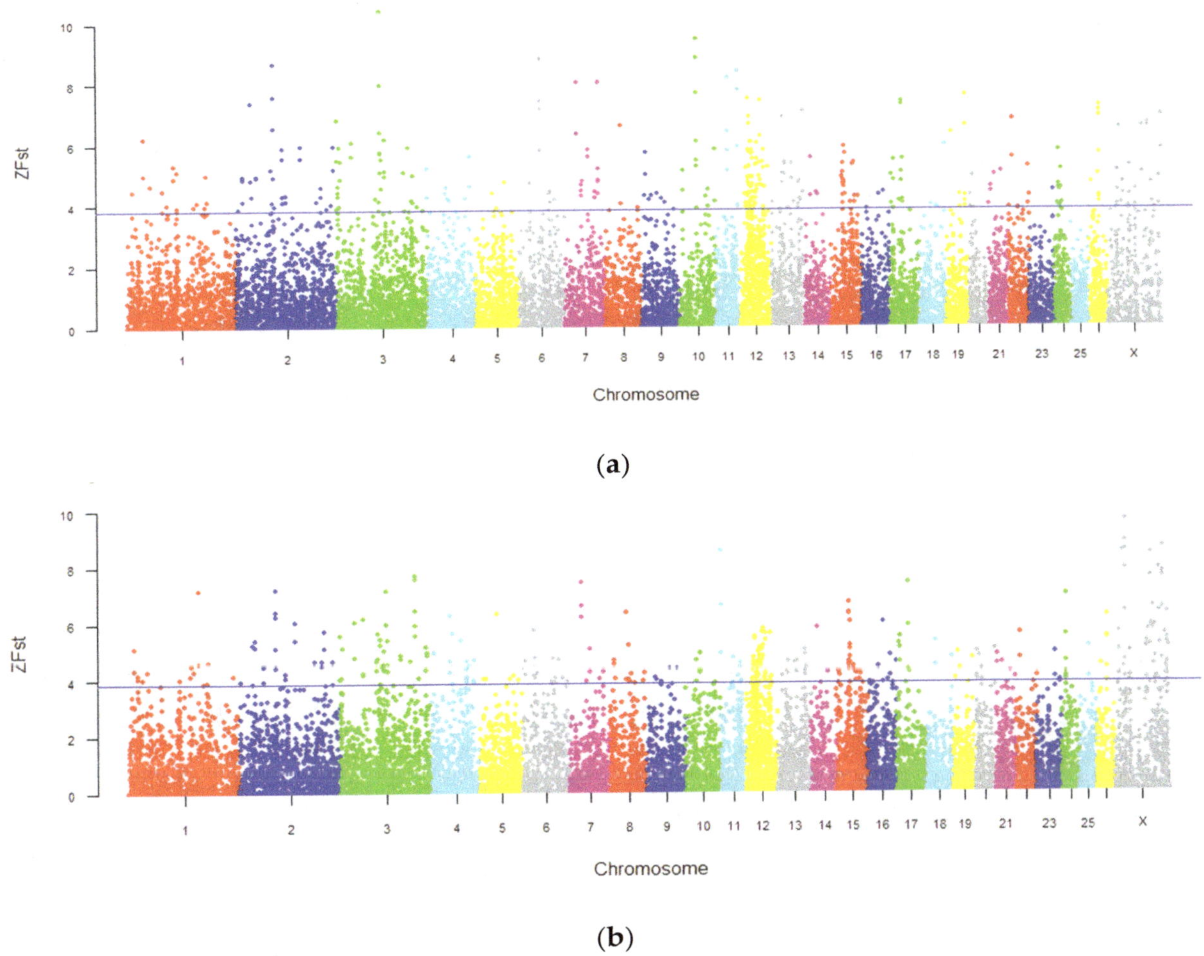

Figure 3. The detection of genome-wide selection signals in intersex and normal populations. (**a**) The genome-wide distribution of *ZFst* between intersex sheep and normal sheep (including normal Lanzhou large-tailed sheep and Tan sheep). (**b**) The genome-wide distribution of *ZFst* between intersex and normal individuals of Lanzhou large-tailed sheep. Note: The blue line represents the top 1% of the ZFst value.

A total of 466 genes were obtained by gene annotation (Supplemental Table S7), and then those genes were functionally enriched by KOBAS3.0. A total of 1757 significant entries were found ($p < 0.05$), and 1038 significant entries remained after the false discovery rate (FDR)-correction (corrected p-Value < 0.05), mainly including items, such as muscle development, fat development, and immunity. Furthermore, the pathways were screened and two more significant entries related to female gonadal development (GO: 0008585) and the development of primary female sexual characteristics (GO: 0046545) were found ($p < 0.05$) (Supplemental Table S7). Nevertheless, neither entry was significant after correction.

3.6. Genome-Wide Selection Sweeping Analysis in Intersex LFT Sheep and Normal LFT Sheep

To exclude the effects of SNP locus frequencies between different breeds, the study then compared two intersex individuals and two normal LFT sheep. Consistent with the previous section, the region with the largest *ZFst* value was located on the X chromosome (Figure 3b). By contrast, the second region was also in the X chromosome, rather than chromosome 3 (Figure 3b). Moreover, a total of 451 genes were obtained by annotation (Supplemental Table S8). After functional enrichment analysis, 1680 significant entries were found ($p < 0.05$) and 969 significant terms remained after false discovery rate (FDR)-correction (corrected p-value < 0.05) (Supplemental Table S9). Screening of the pathway revealed five significant entries related to the synthesis and response of the sex hormone ($p < 0.05$). After correction (corrected p-value < 0.05), the genes, such as *SRD5A2*, *SRD5A3*, and *PAWR*, were significantly rich in the androgen biosynthesis process and their responses to follicle stimulating hormones (Supplemental Table S9). Additionally, the genes involved in androgen receptor signaling pathways, androgen metabolism, and the regulation of intracellular estrogen receptor signaling pathways, and gonadotropin response processes, such as *UFM1 specific ligase 1* (*UFL1*), *GTP-binding nuclear protein Ran-like* (*LOC105609617*), *mediator complex subunit 14* (*MED14*), *DEAD-box helicase 5* (*DDX5*), etc. (Supplemental Table S9).

3.7. Detection of Genome-Wide Copy Number Variation (CNV) in Intersex and Normal Populations

As copy number variation regions (CNVRs) can be separated by gaps or poorly assembled regions, the adjacent initial calls were merged if their reads depth were highly correlated. The default parameters were as follows: the distance between the two initial calls was less than 20% of their combined length, and the Pearson's correlation index of the two CNVRs was significant at the $p = 0.01$ level [21]. After calculation and combination through the CNVcaller software, 87,729 CNVRs were obtained, of which 1817 CNVRs were located on the scaffold sequence (not assembled into chromosomes) and 11,170 CNVRs were located on the X chromosome (Supplemental Table S10).

As the number of X chromosomes is different in females and males, the copy number variation on the scaffold and X chromosomes was not considered in the results. Therefore, 74,302 CNVRs located on autosomes were used for the subsequent analysis. As shown in Supplemental Table S10, the smallest proportion of CNVRs was chromosome 26 (5.8%), and the largest was chromosome 11 (9.92%). In addition, the number of CNVRs distributed on chromosome 1 ($n = 8267$) was the highest with a total length of 19,584,800 bp, while the smallest was on chromosome 26 ($n = 1116$) with 2,556,800 bp. The longest CNVR was 380,800 bp and located on chromosome 13 (Supplemental Table S10).

The copy number of the normal and intersex populations was screened with variation length >2000 bp and Vst value >0.25, and a total of 238 candidate regions were obtained. Gene annotation of the above 238 candidate CNVRs revealed that 140 were located in the intergenic region, and the remaining 98 overlapped with the genes (Supplemental Table S11). Functional enrichment analysis was performed on the annotated genes, revealing a total of 1838 significant entries ($p < 0.05$) and 1039 significant entries after FDR-correction (corrected p-value < 0.05) (Supplemental Table S12).

Through further GO enrichment analysis of CNVRs, four GO items related to female gonad development were found. Based on functional enrichment analysis, the enriched genes were mainly *ZFPM2*, *LHX8* (located at 43,507 nt downstream of its corresponding copy number region), IMMP2L (located at 400835 nt upstream of its corresponding copy number region), and *SLIT3* (Supplemental Table S12). The above four genes corresponded to four CNVRs, respectively. Furthermore, in the intersex individuals, the copy number region associated with the *LHX8*, *IMMP2L*, and *ZFPM2* genes were gained, while the copy number region associated with the *SLIT3* gene was lost (Table 1).

Table 1. The information of the four candidates copy number variation region and the genotype of eight samples.

CNV Regions			Related Genes	*V*st-Values	Sample Genotype							
Chromosome	Start Position	End Position			LZ1	LZ2	LZ3	LZ4	Tan1	Tan2	Tan3	Tan4
1	50776001	50778000	*LHX8*	0.5713	AB	AB	AA	AA	AA	AA	AA	AA
4	58119201	58121600	*IMMP2L*	0.7097	AB	AB	AA	AA	AA	AA	AA	AA
9	71660801	71662800	*ZFPM2*	0.8611	AB	AB	AA	AA	AA	AA	AA	AA
16	778801	780800	*SLIT3*	0.4357	Ad	Ad	AA	AA	AA	AA	AA	AA

Note: AA means two copies; AB means three copies; Ad means just one copy. *LHX8, LIM homeobox 8* gene; *IMMP2L, inner mitochondrial membrane peptidase subunit 2* gene; *ZFPM2, zinc finger protein FOG family member 2* gene; *SLIT3, slit guidance ligand 3* gene. The *V*st-values measure the difference in the size of each copy number variation between different groups.

4. Discussion

It is well-known that the mutation of the goat PIS region contributes to the absence of horns and sex-reversal [4]. Herein, through the reads depth and the PCR amplification experiments, the PIS homologous segments of two intersex sheep and normal sheep were not in a missing state, which indicated that the intersex trait of LFT sheep may not be caused by the absence of this region. The intersexuality of goats was always accompanied by hornlessness, manifested as non-interval syndrome, and the probability of the intersex appearance in the hornless goat population was 3% to 10% [32].

Genetic variations or regulatory regions may affect an individual's phenotypic traits by affecting the transcription or transition of key genes. We speculated that some mutations may lead to the abnormal expression of certain genes that affect sex formation, leading to the appearance of intersex. Furthermore, a previous study reported that the replication of the *SRY-box transcription factor 3* (*SOX3*) gene may also cause human developmental disorders [33]. An increased copy number of the *SRY-box transcription factor 9* (*SOX9*) gene may trigger the probability of intersex individuals [34], so it is suspected that the intersexuality of the sheep may be due to other reasons, such as genetic variations.

Functional enrichment analysis revealed significant entries for the androgen biosynthesis processes and follicle stimulating hormone responses, including *SRD5A2*, *SRD5A3*, and *PAWR* genes. Among them, mutations of the *SRD5A2*, which were closely related to testicular decline, could affect the formation of the urethra and external genitalia, leading to hypoplasia of the male reproductive organs [35]. Therefore, polymorphisms of the *SRD5A2* gene may be a key point leading to intersexuality in sheep.

Functional enrichment of the sequencing data for intersex sheep and normal sheep populations (including Tan sheep) did not find significant entries related to gonadal development or sex hormone metabolisms. A previous study reported that testicular tissue dysplasia was a key cause of human gender developmental disorders [35]. Additionally, the excessive synthesis of estrogen in vivo also affected the formation and development of female reproductive organs. Therefore, it was speculated that various mutations of genes related to the synthesis and secretion of androgen led to the fact that the testis and its accessory reproductive organs could not be maintained.

As hermaphroditism is not conducive to animal reproduction, it is speculated that intersexual individuals are selected to be eliminated in evolution, so the occurrence in the current group is low. A major limitation of this study is that there were only two intersexual individuals sequenced, which may result in a certain number of false positives in the sequencing results. If the limitation of the sample size is eliminated, the study may obtain more mutation regions or copy number variation regions that are more reliable than in this paper, and may even lock in the major genes that lead to intersex traits. It is undeniable that this study provides a direction and reference basis for further in-depth exploration of the molecular mechanism of sheep intersex traits.

5. Conclusions

This study was the first to locate the homologous sequence of the goat PIS region in sheep and found that the intersex traits of LFT sheep were not caused by the lack of this region. Through detecting the selective sweep regions, the vital genes associated with androgen biosynthesis and the follicle stimulating hormone response entry were found, including *SRD5A2*, *SRD5A3*, and *PAWR*. Additionally, the copy number variations of the four regions on chr9, chr1, chr4, and chr16 may affect the expression of the gonadal development genes, *ZFPM2*, *LHX8*, *IMMP2L*, and *SLIT3*, respectively, which contribute to the appearance of intersex traits.

Supplementary Materials:
944/s1, Table S1: PCR amplification primer information for candidate region on sheep chromosome 1; Table S2: The statistics of resequencing samples from 4 Lanzhou large-tailed sheep; Table S3: The statistics of resequencing samples from 8 sheep; Table S4: Chromosome distribution of SNPs in sheep; Table S5: Goat PIS regional positioning on sheep genome (the top 10 score); Table S6: List of genes in the selected overlapping regions by top 1% highest Z(Fst) between intersex sheep and normal sheep (including normal Lanzhou large-tailed sheep and Tan sheep); Table S7: GO term of the candidate genes associated with the intersex; Table S8: List of genes in the selected overlapping regions by top 1% highest Z(Fst) between intersex and normal individuals of Lanzhou large-tailed sheep; Table S9: GO term of the candidate genes associated with the intersex; Table S10: Autosomal distribution of CNVRs in sheep; Table S11: Gene annotation of the candidate CNVRs; Table S12: Functional enrichment analysis of annotated genes.

Author Contributions: Methodology, H.X.; software, H.X. and X.L. (Xinfeng Liu); validation, H.X.; formal analysis, H.X. and X.L. (Xinfeng Liu); resources, H.X. and Y.C.; writing—original draft preparation, J.L.; writing—review and editing, X.L. (Xianyong Lan); supervision, X.L. (Xianyong Lan) and H.X.; funding acquisition, X.L. (Xianyong Lan) and H.X. All authors have read and agreed to the published version of the manuscript.

Acknowledgments: We greatly thank the staffs of Ruilin Sci-Tech Cluture and Breeding Limit Company Yongjing county, Gansu Province, for collecting samples of Tan sheep and Lanzhou fat-tail sheep. Moreover, we sincerely thank Wang XL and Jiang Y from Northwest A&F University for their data and technical support.

References

1. Marshall Graves, J.A. Weird animal genomes and the evolution of vertebrate sex and sex chromosomes. *Annu. Rev. Genet.* **2008**, *42*, 565–586. [CrossRef] [PubMed]
2. Eaton, O.N. The relation between polled and hermaphroditic characters in dairy goats. *Genetics* **1945**, *30*, 51–61. [PubMed]
3. Pailhoux, E.; Vigier, B.; Chaffaux, S. A 11.7-kb deletion triggers intersexuality and polledness in goats. *Nat. Genet.* **2001**, *29*, 453–458. [CrossRef] [PubMed]
4. Pailhoux, E.; Vigier, B.; Schibler, L. Positional cloning of the PIS mutation in goats and its impact on understanding mammalian sex-differentiation. *Genet. Sel. Evol.* **2005**, *37*, S55–S64. [CrossRef] [PubMed]
5. Simon, R.; Lischer, H.E.L.; Pieńkowska-Schelling, A.; Keller, I.; Häfliger, I.M.; Letko, A.; Schelling, C.; Lühken, G.; Drögemüller, C. New genomic features of the polled intersex syndrome variant in goats unraveled by long-read whole-genome sequencing. *Anim. Genet.* **2020**, *51*, 439–448. [CrossRef]
6. Pannetier, M.; Renault, L.; Jolivet, G. Ovarian-specific expression of a new gene regulated by the goat PIS region and transcribed by a FOXL2 bidirectional promoter. *Gnomics* **2005**, *85*, 715–726. [CrossRef]
7. Alberto, F.J.; Boyer, F.; Orozco-terWengel, P.; Streeter, I.; Servin, B.; de Villemereuil, P.; Benjelloun, B.; Librado, P.; Biscarini, F.; Colli, L.; et al. Convergent genomic signatures of domestication in sheep and goats. *Nat. Commun.* **2018**, *9*, 813. [CrossRef]
8. Wong, K.K.; de Leeuw, R.J.; Dosanjh, N.S.; Kimm, L.R.; Cheng, Z.; Horsman, D.E.; MacAulay, C.; Ng, R.T.; Brown, C.J.; Eichler, E.E.; et al. A comprehensive analysis of common copy-number variations in the human genome. *Am. J. Hum. Genet.* **2007**, *80*, 91–104. [CrossRef]

9. Flisikowski, K.; Venhoranta, H.; Nowacka-Woszuk, J. A novel mutation in the maternally imprinted PEG3 domain results in a loss of MIMT1 expression and causes abortions and stillbirths in cattle (Bos Taurus). *PLoS ONE* **2010**, *5*, e15116. [CrossRef]
10. Meyers, S.N.; McDaneld, T.G.; Swist, S.L. A deletion mutation in bovine SLC4A2 is associated with osteopetrosis in Red Angus cattle. *BMC Genom.* **2010**, *11*, 337. [CrossRef]
11. Elferink, M.G.; Vallée, A.; Jungerius, A.P. Partial duplication of the PRLR and SPEF2 genes at the late feathering locus in chicken. *BMC Genom.* **2008**, *9*, 391. [CrossRef] [PubMed]
12. Bu, G.; Huang, G.; Fu, H. Characterization of the novel duplicated PRLR gene at the late-feathering K locus in Lohmann chickens. *J. Mol. Endocrinol.* **2013**, *51*, 261–272. [CrossRef] [PubMed]
13. Norris, B.J.; Whan, V.A. A gene duplication affecting expression of the ovine ASIP gene is responsible for white and black sheep. *Genome Res.* **2008**, *18*, 1282–1293. [CrossRef] [PubMed]
14. Zhang, S.H.; Sun, K.; Bian, Y.N.; Zhao, Q.; Wang, Z.; Ji, C.N.; Li, C. Developmental validation of an X-Insertion/Deletion polymorphism panel and application in HAN population of China. *Sci. Rep.* **2015**, *5*, 18336. [CrossRef] [PubMed]
15. Wang, X.; Liu, J.; Niu, Y.; Li, Y.; Zhou, S.; Li, C.; Ma, B.; Kou, Q.; Petersen, B.; Sonstegard, T.; et al. Low incidence of SNVs and indels in trio genomes of Cas9-mediated multiplex edited sheep. *BMC Genom.* **2018**, *19*, 397. [CrossRef]
16. Zhou, S.; Cai, B.; He, C.; Wang, Y.; Ding, Q.; Liu, J.; Liu, Y.; Ding, Y.; Zhao, X.; Li, G.; et al. Programmable base editing of the sheep genome revealed no genome-wide off-target mutations. *Front. Genet.* **2019**, *10*, 215. [CrossRef]
17. Bolger, A.M.; Lohse, M.; Usadel, B. Trimmomatic: A flexible trimmer for Illumina sequence data. *Bioinformatics* **2014**, *30*, 2114–2120. [CrossRef]
18. Jiang, Y.; Xie, M.; Chen, W.; Talbot, R.; Maddox, J.F.; Faraut, T.; Wu, C.; Muzny, D.M.; Li, Y.; Zhang, W.; et al. The sheep genome illuminates biology of the rumen and lipid metabolism. *Science* **2014**, *344*, 1168–1173. [CrossRef]
19. Li, H.; Durbin, R. Fast and accurate short read alignment with Burrows-Wheeler transform. *Bioinformatics* **2009**, *25*, 1754–1760. [CrossRef]
20. McKenna, A.; Hanna, M.; Banks, E.; Sivachenko, A.; Cibulskis, K.; Kernytsky, A.; Garimella, K.; Altshuler, D.; Gabriel, S.; Daly, M.; et al. The Genome Analysis Toolkit: A MapReduce framework for analyzing next-generation DNA sequencing data. *Genome Res.* **2010**, *20*, 1297–1303. [CrossRef]
21. Wang, K.; Li, M.; Hakonarson, H. ANNOVAR: Functional annotation of genetic variants from high-throughput sequencing data. *Nucleic Acids Res.* **2010**, *38*, e164. [CrossRef] [PubMed]
22. Wang, X.; Zheng, Z.; Cai, Y.; Chen, T. CNVcaller: Highly efficient and widely applicable software for detecting copy number variations in large populations. *Gigascience* **2017**, *6*, 1–12. [CrossRef] [PubMed]
23. Gao, Y.; Jiang, J.; Yang, S.; Hou, Y.; Liu, G.E.; Zhang, S.; Zhang, Q.; Sun, D. CNV discovery for milk composition traits in dairy cattle using whole genome resequencing. *BMC Genom.* **2017**, *18*, 265. [CrossRef] [PubMed]
24. Redon, R.; Ishikawa, S.; Fitch, K.R.; Feuk, L.; Perry, G.H.; Andrews, T.D.; Fiegler, H.; Shapero, M.H.; Carson, A.R.; Chen, W.; et al. Global variation in copy number in the human genome. *Nature* **2006**, *444*, 444–454. [CrossRef] [PubMed]
25. Sudmant, P.H.; Mallick, S.; Nelson, B.J.; Hormozdiari, F.; Krumm, N.; Huddleston, J.; Coe, B.P.; Baker, C.; Nordenfelt, S.; Bamshad, M.; et al. Global diversity, population stratification, and selection of human copy-number variation. *Science* **2015**, *349*, aab3761. [CrossRef]
26. Kent, W. BLAT—The BLAST-like alignment tool. *Genome Res.* **2002**, *12*, 656–664. [CrossRef]
27. Li, J.; Zhang, S.; Erdenee, S.; Sun, X.; Dang, R.; Huang, Y.; Lei, C.; Chen, H.; Xu, H.; Cai, Y.; et al. Nucleotide variants in prion-related protein (testis-specific) gene (PRNT) and effects on Chinese and Mongolian sheep phenotypes. *Prion* **2018**, *12*, 185–196. [CrossRef]
28. Lai, F.N.; Zhai, H.L.; Cheng, M.; Ma, J.Y.; Cheng, S.F.; Ge, W.; Zhang, G.L.; Wang, J.J.; Zhang, R.Q.; Wang, X.; et al. Whole-genome scanning for the litter size trait associated genes and SNPs under selection in dairy goat (Capra hircus). *Sci. Rep.* **2016**, *6*, 38096. [CrossRef]
29. Guo, J.H.; Tao, H.X.; Li, P.F.; Li, L.; Zhong, T.; Wang, L.J.; Ma, J.; Chen, X.; Song, T.; Zhang, H. Whole-genome sequencing reveals selection signatures associated with important traits in six goat breeds. *Sci. Rep.* **2018**, *8*, 10405. [CrossRef]

30. Zhou, Y.; Connor, E.E.; Wiggans, G.R.; Lu, Y.; Tempelman, R.J.; Schroeder, S.G.; Chen, H.; Liu, G.E. Genome-wide copy number variant analysis reveals variants associated with 10 diverse production traits in Holstein cattle. *BMC Genom.* **2018**, *19*, 314. [CrossRef]
31. Xie, C.; Mao, X.; Huang, J.; Ding, Y.; Wu, J.; Dong, S.; Kong, L.; Gao, G.; Li, C.Y.; Wei, L. KOBAS 2.0: A web server for annotation and identification of enriched pathways and diseases. *Nucleic Acids Res.* **2011**, *39*, W316–W322. [CrossRef] [PubMed]
32. E, G.X.; Jin, M.L.; Zhao, Y.J.; Li, X.L.; Li, L.H.; Yang, B.G.; Duan, X.H.; Hunag, Y.F. Genome-wide analysis of Chongqing native intersexual goats using next-generation sequencing. *3 Biotech* **2019**, *9*, 99. [CrossRef] [PubMed]
33. Moalem, S.; Babul-Hirji, R.; Stavropolous, D.J.; Wherrett, D.; Bägli, D.J.; Thomas, P.; Chitayat, D. XX male sex reversal with genital abnormalities associated with a de novo SOX3 gene duplication. *Am. J. Med Genet.* **2012**, *158*, 1759–1764. [CrossRef]
34. Kropatsch, R.; Dekomien, G.; Akkad, D.A.; Gerding, W.M.; Petrasch-Parwez, E.; Young, N.D.; Altmüller, J.; Nürnberg, P.; Gasser, R.B.; Epplen, J.T. SOX9 duplication linked to intersex in deer. *PLoS ONE* **2013**, *8*, e73734. [CrossRef] [PubMed]
35. Jia, W.; Zheng, D.; Zhang, L.; Li, C.; Zhang, X.; Wang, F.; Guan, Q.; Fang, L.; Zhao, J.; Xu, C. Clinical and molecular characterization of 5α-reductase type 2 deficiency due to mutations (p.Q6X, p. R246Q) in SRD5A2 gene. *Endocr. J.* **2018**, *65*, 645–655. [CrossRef]

PERMISSIONS

All chapters in this book were first published by MDPI; hereby published with permission under the Creative Commons Attribution License or equivalent. Every chapter published in this book has been scrutinized by our experts. Their significance has been extensively debated. The topics covered herein carry significant findings which will fuel the growth of the discipline. They may even be implemented as practical applications or may be referred to as a beginning point for another development.

The contributors of this book come from diverse backgrounds, making this book a truly international effort. This book will bring forth new frontiers with its revolutionizing research information and detailed analysis of the nascent developments around the world.

We would like to thank all the contributing authors for lending their expertise to make the book truly unique. They have played a crucial role in the development of this book. Without their invaluable contributions this book wouldn't have been possible. They have made vital efforts to compile up to date information on the varied aspects of this subject to make this book a valuable addition to the collection of many professionals and students.

This book was conceptualized with the vision of imparting up-to-date information and advanced data in this field. To ensure the same, a matchless editorial board was set up. Every individual on the board went through rigorous rounds of assessment to prove their worth. After which they invested a large part of their time researching and compiling the most relevant data for our readers.

The editorial board has been involved in producing this book since its inception. They have spent rigorous hours researching and exploring the diverse topics which have resulted in the successful publishing of this book. They have passed on their knowledge of decades through this book. To expedite this challenging task, the publisher supported the team at every step. A small team of assistant editors was also appointed to further simplify the editing procedure and attain best results for the readers.

Apart from the editorial board, the designing team has also invested a significant amount of their time in understanding the subject and creating the most relevant covers. They scrutinized every image to scout for the most suitable representation of the subject and create an appropriate cover for the book.

The publishing team has been an ardent support to the editorial, designing and production team. Their endless efforts to recruit the best for this project, has resulted in the accomplishment of this book. They are a veteran in the field of academics and their pool of knowledge is as vast as their experience in printing. Their expertise and guidance has proved useful at every step. Their uncompromising quality standards have made this book an exceptional effort. Their encouragement from time to time has been an inspiration for everyone.

The publisher and the editorial board hope that this book will prove to be a valuable piece of knowledge for researchers, students, practitioners and scholars across the globe.

LIST OF CONTRIBUTORS

Guoyu Hu, Duy Ngoc Do, Janine Gray and Younes Miar
Department of Animal Science and Aquaculture, Dalhousie University, Truro, NS B2N 5E3, Canada

Ellen Lai, Alexa L. Danner, Thomas R. Famula and Anita M. Oberbauer
Department of Animal Science, University of California, Davis, CA 95616, USA

Sara González-Ruiz
Doctorado en Ciencias Biológicas, Universidad Autónoma de Querétaro, Avenida de las Ciencias S/N Juriquilla, Delegación Santa Rosa Jáuregui, Querétaro C.P. 76230, Mexico

Maria G. Strillacci and Alessandro Bagnato
Department of Veterinary Medicine, Università degli Studi di Milano, Via Trentacoste, 2, 20134 Milano, Italy

Marina Durán-Aguilar, Feliciano Milián-Suazo and Germinal J. Cantó-Alarcón
Facultad de Ciencias Naturales, Universidad Autónoma de Querétaro, Avenida de las Ciencias S/N Juriquilla, Delegación Santa Rosa Jáuregui, Querétaro C.P. 76230, Mexico

Sara E. Herrera-Rodríguez
Centro de Investigación y Asistencia en Tecnología y Diseño del Estado de Jalisco A.C., Guadalajara C.P. 44270, Mexico

Luis F. Guzmán
Centro Nacional de Recursos Genéticos, INIFAP, Tepatitlán de Morelos 47600, Mexico

Sergio I. Román-Ponce
Centro Nacional de Investigación Disciplinaria en Fisiología y Mejoramiento animal, INIFAP, SAGARPA, Km. 1 Carretera a Colón, Ajuchitlán, Colón, Querétaro C.P. 76280, Mexico

Paweł Solarczyk, Marcin Gołębiewski, Jan Slósarz, Monika Łukasiewicz, Tomasz Przysucha and Kamila Puppel
Institute of Animal Science, Warsaw University of Life Sciences, Ciszewskiego 8, 02-786 Warsaw, Poland

Md. Aminul Islam
Department of Medicine, Faculty of Veterinary Science, Bangladesh Agricultural University, Mymensingh 2202, Bangladesh
Food and Feed Immunology Group, Graduate School of Agricultural University Science, Tohoku University, Sendai 980-8572, Japan
Livestock Immunology Unit, International Research and Education Centre for Food and Agricultural Immunology (CFAI), Graduate School of Agricultural Science, Tohoku University, Sendai 980-8572, Japan

Haruki Kitazawa
Food and Feed Immunology Group, Graduate School of Agricultural University Science, Tohoku University, Sendai 980-8572, Japan
Livestock Immunology Unit, International Research and Education Centre for Food and Agricultural Immunology (CFAI), Graduate School of Agricultural Science, Tohoku University, Sendai 980-8572, Japan

Sharmin Aqter Rony
Department of Parasitology, Faculty of Veterinary Science, Bangladesh Agricultural University, Mymensingh 2202, Bangladesh

Mohammad Bozlur Rahman
Department of Livestock Services, Krishi Khamar Sarak, Farmgate, Dhaka 1215, Bangladesh

Mehmet Ulas Cinar
Department of Animal Science, Faculty of Agriculture, Erciyes University, 38039 Kayseri, Turkey
Department of Veterinary Microbiology & Pathology, College of Veterinary Medicine, Washington State University, Pullman, WA 99164, USA

Julio Villena
Food and Feed Immunology Group, Graduate School of Agricultural University Science, Tohoku University, Sendai 980-8572, Japan
Laboratory of Immunobiotechnology, Reference Centre for Lactobacilli, (CERELA), Tucuman 4000, Argentina

Muhammad Jasim Uddin
Department of Medicine, Faculty of Veterinary Science, Bangladesh Agricultural University, Mymensingh 2202, Bangladesh
School of Veterinary Science, Gatton Campus, The University of Queensland, Brisbane 4072, Australia

Liliana Di Stasio, Alfredo Pauciullo and Giustino Gaspa
Department of Agricultural, Forest and Food Sciences, University of Torino, Largo Baccini 2, 10095 Grugliasco (TO), Italy

Andrea Albera
Associazione Nazionale Allevatori Bovini di Razza Piemontese, strada provinciale Trinita' 31/A, 12061 Carrù (CN), Italy

Alberto Cesarani and Nicolò P. P. Macciotta
Department of Agriculture, University of Sassari, Via De Nicola 9, 07100 Sassari, Italy

Khaled M. M. Saleh and Amneh H. Tarkhan
Department of Applied Biological Sciences, Faculty of Science and Arts, Jordan University of Science and Technology, Irbid 22110, Jordan

Mohammad Borhan Al-Zghoul
Department of Basic Medical Veterinary Sciences, Faculty of Veterinary Medicine, Jordan University of Science and Technology, Irbid 22110, Jordan

Valerio Bronzo, Federica Riva, Giulio Curone and Maria Filippa Addis
Dipartimento di Medicina Veterinaria, Università degli Studi di Milano, 26900 Lodi, Italy

Erminio Trevisi and Vincenzo Lopreiato
Dipartimento di Scienze animali, Alimentazione e Nutrizione, Facoltà di Agraria, Scienze Alimentari e Ambientali, Università Cattolica del Sacro Cuore, 29122 Piacenza, Italy

Massimo Amadori
Rete Nazionale di Immunologia Veterinaria, 25125 Brescia, Italy

Paola Cremonesi and Bianca Castiglioni
Institute of Biology and Biotechnology in Agriculture, National Research Council (CNR), 26900 Lodi, Italy

Paolo Moroni
Dipartimento di Medicina Veterinaria, Università degli Studi di Milano, 26900 Lodi, Italy
Quality Milk Production Services, Animal Health Diagnostic Center, Cornell University, 240 Farrier Road, Ithaca, NY 14850, USA

Bryan Irvine Lopez
Division of Animal Genomics and Bioinformatics, National Institute of Animal Science, Rural Development Administration, Wanju 55365, Korea

Kier Gumangan Santiago
Department of Animal Science and Technology, Sunchon National University, Suncheon 57922, Korea
Department of Animal Science, College of Agriculture, Central Luzon State University, Science City of Muñoz 3120, Philippines

Donghui Lee and Kangseok Seo
Department of Animal Science and Technology, Sunchon National University, Suncheon 57922, Korea

Seungmin Ha
Dairy Science Division, National Institute of Animal Science, Rural Development Administration, Cheonan 31000, Korea

Anna Migdał and Łukasz Migdał
Department of Genetics, Animal Breeding and Ethology, Faculty of Animal Sciences, University of Agriculture in Krakow, al. 29 Listopada 46, 31-425 Kraków, Poland

Maria Oczkowicz
Department of Animal Molecular Biology, National Research Institute of Animal Production, Krakowska 1, 32-083 Balice, Poland

Adam Okólski
Institute of Veterinary Science, University Centre of Veterinary Medicine UJ-UR, University of Agriculture in Krakow, al. Mickiewicza 24/28, 30-059 Kraków, Poland

Anna Chełmońska-Soyta
Laboratory of Reproductive Immunology, Hirszfeld Institute of Immunology and Experimental Therapy, Polish Academy of Sciences, Weigla 12 Street, 53-114 Wroclaw, Poland
Department of Immunology, Pathophysiology and Veterinary Preventive Medicine, Division of Immunology and Veterinary Preventive Medicine, Faculty of Veterinary Medicine, Wroclaw University of Environmental and Life Sciences, Norwida 31 Street, 50-375 Wroclaw, Poland

Adnan Khan
Key Laboratory of Animal Genetics, Breeding, and Reproduction, Ministry of Agriculture & National Engineering Laboratory for Animal Breeding, College of Animal Science and Technology, China Agricultural University, Beijing 100193, China

Jian Gao
Department of Clinical Veterinary Medicine, College of Veterinary Medicine, China Agricultural University, Beijing 100193, China

Francesco Tiezzi
Department of Animal Science, North Carolina State University, Raleigh, NC 27695, USA

Antonio Marco Maisano
Istituto Zooprofilattico Sperimentale Lombardia Emilia Romagna "Bruno Ubertini"—I.Z.S.L.E.R. Territorial Section of Lodi and Brescia Sector Diagnostic, Animal Health and Welfare, 26900 Lodi, Italy

Stefania Chessa
Dipartimento di Scienze Veterinarie, Università degli Studi di Torino, 10095 Grugliasco, Italy

Mario Luini
Istituto Zooprofilattico Sperimentale Lombardia Emilia Romagna "Bruno Ubertini"—I.Z.S.L.E.R. Territorial Section of Lodi and Brescia Sector Diagnostic, Animal Health and Welfare, 26900 Lodi, Italy
Consiglio Nazionale delle Ricerche (CNR), Istituto di biologia e biotecnologia agraria (IBBA), Via Edoardo Bassini, 20133 Milano, Italy

Stefano Biffani
Consiglio Nazionale delle Ricerche (CNR), Istituto di biologia e biotecnologia agraria (IBBA), Via Edoardo Bassini, 20133 Milano, Italy

Jiahao Shao, Xue Bai, Yanhong Li, Xianbo Jia, Jie Wang and Songjia Lai
College of Animal Science and Technology, Sichuan Agricultural University, Chengdu 611130, China

Ting Pan
College of Veterinary Medicine, Sichuan Agricultural University, Chengdu 611130, China

Muhammad Zahoor Khan, Jianxin Xiao, Jiaying Ma, Yulin Ma, Tianyu Chen and Zhijun Cao
State Key Laboratory of Animal Nutrition, Beijing Engineering Technology Research Center of Raw Milk Quality and Safety Control, College of Animal Science and Technology, China Agricultural University, Beijing 100193, China

Dafu Shao
Institute of Agricultural Information of CAAS, Beijing 100081, China

Jie Li, Xinfeng Liu and Xianyong Lan
Animal Genome and Gene Function Laboratory, College of Animal Science and Technology, Northwest A&F University, Yangling 712100, China

Han Xu
Animal Genome and Gene Function Laboratory, College of Animal Science and Technology, Northwest A&F University, Yangling 712100, China
School of Medicine, Sun Yat-sen University, Guangzhou 510275, China

Hongwei Xu
College of Life Science and Engineering, Northwest Minzu University, Lanzhou 730030, China
Gansu Tech Innovation Center of Animal Cell, Biomedical Research Center, Northwest Minzu University, Lanzhou 730030, China

Yong Cai
Science Experimental Center, Northwest Minzu University, Lanzhou 730030, China
Key Laboratory of Biotechnology and Bioengineering of State Ethnic Affairs Commission, Biomedical Research Center, Northwest Minzu University, Lanzhou 730030, China

Index

www.ingramcontent.com/pod-product-compliance
Lightning Source LLC
LaVergne TN
LVHW080952210926
848485LV00004B/826